Osseointegration
and Dental Implants

Osseointegration
and Dental Implants

Edited by Asbjorn Jokstad, DDS, PhD

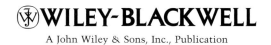

A John Wiley & Sons, Inc., Publication

Asbjorn Jokstad, DDS, PhD, is Professor and Head of the Discipline of Prosthodontics, Faculty of Dentistry at the University of Toronto in Toronto, Ontario, Canada. He is also the Director of the prosthodontic speciality training and holds the Nobel Biocare Chair in Prosthodontics at the University of Toronto.

Edition first published 2009
© 2009 Wiley-Blackwell

Blackwell Munksgaard, formerly an imprint of Blackwell Publishing, was acquired by John Wiley & Sons in February 2007. Blackwell's publishing programme has been merged with Wiley's global Scientific, Technical, and Medical business to form Wiley-Blackwell.

Editorial Office
2121 State Avenue, Ames, Iowa 50014-8300, USA

For details of our global editorial offices, for customer services, and for information about how to apply for permission to reuse the copyright material in this book please see our website at www.wiley.com/wiley-blackwell.

Authorization to photocopy items for internal or personal use, or the internal or personal use of specific clients, is granted by the publisher, provided that the base fee is paid directly to the Copyright Clearance Center, 222 Rosewood Drive, Danvers, MA 01923. For those organizations that have been granted a photocopy license by CCC, a separate system of payments has been arranged. The fee code for users of the Transactional Reporting Service is ISBN-13: 978-0-8138-1341-7/2009.

Designations used by companies to distinguish their products are often claimed as trademarks. All brand names and product names used in this book are trade names, service marks, trademarks, or registered trademarks of their respective owners. The publisher is not associated with any product or vendor mentioned in this book. This publication is designed to provide accurate and authoritative information in regard to the subject matter covered. It is sold on the understanding that the publisher is not engaged in rendering professional services. If professional advice or other expert assistance is required, the services of a competent professional should be sought.

Library of Congress Cataloguing-in-Publication Data

Toronto Osseointegration Conference Revisited (2008 : Toronto, Canada)
  Osseointegration and dental implants / [edited by] Asbjorn Jokstad.
    p. ; cm.
  Based on the proceedings of the Toronto Osseointegration Conference Revisited, which took place on May 8–10, 2008.
  Includes bibliographical references and index.
  ISBN-13: 978-0-8138-1341-7 (alk. paper)
  ISBN-10: 0-8138-1341-7 (alk. paper)
  1. Dental implants–Congresses. 2. Osseointegration–Congresses. I. Jokstad, Asbjorn. II. Title.
  [DNLM: 1. Dental Implantation–methods–Congresses. 2. Osseointegration–Congresses. 3. Dental Implants–Congresses. WU 640 T686o 2008]
   R667.I45T67 2009
  617.6′92–dc22

                                                         2008033209

A catalogue record for this book is available from the U.S. Library of Congress.

Set in 10 on 12 pt Sabon by SNP Best-set Typesetter Ltd., Hong Kong
Printed in Singapore by Fabulous Printers Pte Ltd

Disclaimer
The contents of this work are intended to further general scientific research, understanding, and discussion only and are not intended and should not be relied upon as recommending or promoting a specific method, diagnosis, or treatment by practitioners for any particular patient. The publisher and the author make no representations or warranties with respect to the accuracy or completeness of the contents of this work and specifically disclaim all warranties, including without limitation any implied warranties of fitness for a particular purpose. In view of ongoing research, equipment modifications, changes in governmental regulations, and the constant flow of information relating to the use of medicines, equipment, and devices, the reader is urged to review and evaluate the information provided in the package insert or instructions for each medicine, equipment, or device for, among other things, any changes in the instructions or indication of usage and for added warnings and precautions. Readers should consult with a specialist where appropriate. The fact that an organization or Website is referred to in this work as a citation and/or a potential source of further information does not mean that the author or the publisher endorses the information the organization or Website may provide or recommendations it may make. Further, readers should be aware that Internet Websites listed in this work may have changed or disappeared between when this work was written and when it is read. No warranty may be created or extended by any promotional statements for this work. Neither the publisher nor the author shall be liable for any damages arising herefrom.

Contents

Foreword

The 2008 Toronto Osseointegration Conference Revisited and this book would not have been possible without the enthusiastic support of everyone involved.

We are grateful to our conference speakers and especially the individuals who spent time putting on paper what they consider are the important messages to be conveyed.

We thank our industry sponsors for supporting the conference, and our participating associations and journals for their cooperation in selecting speakers and program themes. We also express gratitude to everybody who shared our ambition to organize a conference with a main purpose to critically appraise where we have come from and where we are heading within the field of implant dentistry.

Enormous thanks is extended to my husband and editor of this book, Asbjorn Jokstad. This book would never have been written without his indefatigable energy and desire to share scientific knowledge with dentists and researchers throughout the world.

Dr. Anne M. Gussgard, DDS
Steering Committee Chair
Toronto Osseointegration Conference
Revisited, May 9–10, 2008

Preface

Osseointegration and implant dentistry research are at an unprecedented peak. More than one million dentists worldwide are ready to learn more about implant practices and eager to offer implant solutions to their patients. The consequence is that the market today is saturated with new implant manufacturers, new implant brands, new surfaces, and new marketing strategies. Some say this is history repeating itself, that the field has regressed to the implant dentistry practices and research preceding the first Toronto Osseointegration Conference, which was organized by Professor Emeritus George A. Zarb in 1982.

A 25-year mark is a good point to call a time-out, to take stock of our accomplishments, and to question where we have come from, where we are, and where we seem to be heading. By learning from our past mistakes, we may better be able to meet the future. What have we achieved over the last 25 years and what are emerging as new and innovative developments in the field of osseointegration? This textbook attempts to answer these questions by reflecting on the many significant developments of the current and future application of implants to support intra and extraoral prostheses. A sincere thank you to all colleagues who have shared this vision and contributed to the Toronto Osseointegration Conference Revisited and to this textbook.

Asbjorn Jokstad, DDS, Dr. Odont.
Toronto, May 10, 2008

Contributing Authors

James D. Anderson, DDS, MSD
Professor, Discipline of Prosthodontics, University of Toronto, Toronto, Ontario, Canada

Jay R. Beagle, DDS, MSD
Certified Periodontist, specialty private practice, Indianapolis, Indiana, United States

Birgitta Bergendal, DDS, Odont. Dr.
Head and Senior Consultant, National Oral Disability Centre, the Institute for Postgraduate Dental Education, Jönköping, Sweden

John B. Brunski, PhD
Professor, Department of Biomedical Engineering, Rensselaer Polytechnic Institute, Troy, New York, United States

Lyndon Cooper, DDS, PhD
Professor, Department of Prosthodontics, University of North Carolina, Chapel Hill, North Carolina, United States

Luca Cordaro, MD, DDS, PhD
Professor and Head, Department of Periodontology and Implant Dentistry, Eastman Dental Hospital, Rome, Italy

Paul Coulthard, BDS, MDS, PhD
Professor, Oral and Maxillofacial Surgery School of Dentistry, University of Manchester, Manchester, United Kingdom

Jennifer A. Currey, PhD
Visiting Assistant Professor, Department of Mechanical Engineering Union College, Schenectady, New York, United States

Shadi Daher, DMD
Assistant Clinical Professor, Boston University Goldman School of Dental Medicine, Boston, Massachusetts, United States

John E. Davies, BDS, PhD, DSc
Professor, Institute of Biomaterials and Biomedical Engineering, University of Toronto, Toronto, Ontario, Canada

Nikolaos Donos, DDS, MS, PhD
Professor and Head, Periodontology, UCL Eastman Dental Institute, London, United Kingdom

Joke Duyck, DDS, PhD
Post doc. Fellow, Department of Prosthetic Dentistry / BIOMAT Research Group, School

of Dentistry, Faculty of Medicine, KU. Leuven, Leuven, Belgium

Steven E. Eckert, DDS, MS
Professor, Division of Prosthodontics, College of Medicine, Mayo Clinic, Rochester, Minnesota, United States

Marco Esposito, DDS, PhD
Senior Lecturer in Oral and Maxillofacial Surgery, School of Dentistry, University of Manchester, Manchester, United Kingdom

Øystein Fardal, BDS, MDS, PhD
Certified Periodontist, specialty private practice, Egersund, Norway

Jocelyne S. Feine, DDS, MS, HDR
Professor and Director of Graduate Studies, McGill University, Montreal, Quebec, Canada

David A. Felton, DDS, MS
Professor, Department of Prosthodontics, University of North Carolina, Chapel Hill, North Carolina, United States

Stuart J. Froum, DDS
Clinical Professor, Department of Periodontology and Implant Dentistry, New York University Dental Center, New York, New York, United States

Scott D. Ganz, DMD
Maxillofacial Prosthodontist, specialty private practice, Fort Lee, New Jersey, United States

Roland Glauser, DMD
Certified Prosthodontist, specialty private practice, Zurich, Switzerland

Michael Glogauer, DDS, PhD
Associate Professor, Discipline of Periodontology, Faculty of Dentistry, University of Toronto, Toronto, Ontario, Canada

Michael Goldberg, DDS, MSc
Assistant Professor, Discipline of Periodontology, Faculty of Dentistry, University of Toronto, Toronto, Ontario, Canada

Klaus Gotfredsen, DDS, Odont. Dr.
Professor, Department of Oral Rehabilitation, University of Copenhagen, Copenhagen, Denmark

Jan Gottlow, DDS, Odont. Dr.
Department of Biomaterials, University of Göteborg, Göteborg, Sweden

Maria Gabriella Grusovin, DDS
Cochrane Oral Health Group, the University of Manchester, Manchester, United Kingdom

Jill A. Helms, DDS, PhD
Associate Professor, Department of Surgery, Stanford University, Stanford, California, United States

Asbjorn Jokstad, DDS, Dr. Odont.
Professor and Head, Division of Prosthodontics, University of Toronto, Toronto, Ontario, Canada

Kenneth W.M. Judy, DDS
Director, International Congress of Oral Implantologists and private practice, New York, New York, United States

Karl-Erik Kahnberg, DDS, Odont. Dr.
Professor and Chair, Department of Oral and Maxillofacial Surgery, Institute of Odontology, the Sahlgrenska Academy and Hospital, University of Göteborg, Göteborg, Sweden

David M. Kim, DDS, DMSc
Assistant Professor, Department of Oral Medicine, Infection and Immunity, Division of Periodontics, Harvard School of Dental Medicine, Boston, Massachusetts, United States

Iven Klineberg, BDS, BSc, PhD
Professor and Head, Jaw Function and Orofacial Pain Research Unit, University of Sydney, Sydney, Australia

Kent Knoernschild, DDS, MS
Co-director, Comprehensive Dental Implant Center, University of Illinois, Chicago, Illinois, United States

Burton Langer, DMD
Certified Periodontist, specialty private practice, New York, New York, United States

Michael Landzberg, DDS
Graduate Student, Discipline of Periodontology, Faculty of Dentistry, University of Toronto, Toronto, Canada

Philipp Leucht, MD
Department of Orthopaedic Surgery, Stanford University School of Medicine, Stanford, United States

Gerard James Linden, BDS, BSc, PhD
Professor of Periodontology, Head of Department of Restorative Dentistry, School of Medicine and Dentistry, Queen's University, Belfast, United Kingdom

Rainer Lutz, Dr. med. dent.
Assistant Physician, Department of Oral and Cranio-Maxillofacial Surgery, Erlangen-Nuremberg University Dental School, Erlangen, Germany

Albert H. Mattia, DMD
Associate Professor, Department of Periodontics, University of Alabama at Birmingham, School of Dentistry

Carl E. Misch, DDS, MDS
Clinical Professor, Oral Implantology, Temple University School of Dentistry, Philadelphia, Pennsylvania, United States

Craig M. Misch, DDS, MDS
Certified Oral and Maxillofacial Surgeon and Prosthodontist, Sarasota, Florida, United States

Peter K. Moy, DMD
Associate Clinical Professor, Department of Oral and Maxillofacial Surgery, University of California, Los Angeles, California, United States

Frauke Müller, Dr. med. dent.
Professor, Division of Gerodontology and Removable Prosthodontics, University of Geneva, Switzerland

Ignace Naert, DDS, PhD
Chairman, Department of Prosthetic Dentistry/BIOMAT Research Group, School of Dentistry, Faculty of Medicine, KU. Leuven, Leuven, Belgium

Antonio Nanci, PhD
Professor and Director of the Stomatology Department, Faculty of Dentistry, University of Montreal, Quebec, Canada

Friedrich W. Neukam, Dr. med., Dr. med. dent., PhD
Chairman and Head, Department of Oral and Cranio-Maxillofacial Surgery, Erlangen-Nuremberg University Dental School, Erlangen, Germany

Myron Nevins, DDS
Associate Clinical Professor, Department of Oral Medicine, Infection and Immunity, Division of Periodontics, Harvard School of Dental Medicine, Boston, Massachusetts, United States

Emeka Nkenke, Dr. med., Dr. med. dent., PhD
Chief Physician, Department of Oral and Cranio-Maxillofacial Surgery, Erlangen-Nuremberg University Dental School, Erlangen, Germany

Bjarni Elvar Pætursson, DDS, Dr. med. dent.
Professor, Department of Prosthodontics, University of Iceland, Reykjavik, Iceland

Michael A. Pikos, DDS
Certified Oral and Maxillofacial Surgeon, Pikos Implant Institute, Palm Harbor, Florida, United States

Robert M. Pilliar, PhD
Professor Emeritus, Faculty of Dentistry and Institute of Biomaterials and Biomedical

Engineering, University of Toronto, Toronto, Ontario, Canada

Lars Rasmusson, DMD, Med. Dr.
Professor, Department of Oral and Maxillofacial Surgery, Institute of Odontology, the Sahlgrenska Academy and Hospital, University of Göteborg, Göteborg, Sweden

Michael S. Reddy, DMD, DMSc
Professor and Chairman, Department of Periodontology, University of Alabama School of Dentistry, Birmingham, Alabama, United States

Mario Roccuzzo, DDS
Lecturer in Periodontology, University of Torino, Torino, Italy

Georgios E. Romanos, DDS, Dr. med. dent., PhD
Professor of Clinical Dentistry, Divisions of Periodontology and General Dentistry, Eastman Department of Dentistry, Rochester, New York, United States

George K.B. Sándor, MD, DDS, PhD, Dr. habil.
Professor and Head, Oral Maxillofacial Surgery, University of Toronto, Canada

Antonio Sanz Ruiz, DDS
Professor, Periodontal and Implant Department, University de los Andes, Santiago, Chile

E. Todd Scheyer, DDS, MS
Certified Peridontist, specialty private practice, Houston, Texas, United States

John K. Schulte, DDS, MSD
Associate Professor, Department of Restorative Sciences, University of Minnesota School of Dentistry, Minneapolis, Minnesota, United States

Peter Schüpbach, PhD
Research Laboratory for Microscopy and Histology, Horgen, Switzerland

Barry J. Sessle, MDS, PhD
Professor and Canada Research Chair, Faculties of Dentistry and Medicine, University of Toronto, Toronto, Ontario, Canada

Massimo Simion, MD, DDS
Professor, Department of Periodontology and Implant Restoration, University of Milan, Milan, Italy

Clark M. Stanford, DDS, PhD
Professor, Dows Institute for Dental Research, University of Iowa, Iowa City, Iowa, United States

Jörg-R. Strub, DDS, Dr. med. dent. habil.
Professor and Chair, Department of Prosthodontics, Albert-Ludwig University, Freiburg, Germany

Peter Svensson, DDS, Dr. Odont.
Professor and Chair, Department of Clinical Oral Physiology, University of Aarhus, Aarhus, Denmark

Thomas D. Taylor, DDS, MSD
Professor and Head, Department of Reconstructive Sciences, Skeletal Development and Biomaterials, University of Connecticut, Farmington, Connecticut, United States

Howard Tenenbaum, DDS, PhD
Professor, Discipline of Periodontology, Faculty of Dentistry, University of Toronto, Toronto, Canada

J. Mark Thomason, BDS, PhD
Chair of Prosthodontics and Oral Rehabilitation, Newcastle University, Newcastle, United Kingdom

Katleen Vandamme, DDS, PhD
Post doc. Fellow, Department of Prosthetic Dentistry/BIOMAT Research Group, School of Dentistry, Faculty of Medicine, KU. Leuven, Leuven, Belgium

Stephen S. Wallace, DDS
Associate Professor, Department of Implant Dentistry, New York University, New York, New York, United States

Rima Wazen, BSc
Post Doctoral Associate, Department of Stomatology, Faculty of Dentistry, University of Montreal, Quebec, Canada

Hans-Peter Weber, Dr. med. dent.
Raymond J. and Elva Pomfret Nagle Professor of Restorative Dentistry and Biomaterials Sciences, Harvard School of Dental Medicine, Boston, Massachusetts, United States

Paul Weigl, DDS
Assistant Professor, Department of Prosthetic Dentistry, J.W. Goethe-University, Frankfurt am Main, Germany

Ulf M.E. Wikesjö, DDS, DMD, PhD
Professor of Periodontics, Oral Biology, and Graduate Studies, Medical College of Georgia, Augusta, Georgia, United States

Daniel Wismeijer, DDS, PhD
Professor, Oral Implantology and Implant Prosthodontics, ACTA, Amsterdam, the Netherlands

Siegbert Witkowski, MDT, CDT
Chief of Dental Technology, University Hospital Freiburg, School of Dentistry, Department of Prosthodontics, Albert-Ludwig University, Freiburg, Germany

Helen Worthington, C. Stat., PhD
Professor, Cochrane Oral Health Group, the University of Manchester, Manchester, United Kingdom

Homah Zadeh, DDS, PhD
Associate Professor, University of Southern California, Los Angeles, California, United States

Introduction

Asbjorn Jokstad

The improvements in implant technology and its practical application in the clinic are not a function primarily of one specific implant surface, a treatment procedure, or some particular loading protocol. Rather it can be understood by conceptualizing the individual elements involved in placing one or more endosseous implants to support an intraoral prosthesis. It is the refinement of each of these individual elements that has contributed to the understanding of osseointegration itself, and improved the technology to solve our patients' problems even further. The chapters that have been included in this collection reflect these elements. Three intertwined treatment planning phases can be identified in the practical application process: a total treatment planning strategy (chapters 2, 3, and 4); a surgery planning strategy (chapter 5); and a restorative planning strategy (chapters 15 and 16). These planning phases take into account patient-centered considerations, for example, risk factors (chapters 3 and 4), healing predictability (chapters 11, 12, and 13), and consideration of the probabilities of possible outcomes of implant interventions (chapters 18, 19, 20, 21, and 22). The actual interventions fall into four categories, that is, the diagnostic and pre-surgical (chapters 6, 7, and 8), the surgical (chapter 10), and the restorative (chapter 14), although at times some of these converge. Each intervention involves the use of different biomaterials for possible site optimizing (chapter 9) and ultimately for the different components of the supra-construction (chapter 17). The observant reader may recognize that the chapter theme order follows the natural progression in the everyday clinical treatment situation. Complementing these practical elements of implant therapy are the three remaining chapters on the assessment of technology in implant therapy (chapter 1), educational requirements for practice (chapter 24), and use of craniofacial and dental implants in adolescent children (chapter 23).

Chapter 1: Any 4-year-old child is able to ask the three essential questions in life—what do we know?, how can you say?, and why should I? More learned scholars would categorize these questions using the more philosophical terms ontology, epistemology, and ethics. The chapter describes what we know about implant therapy outcomes, how we should interpret the claims in the literature, and on which theoretical basis the practicing community should be guided.

Chapter 2: The comprehensive treatment planning phase is the most crucial element determining a successful or unsuccessful treatment outcome. Experience has shown us that it is difficult, or at worst impossible, to achieve an optimal result if this essential factor is neglected. This chapter describes how multi-faceted treatment planning needs to be in order to attain a high probability of treatment success.

Chapter 3: Patients with complex rehabilitation problems remain a challenge for the clinician, whether their condition is due to medical factors, multimorbidity, or old age. This chapter describes how acceptable treatment results from a functional, psychological, and psychosocial aspect can be achieved in sometimes very difficult situations.

Chapter 4: Do periodontal inflammation and/or infection increase the risks for systemic medical conditions? If drawing a parallel with patients with multiple implants, can it be inferred that inflammatory disease in gingival tissues surrounding endosseous implants might also affect the patient's systemic health? This chapter presents new knowledge that needs to be considered when planning treatment in patients with current or past history of refractory periodontitis and/or peri-implantitis.

Chapter 5: Placing an endosseous dental implant always involves some element of risk of adverse events. One important role of the surgeon is to be cognizant of the factors associated with risks, to assess to which extent they apply to the particular patient at hand, and to convey the estimated risk to the patient before commencing treatment. This chapter presents recent findings that challenge our perceptions of risk associated with implant surgery. Do we still have to avoid placing implants in infected sites at all costs? Moreover, are the margins of operator error reduced in special circumstances, for example, by using computer-assisted implant surgery when there is questionable bone volume or

bone quality or proximity to vital anatomical structures?

Chapter 6: In most cases optimal aesthetics and function with implant-supported prosthetics can be achieved after a vertical and/or horizontal regeneration of damaged hard and soft tissues. We have moved from using solely autologous bone and soft-tissue transplants from remote sites to adopting new alloplastic materials, either used alone or in combination with autologous bone and various cell constituents, with the ultimate aim of improving biomimetics. This chapter describes the current state of the science and suggestions for clinical practice.

Chapter 7: For the patient with the atrophic jaw more invasive surgical grafting procedures are needed to reconstruct the resorbed bone. Both inlay and onlay grafts as well as interpositional bone grafts are common techniques that are used in individual situations where the benefit is weighed against possible added treatment length and morbidity. Hard tissue augmentation needs in implant dentistry are also influenced by upcoming new products and applications. This chapter describes how advances in bioengineering now enable new treatment concepts for the reconstruction of atrophic jaws in combination with implants.

Chapter 8: It has always been a challenge to restore the edentulous posterior maxilla with implant-supported prostheses. The advent of implants with new surfaces has only partially improved the situation. Various innovative approaches for grafting into and onto the sinus have been developed and this chapter describes the current surgical techniques, new bioengineering materials, and new research avenues.

Chapter 9: The enormous advances made in developing innovative recombinant-DNA techniques enable us today to use extracellular matrix proteins. Although their exact role in the healing process cascade is currently not fully understood, it appears that they have an important therapeutic utility. This chapter describes the state of the science on regeneration techniques related to dental implant technologies.

Chapter 10: Computer-assisted tools for diagnosis and surgical placement were relatively rapidly adopted by implant surgeons. These digital technologies have now evolved even further and can be applied in treatment planning both to the implant placement and the complete temporary or permanent restoration. This chapter describes how these new digital technologies can be applied, and their potential to improve surgical and restorative treatment outcomes.

Chapter 11: Implant micromotion has an effect on bone healing, but the relationship between the two is complex. For example, do variations in the macro- and micromorphology of the implant influence this relationship? This chapter presents new experimental data that underpin what the leading authorities today believe is the current understanding of the association between implant morphology, micromotion, and healing responses of the bone.

Chapter 12: We are bombarded with "improved" implants with "improved" surfaces. How much of the endless focus on morphological differences is hype and how much is substantiated by sound research? The association between implant surfaces and osteogenesis remains elusive. Surface modifications are motivated by findings from advanced molecular and cellular biology research, combined with advanced bioengineering experiments. This chapter provides perspectives on which implant surfaces will most likely continue to evolve over the next few years and which will falter.

Chapter 13: Many clinicians today believe that the first generation of titanium implants with a turned surface demonstrate less favorable and predictive clinical outcomes compared to implants with other surface geometries, especially in specific intraoral locations. It is intriguing that we are not really sure why, whether it is due to biological width, osteoinduction or -conduction, stress transfer to cortical bone, or other explana-

tions. This chapter describes the current understanding of how the geometries and surface topographies of dental implants can be related to bone responses.

Chapter 14: Have we arrived at the stage where improved grafting materials, implant design and surfaces, and innovative surgical approaches can accelerate the biological responses or is this just wishful thinking? Does it carry any significance that such results can be demonstrated in, for example, rabbits or rats, and should we take it for granted that we can generalize what will happen clinically from laboratory and animal experiments? This chapter examines what is imagination and what is the clinical reality.

Chapter 15: Planning the right technical solution for the right patient, one that will not fail in the foreseeable future, requires more than a clinician's delicate touch. This chapter presents two different, but complementary, principles for restorative treatment planning that have been shown to minimize the risk of adverse biological and mechanical events.

Chapter 16: The finer details of the planning and execution of interventions may result in treatment success or failure. Particularly when shortened clinical loading protocols are used, seemingly minor clinical factors need to be taken into consideration, while making us reconsider some tenets of implant-abutment connection and immediate and early loading in osseointegration that have remained unchallenged.

Chapter 17: New prosthetic components to attach between the endosseous implant and the supra-construction, as well as the supra-construction itself, are developed using a wide range of biomaterials, and by using computer-assisted design and/or manufacture. The benefits for the patient are more individualized technical solutions with optimal aesthetic results, and custom-designed three-dimensional form with improved fit between the components, adapted to functional requirements. The chapter details the merits and disadvantages of current technologies as well as the history and future of this development.

Chapter 18: When the bone mass is limited or of a quality that does not allow the placement of routine dental implants, the clinician is faced with the option to create bone by grafting. Cost-benefit considerations and perceived risks of associated morbidity caused by invasive surgery may exclude this treatment option. Fortunately, specially designed implants can be used in clinical situations where the placement of standard implants will be contraindicated. This chapter presents data that underpins an association between implant design and clinical outcomes.

Chapter 19: Before Brånemark, oral implants were commonly loaded at placement because it was believed that an immediate loading stimulation resulted in less crestal bone loss. The idea never disappeared completely and in fact has gained acceptance in the last few years. This chapter presents and debates the scientific foundation and clinical risks and benefits as reflected from basic, translational animal, and clinical studies.

Chapter 20: We are aware of the importance of somatosensory nerve fibers for recognizing potentially damaging thermal, mechanical, and painful stimuli. In addition, periodontal mechanoreceptors respond to occlusal loads and enable a fine motor control of tooth contacts through complex central and peripheral neural interactions. Implants supporting various forms of suprastructures induce different regulation mechanisms. Moreover, the neurophysiological consequences of the actual implant placement in terms of postoperative sensitivity and pain remain an active focus of research. This chapter presents the relationships between elements of the implant suprastructure occlusion, function and dysfunction, pain, and basic CNS mechanisms.

Chapter 21: There are no medical interventions that can be called truly predictive, nor is it obvious which outcomes best describe the efficacy of interventions. Some outcomes are of great significance for many patients but do not necessarily concern others. While the clinical researchers have slowly moved from recording and reporting surrogate outcomes of implant therapies, modern clinical research focuses more on patient-centered outcomes that matter both to the individual patients and those responsible for public health planning. This chapter reviews how treatment outcomes were evaluated earlier, and how these are being gradually replaced by novel ways of appraising outcomes that are more meaningful for our patients.

Chapter 22: The term "implant therapy" is regarded by many as a misnomer since one does not cure nor manage diseases or disorders with an implanted object. Implants are only adjuncts, albeit very effective, to securely retain dental (i.e., intraoral) or maxillofacial (i.e., extraoral) prostheses. These prostheses in turn are made to enable patients with various amounts of tissue loss to regain a certain degree of oral function, acceptable appearance, and for some socially dysfunctional patients, even their confidence to the extent that they are able to return to a normal social life. A common denominator for many patients receiving implant-supported prostheses is improved quality of life, which does not necessarily depend on the sophistication of the technical solution that the dentist offers. This chapter elaborates on how these factors are interdependent and are of importance for both provider and patients.

Chapter 23: Maxillofacial deformities, whether due to ablative surgery, congenital defects, or trauma, can be masked or restored by artful design and skillful manufacturing of highly individualized prostheses and by using a wide range of biomaterials. Nevertheless, the advent of oral and craniomandibular implants has dramatically increased even further the possibilities of achieving optimal results from functional and aesthetic perspectives. The outcomes are especially critical when treating children and adolescents, and this chapter presents an outstanding panorama of challenges, solutions, and experiences with these patients.

Chapter 24: Implant therapy is usually not a component in the undergraduate curriculum in most dental faculties worldwide. The new graduate as well as the experienced practitioner has to identify and deduce which implant course provider can supply the essential information and basic knowledge required for the clinician to provide safe and efficacious implant therapy. The question is, where can you learn enough to place implants? And what is "enough"?

Osseointegration and Dental Implants

Implant Dentistry: A Technology Assessment

HOW MANY IMPLANT SYSTEMS DO WE HAVE AND ARE THEY DOCUMENTED?

Asbjorn Jokstad

Introduction

We have today close to 600 different implant systems produced by at least 146 different manufacturers located in all corners of the globe. Last year alone, at least 27 new dental implant companies surfaced in the market (Table 1.1).

Is anybody troubled? At least some representatives of the profession have expressed their concern about the seemingly unstoppable avalanche of new implants. Alarm was raised in the United States in 1988 about the heterogeneity of implant designs and the effectiveness of the then 45 different implant systems (English 1988). One of the world's foremost experts in the field, Dr. Patrick Henry, in 1995 challenged the profession and the industry and asked whether implant hardware changes should be regarded as science or just commodity development. He may

perhaps have succeeded in slowing down the output of new products, at least for a few years, since by the year 2000 the number of implant systems had increased "only" to 98 (Binon 2000). Not only did the quantitative issue cause concern, but also the qualitative aspects. Were these new implants really clinically documented? No, according to Albrektsson and Sennerby (1991); no, according to the American Dental Association (ADA 1996); no, according to Eckert and colleagues (1997); and no, according to several other investigators publishing at the time. Around the turn of the millennium the FDI World Dental Federation was alarmed by the apparent rapid increase in the number of implants and implant systems worldwide, and questions were raised about the quality of all the new implants that were being marketed. The FDI Science Committee was asked to investigate the issue and the findings were rather alarming (Jokstad et al. 2003). The investigators identified 225 implant brands from 78 manufacturers, but also discovered that about 70 implant brands were no longer being manufactured. Of the 78 manufacturers, 10 could support their implant system with more than four clinical trials, 11 could support their

Table 1.1. Implant producers of the world.

1. ACE Surgical Supply Company	USA
2. Adaptare Sistema de Implantate	Brazil
3. Advance Company	Japan
4. Allmed S.r.l.	Italy
5. Almitech Incorporated	USA
6. Alpha Bio GmbH	Germany
7. Alpha Bio Implant Limited	Israel
8. Altiva Corporation	USA
9. Anthogyr	France
10. AQB Implant System	Japan
11. AS Technology	Brazil
12. Astra Tech	Sweden
13. Basic Dental Implants LLC	USA
14. BEGO Implant Systems GmbH & Co. KG	Germany
15. Bicon Dental Implants	USA
16. BioHex Corporation (previous name: Biomedical Implant Technology)	Canada
17. BioHorizons Implant Systems Incorporated	USA
18. Bio-Lok International Incorporated (subsidiary of Orthogen Corporation)	USA
19. Biomaterials Korea	South Korea
20. Biomedicare Company	USA
21. Biomet 3i Implant Innovations Incorporated	USA
22. Bionnovation	Brazil
23. Biost S.n.c.	Italy
24. Biotech International	France
25. Blue Sky Bio LLC	USA
26. Bone System	Italy
27. BPI Biologisch Physikalische Implantate GmbH	Germany
28. BrainBase Corporation	Japan
29. Brasseler Group (Gebr. Brasseler GmbH & Co. KG)	Germany
30. Bredent Medical	Germany
31. BTI Biotechnology Institute S.L.	Spain
32. Btlock S.r.l.	Italy
33. Buck Medical Research	USA
34. Camlog Group (previous name: Altatec)	Switzerland
35. Ceradyne Incorporated	USA
36. CeraRoot	Spain
37. Clinical House Europe GmbH	Switzerland
38. Conexão Implant System	Brazil
39. Cowell Medi Company Limited	South Korea
40. CSM Implant	South Korea
41. Curasan AG	Germany
42. De Bortoli ACE	Brazil
43. Dental Ratio Systems GmbH	Germany
44. Dental Tech	Italy
45. Dentatus	Sweden
46. Dentaurum J.P. Winkelstroeter KG	Germany
47. Dentium	South Korea
48. Dentoflex Comércio e Indústria de Materiais Odontológicos	Brazil
49. Dentos Incorporated	South Korea
50. Dentsply Friadent Ceramed Incorporated (Friadent GmbH Germany)	USA
51. DIO Implant	South Korea
52. Dr Ihde Dental GmbH	Germany
53. Dyna Dental Engineering b.v.	Netherlands
54. Eckermann Laboratorium	Spain
55. Elite Medica	Italy
56. Europäische Akademie für Sofort-Implantologie	Germany
57. Euroteknika	France

Table 1.1. *Continued*

58. GC Implant System	Japan
59. General Implant Research System	Spain
60. Global Dental Corporation	USA
61. Hi-Tec Implants Limited	Israel
62. Impladent Limited	USA
63. Implamed S.r.l.	Italy
64. Implant Direct LLC	USA
65. Implant Logic Systems	USA
66. Implant Media S.A. (outsourcing manufacturing plant)	Spain
67. Implant Microdent System S.L.	Spain
68. Implantkopp	Brazil
69. IMTEC Corporation	USA
70. Institut Straumann AG	Switzerland
71. Interdental S.r.l.	Italy
72. International Defcon Group	Spain
73. Intra-Lock System International	USA
74. Ishifu Metal Industry Incorporated	Japan
75. Japan Medical Materials Corporation	Japan
76. Jeil Medical Corporation	South Korea
77. jmp dental GmbH	Germany
78. JOTA AG	Switzerland
79. Klockner Implants	Spain
80. LASAK Limited	Czech Republic
81. Leader Italy S.r.l.	Italy
82. Leone S.p.A.	Italy
83. Lifecore Biomedical Incorporated	USA
84. Maxon ceramic	Germany
85. Medentis Medical	Germany
86. Megagen	South Korea
87. MIS Implant Technologies Limited Company (MIS)	Israel
88. Mozo-Grau	Spain
89. Neobiotech Company Limited	South Korea
90. Neodent	Brazil
91. Neoss Dental Implant System	UK
92. Nobel Biocare	Sweden
93. OCO Biomedical (previous name: O Company Incorporated)	USA
94. Odontit S.A.	Argentina
95. OGA implant	Japan
96. o.m.t (previous name: Biocer)	Germany
97. Oral implant S.r.l.	Italy
98. Osfix Limited	Finland
99. Ospol AB	Sweden
100. Osstem Company Limited	South Korea
101. Osteocare Implant System Limited	UK
102. Osteo-Implant Corporation	USA
103. Osteoplant	Poland
104. Osteo-Ti	UK
105. PACE™ Dental Technologies Incorporated (Renick Enterprises Incorporated)	USA
106. Paraplant 2000	Germany
107. Paris implants	France
108. Park Dental Research Corporation	USA
109. Pedrazzini Dental Technologie	Germany
110. PHI S.r.l.	Italy
111. Poligono Industrail MasD'En Cisa	Spain
112. Qualibond Implantat GmbH	Germany
113. Quantum Implants	USA
114. Renew Biocare	USA

Table 1.1. *Continued*

115. Reuter Systems GmbH	Germany
116. RT Medical Research & Technologies	Italy
117. Sargon Enterprises Incorporated	USA
118. Schrauben-Implantat-Systeme GmbH	Germany
119. Schütz-Dental	Germany
120. SERF (Société d'Etudes de Recherches et de Fabrications)	France
121. Sic Implants	Switzerland
122. Simpler Implants Incorporated	Canada
123. Sistema de Implante Nacional	Brazil
124. Southern Implants (Pty) Limited	South Africa
125. Star Group International Implant Developments & Technology GmbH	Germany
126. Sterngold Implamed Dental Implant Systems	USA
127. Sweden & Martina S.p.A.	Italy
128. Swiss Implants Incorporated	USA
129. Sybron Implant Solutions (merge from: Innova—Canada & Oraltronics—Germany)	USA
130. Tatum Surgical	USA
131. T.B.R.® Group (previous name: Sudimplant)	France
132. Tenax Dental Implant Systems	Canada
133. TFI System	Italy
134. Thommen Medical	Switzerland
135. Timplant	Czech Republic
136. Tiolox Implants GmbH (previous name: Dentaurum Implants GmbH)	Germany
137. Titan Implants	USA
138. Tixxit GmbH	Germany
139. Trinon Titanium GmbH	Germany
140. Victory-med GmbH	Germany
141. Wieland Dental Implants GmbH	Germany
142. Wolf GmbH	Germany
143. Zimmer Dental (previous names: Centerpulse & Sulzer Dental & Calcitek)	USA
144. Ziterion GmbH	Germany
145. ZL-Microdent-Attachment GmbH & Co. KG	Germany
146. Z-systems AG (Drachenfels AG)	Germany

implant system with less than four trials, but of good methodological quality, and 29 had limited published clinical documentation. It was considered quite troublesome that 28 manufacturers sold implant systems without any form of published clinical documentation. Also worrying was that many manufacturers did not appear to follow international standards for manufacturing their products. The FDI General Assembly in 2004 declared that "Implants are manufactured and sold in some parts of the world without compliance to international standards. It would seem prudent to only use dental implants supported by sound clinical research documentation and which conform to the general principles of good manufacturing practice in compliance with the ISO Standards or FDA (Food and Drug Administration) and other regulatory bodies" (FDI 2004).

The major reason for the chaos reigning today is that in 1998 the U.S. FDA decided to reassign implants made from titanium from class III to class II medical devices. Simply put, this signifies that in order to have a new titanium implant approved in the United States there are no requirements to document clinical performance. It should be stated that this decision was made following massive lobbying by the implant industry at the time. One may wonder whether the implant companies that lobbied for the changes at the time (several of which have since disappeared from the market) are happy today. To be fair, though, nobody could have anticipated the anarchy this would cause today. What can be agreed on is that it is really difficult to see who benefits from this seemingly unstoppable flood of new implant brands. It can't be the dental profession, who will spend time in the future repairing and maintaining the implants. It will not be the patient because they won't be able to locate the dentist who will have the specific required hardware inventory and the knowledge about the particular implant placed, say, 10 years previously. The established implant companies will not benefit because they will need to fend off the often aggressive new companies who under the circumstances market the virtues of their products by extrapolation from bench and animal study data. The regulators are also in a problematic situation, as demonstrated by the recent dramatic failures of one particular single-piece implant carrying the European "CE" mark, indicating that it was an approved product in Europe, and was also approved by the FDA. Thus, in spite of the fact that the implant had been made from the "magical" titanium, and assuming approval based on bench and/or animal models, implant therapy can go horribly wrong in the everyday clinical situation. Who under the circumstances is to blame in the chain between patient, clinician, distributor, manufacturer, and regulators?

Clinical Documentation of Implant Systems

The FDI report published in 2003 summarized the clinical research that validated claims of implant superiority and documented the relationship between particular implant design characteristics and clinical outcomes. In general, the scientific literature until then did not provide any clear directives regarding claims of alleged benefits of specific morphological characteristics of root-formed dental implants (Jokstad et al. 2003). Since then, about 530 new clinical trials involving more than n = 1 patients have been published (Fig 1.1).

These studies form the bulk of scientific evidence for claims of differences in clinical performance of today's various dental implant systems. Unfortunately, the situation is not very different from 2003 in that more than 50% of all trials report on implants manufactured by either Nobel Biocare or Straumann, and 80% of all trials are limited to reports on implants from only six manufacturers (Table 1.2).

Thus, the vast majority of the implant brands on the market today have zero clinical documentation. It is not unreasonable to assume that the manufacturers will not spend time and resources conducting clinical research as long as the current regulations for

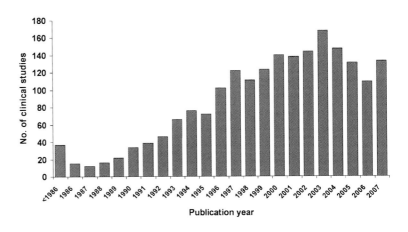

Figure 1.1. Number of clinical trials on implant therapy published in the scientific literature since 1967 sorted according to year of publication (n = 2,029).

Table 1.2. Clinical trials published since 2003 (n = 530), sorted according to implant brand.

Implant Brand	No. of Studies	%	Cumulative %
Nobel Biocare: Brånemark / Replace / Nobeldirect / Nobelperfect / SteriOss, etc.	176	33	33
Straumann / ITI	101	19	52
Dentsply: Frialit / Frialit2 / Frialit+ / Friadent / Frialoc / Frios / Xive / Ankylos	53	10	62
Biomet 3i: Osseotite / Nanotite	41	8	70
Astra	23	4	74
Zimmer: Calcitek / Integral / Omniloc / ScrewVent / Spline / Swissplus, etc.	22	4	78
IMZ	16	3	81
Camlog	7	1	83
Biohorizons/Maestro	6	1	84
Southern Implants	5	1	85
Bicon	5	1	86
Defcon	4	1	87
Sweden&Martina	4	1	88
Other or Not stated	67	13	100%

approval of new implants in the United States do not require any clinical studies at all. "In accordance with the least burdensome provisions of the FDA Modernization Act of 1997, the agency will rely on well-designed bench and/or animal testing rather than requiring clinical studies for new devices unless there is a specific justification for asking for clinical information to support a determination of substantial equivalence" (U.S. Dept. of Health and Human Services 2008). This raises the question of how well the clinical realities are reflected by "well-designed bench and/or animal testing." The current scientific evidence of this assumed correlation is confusing, which may indicate that it is rather weak.

Validity and Value of Animal Studies

It can be established that data from animal models cannot be directly extrapolated to predict longitudinal trial results (Jokstad

et al. 2003). For example, the relationship between the implant surface roughness on bone healing, as measured by biomechanical tests and/or histology, has been reported to correlate (Buser et al. 1998), and not to correlate (London et al. 2002; Novaes et al. 2002; Vercaigne et al. 1998, 2000). Another hypothesis is that such measurements may offer some indications within a midrange of roughness (Wennerberg and Albrektsson 2000). Part of the confusion stems from the variability of (1) surface topography description; (2) animal model used; (3) measuring devices used for roughness characterization; (4) lack of consistency of results; and (5) unknown surgical technique for implant placement.

Regarding surface topography description, Wieland et al. (2001) describe several standards for 2-D and 3-D roughness parameters with respect to amplitude, spacing, or combined amplitude and spacing characteristics. It is not apparent which one is the most appropriate to use, that is, which one best correlates with clinical data from humans.

Animal models that have been used range from implants placed in the mandible, maxilla, tibia, knee, femur, or humerus in goats, canines, rats, rabbits, ewes, miniature pigs, baboons, and rhesus monkeys (Sykaras et al. 2000). What is clear is that no species fulfills all of the requirements of an ideal model (Pearce et al. 2007). Adding to the confusion is the variation of the dimensions of the test implants as well as the observation times, usually varying between 2 weeks and 3 months. It is in fact remarkable that regulatory agencies and clinicians believe in results from "well-designed bench and/or animal testing," given the fact that histological and biomechanical data are affected by a multitude of experimental variables. Some that have been identified as confounders are implant length, implant diameter, implant design, implant material, surface topography, animal model, implantation time, implantation site, biomechanical loading speed, functional loading conditions, analyzed length and thickness, and orientation of the histological section (Sykaras et al. 2000).

Techniques used to characterize surface topographies have all the same advantages and limitations and have the potential to confound meta-analyses if not properly accounted for. The most commonly used, that is, noncontact laser profilometry, interference microscopy, scanning electron microscopy (SEM), stereo-SEM, focused ion beam, transmission electron microscopy, and atomic force microscopy, give different resolution in lateral and vertical directions, and different depths of focus and presence of artifacts (Jarmar et al. 2008; Wieland et al. 2001). It is therefore perhaps not surprising that when the literature on implant surface roughness and bone healing has been critically appraised, it is very difficult to draw statistical inferences from the heterogeneous data (Shalabi et al. 2006).

Finally, the details that most clinicians identify as the most influential variables on implant success—i.e., how the implant bed in the bone was prepared, the relative dimension of the prepared bed to the actual implant diameter or size, and how the implant was actually handled, inserted, angulated, and torqued—are seldom described in detail in "well-designed bench and/or animal testing." It is surprising that without this crucial information, regulatory agencies and many clinicians are prepared to extrapolate in vitro results instead of requesting documentation of realistic clinical performance. It is the author's opinion that it is high time that the regulators worldwide, with FDA as the leading body, attempt to rectify the situation.

WHAT HAVE WE LEARNED FROM RANDOMIZED CONTROLLED CLINICAL TRIALS ON ORAL IMPLANTS?

Marco Esposito, Maria Gabriella Grusovin, Paul Coulthard, and Helen Worthington

The aim of this chapter is to present a brief summary of findings presented in 13 Cochrane *Systematic Reviews* (www.cochrane.org) on the efficacy and safety of various materials and interventions on oral implants.

Methods

Types of studies: Randomized controlled clinical trials (RCTs).

Types of participants: Patients with missing teeth who may require oral rehabilitation with osseointegrated oral implants.

Types of interventions and time points: Dependent on the clinical question; however, in general, implant-supported prostheses had to be in function for at least 1 year.

Types of outcome measures: Dependent on the clinical question; however, the following outcomes were usually evaluated: prosthesis failures, implant failures, complications, patient satisfaction or preference including aesthetics; peri-implant bone-level changes over time; aesthetics evaluated by a dentist; treatment duration and costs.

Search strategy for identification of studies: The following databases were searched— the Cochrane Oral Health Group's Trials Register; the Cochrane Central Register of Controlled Trials (CENTRAL); MEDLINE; EMBASE. There were no language restrictions. We wrote to all the authors of the identified RCTs, we checked the bibliographies of all identified RCTs and relevant review articles, and we used personal contacts in an attempt to identify unpublished or ongoing RCTs. We also wrote to more than 55 oral implant manufacturers and we requested information on trials through an Internet discussion group (implantology@ yahoogroups.com); however, we discontinued this due to poor yield. Several dental journals were hand-searched.

Study selection: The titles, abstracts, and, when necessary, the full report of all identified trials were scanned independently by two review authors to establish whether the studies met the inclusion criteria. Disagreements were resolved by discussion. Where resolution was not possible, a third review author was consulted. All studies meeting the inclusion criteria underwent validity assessment and data extraction. Studies rejected at this or subsequent stages were recorded and reasons for exclusion explained.

Quality assessment: Undertaken independently and in duplicate by two review authors. Three main quality criteria were examined: (1) allocation concealment, recorded as adequate, unclear, or inadequate; (2) treatment blind to outcome assessors, recorded as yes, no, unclear, or not possible; (3) completeness of follow-up (is there a clear explanation for withdrawals and drop-outs in each treatment group?), assessed as yes or no.

After taking into account the additional information provided by the authors of the trials, studies were judged at low risk of

bias (plausible bias unlikely to seriously alter the results) if all criteria were met, or at high risk of bias (plausible bias that seriously weakens confidence in the results) if one or more criteria were not met.

Data extraction: Data were extracted by two review authors independently using specially designed data extraction forms. Any disagreement was discussed and a third review author consulted where necessary. All authors were contacted for clarification or missing information. Data were excluded until further clarification was available if agreement could not be reached.

Data synthesis: For dichotomous outcomes, the estimate of the effect of an intervention was expressed as relative risks (RRs) or odds ratios (ORs) together with 95% confidence intervals (CIs). For continuous outcomes, weighted mean differences and standard deviations were used to summarize the data for each group using mean differences and 95% CIs. The statistical unit was the patient and not the procedure or the implant. Only if there were studies of similar comparisons reporting the same outcome measures was meta-analysis done. Odds ratios were combined for dichotomous data, and mean differences for continuous data, using random-effects models.

Clinical Hypotheses and Main Findings

The following clinical hypotheses were tested:

1. What is more effective for patients, pre-prosthetic surgery and a denture or an implant-retained prosthesis? (1 included RCT) (Coulthard et al. 2002). Last search: January 2008.

2. (a) Are prophylactic antibiotics effective in reducing postoperative infections and failures? (2 included RCTs); (b) Which is the most effective antibiotic, at what dose and duration? (0 RCTs) (Esposito et al. 2008c). Last search: January 2008.

3. Is there a difference in clinical performance between various implants? (16 included and 24 excluded trials). Is there a difference in the occurrence of early failures between turned and roughened dental implants? Is there a difference in the occurrence of peri-implantitis between turned and roughened dental implants? (Esposito et al. 2007e). Last search: June 2007.

4. Whether and when is flap elevation necessary? (2 included RCTs). Which is the most effective flap design or technique for specific clinical indications? (3 included RCTs). Whether and when are soft tissue correction or augmentation procedures necessary? (1 excluded RCT). Which is the most effective soft tissue correction or augmentation technique for specific clinical indications? (0 RCT). Whether and when the peri-implant attached or keratinized mucosa has to be increased? (0 RCT). Which is the most effective technique to increase the attached or keratinized mucosa for specific clinical indications? (1 excluded RCT). Which are the most effective suturing techniques or materials? (1 excluded RCT) (Esposito et al. 2007a). Last search: June 2007.

5. Is it better to place implants immediately after tooth extraction? To wait for a few weeks for the soft tissue to heal? Or to wait for complete bony healing? (2 included RCTs) (Esposito et al. 2006). Last search: January 2008.

6. How many implants are needed to support different types of prostheses? (2 included RCTs) (Coulthard et al. 2003). Last search: June 2007.

7. Is it better to load the implants immediately, early, or after a conventional healing period? (11 included and 9 excluded RCTs) (Esposito et al. 2007d). Last search: June 2007.

8. Is a one-stage implant placement procedure as effective as a two-stage procedure submerging the implants under soft tissue for undisturbed healing? (2 included and 1 excluded RCTs) (Esposito et al. 2007b). Last search: January 2008.

9. Whether and when are bone augmentation procedures necessary? Which is the most effective augmentation technique for specific clinical indications? (17 included and 23 excluded RCTs) (Esposito et al. 2008b). Last search: January 2008.

10. Are zygomatic implants with and without bone augmenting procedures more effective than conventional dental implants in augmented bone for severely resorbed maxillae? (no RCT) (Esposito et al. 2005). Last search: January 2008.

11. Which are the most effective interventions for maintaining and recovering soft tissue health around osseointegrated dental implants? (9 included and 9 excluded RCTs) (Grusovin et al. 2008). Last search: June 2007.

12. Which are the most effective interventions for treating peri-implantitis? (7 included and 3 excluded RCTs) (Esposito et al. 2008a). Last search: January 2008.

13. Is hyperbaric oxygen therapy (HBO) beneficial for patients requiring dental implants who were irradiated in the head and neck? (1 included RCT) (Esposito et al. 2007c). Last search: January 2008.

Conclusions and Main Clinical Implications

1. There is weak evidence from the results of 1 RCT with 60 subjects that patients are generally less satisfied with preprosthetic surgery and a conventional denture than with an implant-retained overdenture.

2. A meta-analysis of two trials suggested that 2 g of amoxicillin given 1 hour preoperatively significantly reduces early failures of dental implants placed in ordinary conditions. More specifically, giving antibiotics to 25 patients will avoid 1 patient experiencing early implant losses.

No statistically significant differences in postoperative infections and adverse events were observed. No major adverse events were reported. Therefore it might be sensible to suggest the routine use of one dose of prophylactic amoxicillin just before placing dental implants. It remains unclear whether an adjunctive use of postoperative antibiotics is beneficial.

3. There is no evidence showing that any particular type of dental implant has superior long-term success. There is limited evidence showing that implants with relatively smooth (turned) surfaces are less prone to lose bone due to chronic infection (peri-implantitis) than implants with rougher surfaces. There is a tendency for implants with a turned surface to fail early more often than implants with roughened surfaces. No trial described implants made or coated with materials other than titanium. These conclusions are based on RCTs with relatively short follow-up periods, few patients, and at high risk of bias. So we do not know if there are implant characteristics or an implant system superior to others due to the scarcity of reliable scientific research.

4. There is evidence suggesting that flapless or mini-invasive procedures can cause less postoperative pain, edema, and consumption of analgesics than conventional flap elevation. Flapless surgery performed by skillful clinicians in properly selected cases can be as successful and complication-free as conventional flap elevation. However, there is still insufficient evidence regarding a potential increased risk of complications or failures using a flapless approach. Clinicians should select patients for flapless implant placement with a great deal of caution in relation to their own clinical skills and experience. Still needing to be assessed are the safety and efficacy of customized surgical templates created with the help of planning software on CT scans to facilitate placement of dental implants.

There is still a lack of evidence about the most effective incision or suturing techniques or materials, or the most effective techniques to manipulate or augment soft tissues for aesthetic reasons or to increase the width of keratinized or attached mucosa, if the latter is of any benefit for the patients.

5. Post-extractive immediate and immediate-delayed implants are viable treatment options. Immediate-delayed implants may provide a better aesthetic outcome and are preferred by patients when compared to delayed implants, even though they might be associated with increased failure and complication rates. More RCTs are needed to confirm these preliminary findings.

6. Two implants appear to be as effective as four implants to support a mandibular overdenture.

7. It is possible to successfully load implants immediately or early after their placement in selected patients, though not all clinicians may be able to achieve optimal results. A high degree of primary implant stability (high value of insertion torque) seems to be one of the prerequisites for a successful procedure.

8. No relevant clinical differences appear to exist between a one- or a two-stage implant procedure; however, the number of patients included in the trials (45 subjects) was too small to draw definitive conclusions. If these findings are confirmed by larger trials, the major clinical implication will be that the one-stage approach might be preferable since it avoids one surgical intervention and shortens treatment times. However, there might be situations, for instance when an implant has not obtained an optimal primary stability or when barriers are used for guided tissue regeneration, in which a two-stage submerged approach might still be preferable.

9. Three trials investigated whether and when augmentation procedures are necessary: the augmentation of resorbed mandibles of 6–12 mm height with an interposed iliac crest graft resulted in more surgical and prosthetic complica-

tions, and statistically significantly more implant failures, severe pain, days of hospitalization, costs, and longer treatment time than using short implants. Current evidence may not justify major bone grafting procedures for resorbed mandibles. There is evidence that non-resorbable barriers allow statistically significantly more bone regeneration than no barrier at fenestrated implants; however, it is not proven that such newly generated bone is of any use or benefit to the patient. While bone regenerative procedures at exposed implants might be useful, there is not yet reliable evidence regarding which are the proper indications. There is not enough reliable evidence supporting or refuting the need for augmentation procedures at immediate implants placed in fresh extraction sockets.

Fourteen trials investigated the most effective augmentation techniques for specific clinical indications: bone substitutes (Bio-Oss and Cerasorb) might be equally effective as autogenous bone grafts for augmenting atrophic maxillary sinuses. Therefore they might be used as a replacement for autogenous bone grafting, although these preliminary findings need to be confirmed by large multicenter trials. Various augmentation techniques are able to regenerate bone in a vertical direction. There is, however, insufficient evidence to indicate which technique could be preferable. Osteodistraction is of little use in the presence of thin ridges but may allow more vertical regeneration. Complications with GBR techniques are common, and in some cases determined the failure of the augmentation procedure. Clinicians and patients should carefully evaluate the benefits and risks in relation to the desired outcome when deciding whether to use vertical ridge augmentation techniques. Various augmentation techniques are able to regenerate bone horizontally; there is, however, insufficient evidence to indicate which technique is preferable. It appears that a bone substitute (Bio-Oss) can be used with little higher risk of an implant failure. There is no reliable evidence supporting superior success of any of the alternative techniques for augmenting bone at fenestrated implants or at immediate implants placed in fresh extraction sockets. Sites treated with barrier plus Bio-Oss showed a higher position of the gingival margin (1.2 mm) when compared to sites treated with barriers alone. Bone morphogenetic proteins (rhBMP-2) used in conjunction with Bio-Oss and resorbable barriers may promote bone formation at exposed implants with bone fenestration and dehiscence. There is insufficient evidence supporting or confuting the efficacy of various active agents such as platelet-rich plasma in conjunction with implant treatment. Titanium screws might be preferable to resorbable poly (D, L-lactide) acid screws to fix onlay bone blocks. It can be hypothesized that the use of particulated autogenous bone collected from intraoral locations with bone filters attached to suction devices might be associated with an increased risk of infective complications. These findings are based on few trials including few patients, some with short follow-up, and frequently judged to be at high risk of bias.

10. No published or ongoing RCT and controlled clinical trial evaluating the efficacy of zygomatic implants was identified.

11. There is some evidence from one small RCT that Listerine mouthwash, used twice a day for 30 seconds, as an adjunct to routine oral hygiene, is effective in reducing plaque formation and marginal peri-implant bleeding. Evaluation of the other tested maintenance interventions was inconclusive because it was based on trials having too short of follow-up periods (6 months or less) and limited numbers of subjects. There is not any reliable evidence regarding which could be the most effective maintenance regimens from a long-term perspective.

12. The use of adjunctive antibiotic therapy (Atridox) to manual debridement was associated with additional probing attachment level (PAL) and pocket probing depth (PPD) improvements in the range of 0.6 mm after 4 months in patients who had severe forms of peri-implantitis (i.e., having lost at least 50% of the peri-implant bone) in one trial. The use of a bovine-derived xenograft (Bio-Oss) with a resorbable barrier (Bio-Gide) was associated with PAL and PPD improvements of 0.5 mm after 6 months in infrabony defects deeper than 3 mm when compared to nanocrystalline hydroxyapatite (Ostim) in one trial. In four other trials evaluating local antibiotics, the Vector system, and a laser therapy, respectively, no statistically significant differences were observed when compared with subgingival debridement. Smoothening of rough implant surfaces did not show statistically significant differences when compared to implants whose surfaces were not smoothed. However, sample sizes were small, and therefore these conclusions have to be viewed with great caution.

13. It appears that HBO therapy in irradiated patients requiring dental implants may not offer any appreciable clinical benefits.

SYSTEMATIC REVIEWS OF SURVIVAL AND COMPLICATION RATES OF IMPLANT-SUPPORTED FIXED DENTAL PROSTHESES AND SINGLE CROWNS

Bjarni Elvar Pætursson

Introduction

In daily practice, dentists routinely face the challenge of making quick and often difficult decisions. These are mostly influenced by paradigms dictated by basic dental education and many years of clinical practice.

There is still an open question as to whether or not the practice of evidence-based treatment planning is possible in prosthetic dentistry. Ideally, treatment decisions should be based on well-performed systematic reviews of the available evidence and, if possible, on formal quantitative evidence, synthesis, and meta-analysis (Egger and Smith 1997; Egger et al. 2001a, 2001c).

Reviewing the literature involves grading of the available and published studies. Often, such gradings are based on study design. Usually randomized studies are rated higher than observational studies (Grades of Recommendation 2004). Furthermore, the quality of studies and trials is of crucial importance: if the "raw material" is flawed, then the findings of reviews of this material may also be compromised (Egger and Smith 1997; Egger et al. 2001a). The trials and studies included in systematic reviews and meta-analyses should ideally be of high methodological quality and free of bias. As a consequence the differences in study outcomes observed between patients can confidently be attributed to the intervention under investigation. If there are no studies on the highest level of evidence (randomized controlled clinical trials), the systematic review has to be based on the highest level of evidence available (Egger et al. 2001b; Glasziou et al. 2004) and point out what additional research should be conducted to strengthen the evidence base.

The studies in the dental literature reporting on tooth-supported and implant-supported fixed dental prostheses (FDPs) are mostly observational studies and single-center case cohorts. There are no studies available on the highest level of evidence (RCTs) comparing tooth-supported and implant-supported FDPs. In addition, only a few studies have reported on the longevity of reconstructions on implants with the same details.

An RCT to compare tooth-supported and implant-supported FDPs would be best conducted in a multicenter setting with long enough follow-up time and sample sizes to allow the estimation of relevant differences between the outcomes of the treatments.

respectively (Table 1.4). However, it must be remembered that the results for combined tooth-implant-supported FDPs, implant-supported SCs, and RBBs after 10-year follow-up are based on a small number of observations, with 72, 69, and 51 reconstructions, respectively (Table 1.4).

When the studies reporting solely on metal-ceramic reconstructions, excluding gold-resin and all-ceramic reconstruction, were analyzed separately, the lowest annual failure rate was seen for implant-supported FDP (0.66), followed by implant-supported SCs (0.92) (Table 1.5).

Table 1.4. Summary of annual failure rates, relative failure rates, and 10-year survival estimates.

Type of Reconstruction	Total No. of Reconstructions	Total Exposure Time	Mean Follow-Up Time	Estimated Annual Failure Rate	10-Year Survival Summary Estimate (95% CI)
Conventional FDPs	1,218	10,446	11.9	1.14** (0.48–2.73)	89.2%** (76.1–95.3%)
Cantilever FDPs	239	2,229	10.9	2.20* (1.70–2.84)	80.3%* (75.2–84.4%)
Resin Bonded Bridges	51	464	9.1	4.31* (2.63–6.66)	65.0%* (51.4–76.9%)
Implant-Supported FDPs	219	1,889	10	1.43* (1.08–1.89)	86.7%* (82.8–89.8%)
Tooth-Implant-Supported FDPs	72	517	10	2.51* (1.54–4.10)	77.8%* (66.4–85.7%)
Implant-Supported SCs	69	623	10	1.12 (0.45–2.32)	89.4% (79.3–95.6%)

*Based on standard Poisson regression.
**Based on random-effects Poisson regression.

Table 1.5. Summary of annual failure rates, relative failure rates, and 5-year survival estimates for different types of metal-ceramic reconstructions.

Type of Reconstruction	Total No. of Reconstructions	Total Exposure Time	Mean Follow-Up Time	Estimated Annual Failure Rate	5-Year Survival Summary Estimate (95% CI)
Conventional FDPs	1,163	9,301	8.0	1.15** (0.71–1.87)	94.4%** (91.1–96.5%)
Cantilever FDPs	304	1,947	6.4	2.00* (1.44–2.79)	90.5%* (87.0–93.1%)
Implant-Supported FDPs	948	5,014	5.3	0.66* (0.52–0.83)	96.8%* (95.9–97.4%)
Tooth-Implant-Supported FDPs	124	712	5.7	1.37** (0.35–5.32)	93.4%** (76.6–98.2%)
Implant-Supported SCs	259	1,636	6.3	0.92* (0.66–1.27)	95.5%* (93.9–96.7%)

*Based on standard Poisson regression.
**Based on random-effects Poisson regression.

Biological Complications

Peri-implant mucosal lesions were reported in various ways by the different authors. Several studies provided information on soft tissue complications and peri-implantitis, while other studies reported signs of inflammation (pain, redness, swelling, and bleeding) or "soft tissue complications," defined as fistula, gingivitis, or hyperplasia.

In a random-effects Poisson-model analysis, the annual complication rates were 1.79 for implant-supported FDPs, 1.44 for combined tooth-implant-supported FDPs, and 2.03 for implant-supported SCs. This translates into 5-year rates of soft tissue complications of 8.6% for implant-supported FDPs, 7.0% for combined tooth-implant-supported FDPs, and 9.7% for implant-supported SCs (Table 1.6).

For combined tooth-implant-supported FDPs, five studies reported on intrusion of abutment teeth. After a 5-year observation period, intrusion was detected in 5.2% of the abutment teeth (Table 1.6).

Nine studies reported on survival of tooth and implant abutments in combined tooth-implant FDPs. After an observation period of 5 years, 3.2% of the abutment teeth and 3.4% of the functionally loaded implants were lost. At 10 years, this information was available only from two studies (Brägger et al. 2005; Gunne et al. 1999). The corresponding proportions were 10.6% for the abutment teeth compared to 15.6% for the implants. The reasons reported for loss of abutment teeth were tooth fractures, caries, endodontic complications, and periodontitis. Loss of retention was frequently associated with tooth fractures or caries.

For implant-supported SCs, ten studies evaluated changes in marginal bone height over the observation period, evaluated on radiographs. In Poisson-model analysis, the cumulative rate of implants having bone loss exceeding 2 mm after 5 years was 6.3% (Table 1.6).

Multivariable Poisson regression was used to investigate formally whether incidence of soft tissue complications and incidence of bone loss > 2 mm varied between cemented and screw-retained crowns. No significant difference ($p = 0.42$ and $p = 0.84$) was detected regarding influence of crown design on these biological complications.

Six studies on SCs reported on the aesthetic outcome of the treatment. The aesthetic appearance was evaluated either by dental professionals or by patients themselves. In a meta-analysis, the cumulative rate of crowns having unacceptable or semi-optimal aesthetic appearance was 8.7% (Table 1.6).

Technical Complications

The most common technical complication for implant-supported reconstructions was the fracture of a veneer material (acryl, ceramic, and composite). In a Poisson-model analysis, the annual complication rates were 2.53 for implant-supported FDPs, 1.51 for combined tooth-implant-supported FDPs, and 0.92 for implant-supported SCs, translating into 5-year rates of veneer fractures of 11.9% for implant-supported FDPs, 7.2% for combined tooth-implant-supported FDPs, and 4.5% for implant-supported SCs (Table 1.6). When gold-resin reconstructions were excluded and ceramic fractures or chippings analyzed separately for metal-ceramic reconstructions, the 5-year complication rates for implant-supported FDPs decreased to 8.8% and for implant-supported SCs the 5-year rate of fractures decreased to 3.5% (Table 1.6).

Comparing the rate of ceramic fracture or ceramic chipping of conventional tooth-supported FDPs and solely implant-supported FDPs, the tooth-supported FDPs had a significantly ($p = 0.042$) lower 5-year risk of ceramic fracture or chipping of 2.9% compared with 8.8% for the implant-supported FDPs.

With the exception of implant-supported SCs, fracture of the framework of the reconstruction was a rare complication. The annual complication rates were 0.13 for implant-supported FDPs and 0.33 for combined tooth-implant-supported FDPs, translating into

Table 1.6. Summary of complications by implant-supported reconstructions.

Complication	Implant-Supported FDPs			Combined Tooth-Implant-Supported FDPs			Implant-Supported Single Crowns		
	Number of Impl. or Reconst.	Summary Estimate Event Rates (95% CI)	Cumulative 5-Year Complication Rates (95% CI)	Number of Impl. or Reconst.	Summary Estimate Event Rates (95% CI)	Cumulative 5-Year Complication Rates (95% CI)	Number of Impl. or Reconst.	Summary Estimate Event Rates (95% CI)	Cumulative 5-Year Complication Rates (95% CI)
Estimated Rate of Soft Tissue Complications	751	1.79* (1.05–3.03)	8.6%* (5.1%–14.1%)	184	1.44* (0.35–5.96)	7.0%* (1.7–25.8%)	267	2.03* (1.05–3.95)	9.7%* (5.1–17.9%)
Estimated Rate of Bone Loss > 2 mm		n.a.	n.a.		n.a.	n.a.	509	1.31* (0.61–2.79)	6.3%* (3.0–13.0%)
Estimated Rate of Aesthetic Complications		n.a.	n.a.		n.a.	n.a.	418	1.82* (0.64–5.12)	8.7%* (3.2–22.6%)
Estimated Rate of Abutment Tooth Intrusion		n.a.	n.a.	506	1.07* (0.40–2.87)	5.2%* (2.0–13.3%)		n.a.	n.a.
Estimated Rate of Implant Fracture	2,559	0.11* (0.05–0.23)	0.5%* (0.3–1.1%)	530	0.20* (0.08–0.34)	0.8%* (0.4–1.7%)	1,312	0.03* (0.006–0.13)	0.14%* (0.03–0.64%)
Estimated Rate of Abutment or Screw Fracture	2,590	0.30** (0.16–0.57)	1.5%** (0.8–2.8%)	511	0.11* (0.06–0.22)	0.6%* (0.3–1.1%)	510	0.07* (0.018–0.28)	0.35%* (0.09–1.4%)
Estimated Rate of Loose Abutments or Screws	2,453	1.15** (0.76–1.74)	5.6%** (3.7–8.3%)	296	1.44* (0.95–2.17)	6.9%* (4.7–10.3%)	752	2.72** (1.17–6.30)	12.7%** (5.7–27.0%)
Estimated Rate of Lost Access Hole Restorations	169	1.77	8.9%		n.a.	n.a.		n.a.	n.a.
Estimated Rate of Loss of Retention	93	1.18* (0.60–2.34)	5.7%* (3.0–11.0%)	286	1.53* (1.09–2.13)	7.3%* (5.3–10.1%)	374	1.13** (0.44–2.91)	5.5%** (2.2–13.5%)
Estimated Rate of Veneer Fracture	948	2.53** (1.60–4.02)	11.9%** (7.7–18.2%)	125	1.51* (0.98–2.30)	7.2%* (4.8–10.9%)	508	0.92** (0.48–1.75)	4.5%** (2.4–8.4%)
Estimated Rate of Ceramic Chipping or Fracture	521	1.84** (1.03–3.27)	8.8%** (5.0–15.1%)	125	1.51* (0.98–2.30)	7.2%* (4.8–10.9%)	402	0.71** (0.34–1.46)	3.5%** (1.7–7.0%)
Estimated Rate of Framework Fracture	623	0.13* (0.06–0.32)	0.7%* (0.3–1.6%)	120	0.33* (0.12–0.91)	1.6%* (0.6–4.4%)	348	0.61** (0.22–1.73)	3.0%** (1.1–8.3%)

*Based on standard Poisson regression.
**Based on random-effects Poisson regression.

5-year rates of framework fracture of 0.7% and 1.6%, respectively. For implant-supported SCs the fracture of the crown framework (coping) was reported in seven studies, and its annual complication rate was 0.61, translating into a 5-year rate of framework fracture of 3.0%. This technical complication was significantly higher (p = 0.016) in studies reporting on all-ceramic crowns.

The second most common technical complication was abutment or occlusal screw loosening. In a Poisson-model analysis, the annual complication rates were 1.15 for implant-supported FDPs, 1.44 for combined tooth-implant-supported FDPs, and 2.72 for implant-supported SCs, translating into 5-year rates of abutment or occlusal screw loosening of 5.6% for implant-supported FDPs, 6.9% for combined tooth-implant-supported FDPs, and 12.7% for implant-supported SCs (Table 1.6). In this repect one study (Henry et al. 1996), reporting on the first generation of single crowns on Brånemark implants, was a clear outlier. If this study is excluded from the analysis, the cumulative incidence of screw loosening decreases to 5.8%.

Loss of the screw access hole restoration was reported only in one study (Örtorp and Jemt 1999). This occurred in 8.2% of the anchors.

Another technical complication was the loss of retention. From 753 FDPs analyzed, this complication occurred in 45 of the reconstructions. The annual complication rates were 1.18 for implant-supported FDPs, 1.53 for combined tooth-implant-supported FDPs, and 1.13 for implant-supported SCs, translating into 5-year rates of loss of retention of 5.7% for implant-supported FDPs, 7.3% for combined tooth-implant-supported FDPs, and 5.5% for implant-supported SCs (Table 1.6). Two studies reporting on the same cohort of patients (Brägger et al. 2001, 2005) evaluated loss of retention. The cumulative incidence was 2.9% after 5 years but increased to 16.0% after 10 years.

Fractures of components such as implants, abutments, and occlusal screws were rare complications. Out of 3,611 implants analyzed, 21 abutments and occlusal screws fractured. The annual complication rates were 0.30 for implant-supported FDPs, 0.11 for combined tooth-implant-supported FDPs, and 0.07 for implant-supported SCs, translating into 5-year rates of abutment and occlusal screw fractures of 1.5% for implant-supported FDPs, 0.6% for combined tooth-implant-supported FDPs, and 0.35% for implant-supported SCs (Table 1.6).

Out of 4,401 implants analyzed, 21 fractured. The annual failure rates were 0.11 for implant-supported FDPs, 0.20 for combined tooth-implant-supported FDPs, and 0.03 for implant-supported SCs, giving 5-year rates of implant fracture of 0.5% for implant-supported FDPs, 0.8% for combined tooth-implant-supported FDPs, and 0.14% for implant-supported SCs (Table 1.6).

Clinical Implications

When planning prosthetic rehabilitations, conventional end-abutment tooth-supported FDPs, solely implant-supported FDPs, or implant-supported SCs should be the first treatment option. Cantilever tooth-supported FDPs, combined tooth-implant-supported FDPs, or resin bonded bridges should be chosen only as a second option.

For implant-supported reconstructions, the incidence of biological complications such as mucositis and peri-implantitis was similar for solely implant-supported, combined implant-tooth-supported FDPs, and implant-supported SCs. Fractures of the veneer material (ceramic fractures), abutment or screw loosening, and loss of retention were the most frequently encountered technical complications. Fractures of the veneer material were more frequent in studies reporting on gold-acrylic than on metal-ceramic reconstructions.

The incidence of complications is substantially higher in implant-supported than in tooth-supported reconstructions. This, however, does not necessarily imply that the possibilities for corrective measures are more cumbersome.

Although a variety of subjective and objective aspects heavily influences the choice of treatment modalities, the knowledge of survival and complication rates of various reconstructions based on long-term studies certainly helps in optimizing the decision process.

Based on the results of the present systematic review, planning of prosthetic rehabilitations should preferentially include conventional and abutment tooth-supported FDPs, solely implant-supported FDPs, or implant-supported SCs. Only for reasons of anatomical structure or patient-centered preferences, and as a second option, should cantilever tooth-supported FDPs, FDPs supported by combination of implants and teeth, or resin bonded bridges be chosen.

Despite high survival rates of fixed dental prostheses, biological and technical complications were frequent. This, in turn, means that substantial amounts of chair time have to be accepted by the patient, dental services, and society at large following the incorporation of FDPs.

Research Implications

It was evident from the search of the entire dental literature on fixed dental prostheses that there is a need for longitudinal studies with 10 or more years of observation. This is especially evident for implant-supported reconstructions and there is a definitive need for more longitudinal studies addressing such reconstructions.

The present systematic review revealed several shortcomings in the conduct and reporting of clinical studies of fixed dental prostheses resulting in the following recommendations.

Long-term cohort studies on reconstructions should have complete follow-up information, preferably with similar length of follow-up for all patients. This means that data on well-defined time periods should be reported for the entire cohort. Due to various definitions of success authors should report

data on survival in combination with incidence of complications. Survival and success (free of all complications) of the suprastructures should be reported.

Well-defined criteria should be used for the assessment of the biological and technical complications. Data from clinical and radiographic assessments should be described using frequency distributions. Collaborative efforts to conduct a pooled individual patient data analysis of the patients and implants in the various studies would allow the development and use of common definitions of complications and help to obtain a clearer picture of the long-term survival.

Biological complications defined by (1) the threshold level of PPD, (2) the presence/absence of bleeding on probing (BOP)/suppuration assessed at any examination interval, and (3) crestal bone loss over time should be described for implants and neighboring teeth.

Technical complications should be divided into (1) major, such as implant fracture, loss of suprastructures; (2) medium, such as abutment or abutment fracture, veneer or framework fractures, aesthetic and phonetic complications; and (3) minor, such as abutment and screw loosening, loss of retention, loss of screw hole sealing, veneer chipping (to be polished), and occlusal adjustments. The type and number of events of technical complications per time interval as well as time/cost required should also be reported.

References

ADA Council on Scientific Affairs. 1996. Dental endosseous implants: An update. *J Am Dent Assoc* 127(8):1238–1239.

Albrektsson T, Sennerby L. 1991. State of the art in oral implants. *J Clin Periodontol* 18(6):474–481.

Berglundh T, Persson L, Klinge B. 2002. A systematic review of the incidence of biological and technical complications in implant dentistry reported in prospective longitudinal studies of at least 5 years. *J Clin Periodontol* 29:197–212.

Binon PP. 2000. Implants and components: Entering the new millennium. *Int J Oral Maxillofac Implants* 15:76–94.

Brägger U, Aeschlimann S, Bürgi W, Hämmerle CHF, Lang NP. 2001. Biological and technical complications and failures with fixed partial dentures (FDP) on implants and teeth after four to five years of function. *Clin Oral Implants Res* 12:26–34.

Brägger U, Karoussis I, Persso R, Pjetursson BE, Salvi G, Lang NP. 2005. Technical and biological complications and failures with single crowns and fixed partial dentures on implant of the ITI® Dental Implant System: A 10-year prospective cohort study. *Clin Oral Implants Res* 16:326–334.

Buser D, Nydegger T, Hirt HP, Cochran DL, Nolte LP. 1998. Removal torque values of titanium implants in the maxilla of miniature pigs. *Int J Oral Maxillofac Implants* 13(5):611–619.

Coulthard P, Esposito M, Jokstad A, Worthington HV. 2003. Interventions for replacing missing teeth: Surgical techniques for placing dental implants. *Cochrane Database of Systematic Reviews* 2003, Issue 1, article no. CD003606. DOI: 10.1002/14651858.CD003606.

Coulthard P, Esposito M, Worthington HV, Jokstad A. 2002. Interventions for replacing missing teeth: Preprosthetic surgery versus dental implants. *Cochrane Database of Systematic Reviews* 2002, Issue 4, article no. CD003604. DOI: 10.1002/14651858.CD003604.

Eckert SE, Parein A, Myshin HL, Padilla JL. 1997. Validation of dental implant systems through a review of literature supplied by system manufacturers. *J Prosthet Dent* 77(3):271–279.

Egger M, Dickersin K, Smith GD. 2001c. Problems and limitations in conducting systematic reviews. In: *Systematic Reviews in Health Care: Meta-analysis in Context*, 2nd ed. M Egger, GD Smith, and DG Altmann (eds.). London: BMJ.

Egger M, Smith GD. 1997. Meta-analysis: Potentials and promise. *BMJ* 315:1371–1374.

Egger M, Smith GD, Schneider M. 2001b. Systematic reviews of observational studies. In: *Systematic Reviews in Health Care: Meta-analysis in Context*, 2nd ed. M Egger, GD Smith, and DG Altmann (eds.). London: BMJ.

Egger M, Smith GD, Sterne JA. 2001a. Uses and abuses of metaanalysis. *Clin Medicine* 1:478–484.

English CE. 1988. Cylindrical implants. Parts I, II, III. *California Dent Assoc J* 16:17–38.

Esposito M, Grusovin MG, Kakisis I, Coulthard P, Worthington HV. 2008a. Interventions for replacing missing teeth: Treatment of perimplantitis. *Cochrane Database of Systematic Reviews* 2008, Issue 1, article no. CD004970. DOI: 10.1002/14651858.CD004970.pub3.

Esposito M, Grusovin MG, Kwan S, Worthington HV, Coulthard P. 2008b. Interventions for replacing missing teeth: Bone augmentation techniques for dental implant treatment. *Cochrane Database of Systematic Reviews* 2008, Issue 2, article no. CD003607. DOI: 10.1002/14651858.CD003607.pub3.

Esposito M, Grusovin MG, Maghaireh H, Coulthard P, Worthington HV. 2007a. Interventions for replacing missing teeth: Management of soft tissues for dental implants. *Cochrane Database of Systematic Reviews* 2007, Issue 3, article no. CD006697. DOI: 10.1002/14651858.CD006697.

Esposito M, Grusovin MG, Martinis E, Coulthard P, Worthington HV. 2007b. Interventions for replacing missing teeth: 1- vs 2-stage implant placement. *Cochrane Database of Systematic Reviews* 2007, Issue 3, article no. CD006698. DOI: 10.1002/14651858.CD006698.

Esposito M, Grusovin MG, Patel S, Coulthard P, Worthington HV. 2007c. Interventions for replacing missing teeth: Hyperbaric oxygen therapy for irradiated patients who require dental implants. *Cochrane Database of Systematic Reviews* 2007, Issue 4, article no. CD003603. DOI: 10.1002/14651858.CD003603.pub2.

Esposito M, Grusovin MG, Talati M, Coulthard P, Oliver R, Worthington HV. 2008c. Interventions for replacing missing teeth: Antibiotics at dental implant placement to prevent complications. *Cochrane Database of Systematic Reviews* 2008, Issue 2, article no. CD004152. DOI: 10.1002/14651858.CD004152.pub2.

Esposito M, Grusovin MG, Willings M, Coulthard P, Worthington HV. 2007d. Interventions for replacing missing teeth: Different times for loading dental implants. *Cochrane Database of Systematic Reviews* 2007, Issue 1, article no. CD003878. DOI: 10.1002/14651858.CD003878.pub3.

Esposito M, Koukoulopoulu A, Coulthard P, Worthington HV. 2006. Interventions for replacing missing teeth: Dental implants in fresh extraction sockets (immediate, immediate-delayed and delayed implants). *Cochrane Database of Systematic Reviews* 2006, Issue 4, article no. CD005968. DOI: 10.1002/14651858.CD005968.pub2.

Esposito M, Murray-Curtis L, Grusovin MG, Coulthard P, Worthington HV. 2007e. Interventions for replacing missing teeth: Different types of dental implants. *Cochrane Database of Systematic Reviews* 2007, Issue 3, article no. CD003815. DOI: 10.1002/14651858.CD003815.pub3.

Esposito M, Worthington HV, Coulthard P. 2005. Interventions for replacing missing teeth: Dental implants in zygomatic bone for the rehabilitation of the severely deficient edentulous maxilla. *Cochrane Database of Systematic Reviews* 2005, Issue 3, article no. CD004151. DOI: 10.1002/14651858.CD004151.pub2.

FDI World Dental Federation. 2004. FDI Policy Statements. URL: http://www.fdiworldental.org/federation/3_1english.html#D. Accessed March 15, 2008.

Glasziou P, Vandenbroucke JP, Chalmers I. 2004. Assessing the quality of research. *BMJ* 328:39–41.

Grades of Recommendation, Assessment Development and Evaluation (GRADE) Working Group. 2004. Grading quality of evidence and strength of recommendations. *BMJ* 328:1490.

Grusovin MG, Coulthard P, Jourabchian E, Worthington H, Esposito M. 2008. Interventions for replacing missing teeth: Maintaining and recovering soft tissue health around dental implants. *Cochrane Database of Systematic Reviews* 2007, Issue 4, article no. CD003069. DOI: 10.1002/14651858.CD003069.pub3.

Gunne J, Åstrand P, Lindh T, Borg K, Olsson M. 1999. Tooth-implant and implant supported fixed partial dentures: A 10-year report. *Int J Prosthodont* 12:216–221.

Henry PJ. 1995. Implant hardware. Science or commodity development. *J Dent Res* 74(1):301–302.

Henry PJ, Laney WR, Jemt T, Harris D, Krogh PH, Polizzi G, Zarb GA, Herrmann I. 1996. Osseointegrated implants for single-tooth replacement: A prospective 5-year multicenter study. *Int J Oral Maxillofac Implants* 11:450–455.

Jarmar T, Palmquist A, Brånemark R, Hermansson L, Engqvist H, Thomsen P. 2008. Characterization of the surface properties of commercially available dental implants using scanning electron microscopy, focused ion beam, and high-resolution transmission electron microscopy. *Clin Implant Dent Relat Res* 10(1):11–22.

Jokstad A, Braeggger U, Brunski JB, Carr AB, Naert I, Wennerberg A. 2003. Quality of dental implants. *Int Dental J* 53(6 Suppl 2):409–443.

Jung RE, Pjetursson BE, Glauser R, Zembic A, Zwahlen M, Lang NP. 2008. A systematic review of the 5-year survival and complication rates of implant-supported single crowns. *Clin Oral Implants Res* 19:119–130.

Kirkwood BR, Sterne JAC. 2003. *Essential Medical Statistics*. Oxford: Blackwell Science Ltd.

Lang NP, Pjetursson BE, Tan K, Brägger U, Egger M, Zwahlen M. 2004. A systematic review of the survival and complication rates of fixed partial dentures (FDPs) after an observation period of at least 5 years—II: Combined tooth-implant supported FDPs. *Clin Oral Implants Res* 15:643–653.

London RM, Roberts FA, Baker DA, Rohrer MD, O'Neal RB. 2002. Histologic comparison of a thermal dual-etched implant surface to machined, TPS, and HA surfaces: Bone contact in vivo in rabbits. *Int J Oral Maxillofac Implants* 17(3):369–376.

Novaes AB Jr, Souza SL, de Oliveira PT, Souza AM. 2002. Histomorphometric analysis of the bone-implant contact obtained with 4 different implant surface treatments placed side by side in the dog mandible. *Int J Oral Maxillofac Implants* 17(3):377–383.

Örtorp A, Jemt T. 1999. Clinical experiences of implant-supported prostheses with laser-welded titanium frameworks in the partially edentulous jaw: A 5-year follow-up study. *Clin Implant Dent Relat Res* 1:84–91.

Pearce AI, Richards RG, Milz S, Schneider E, Pearce SG. 2007. Animal models for implant biomaterial research in bone: A review. *Eur Cells Materials 2* 13:1–10.

Pjetursson BE, Tan K, Lang NP, Brägger U, Egger M, Zwahlen M. 2004a. A systematic review of the survival and complication rates of fixed partial dentures (FDPs) after an observation period of at least 5 years—I: Implant supported FDPs. *Clin Oral Implants Res* 15:625–642.

Pjetursson BE, Tan K, Lang NP, Brägger U, Egger M, Zwahlen M. 2004b. A systematic review of the survival and complication rates of fixed partial dentures (FDPs) after an observation period of at least 5 years— IV: Cantilever or extensions FDPs. *Clin Oral Implants Res* 15:667–676.

Pjetursson BE, Tan WC, Tan K, Brägger U, Zwahlen M, Lang NP. 2008. A systematic review of the survival and complication rates of resin bonded bridges after an observation period of at least 5 years. *Clin Oral Implants Res* 19:131–141.

Shalabi MM, Gortemaker A, Van't Hof MA, Jansen JA, Creugers NH. 2006. Implant surface roughness and bone healing: A systematic review. *J Dent Res* 85(6):496–500.

Sykaras N, Iacopino AM, Marker VA, Triplett RG, Woody RD. 2000. Implant materials, designs, and surface topographies: Their effect on osseointegration. A literature review. *Int J Oral Maxillofac Implants* 15(5):675–690.

Tan K, Pjetursson BE, Lang NP, Chan ESY. 2004. Systematic review of the survival and complication rates of fixed partial dentures (FDPs) after an observation period of at least 5 years—III: Conventional FDPs. *Clin Oral Implants Res* 15:654–666.

U.S. Dept. of Health and Human Services. 2008. Food and Drug Administration. URL: http://www.fda.gov/cdrh/ode/guidance/1389.html. Accessed March 15, 2008.

U.S Food and Drug Administration. Dental Products Devices. 1998. Reclassification of endosseous dental implant accessories. *Federal Register* 63(194):53859.

Vercaigne S, Wolke JG, Naert I, Jansen JA. 1998. Histomorphometrical and mechanical evaluation of titanium plasma-spray-coated implants placed in the cortical bone of goats. *J Biomed Mater Res* 41(1):41–48.

Vercaigne S, Wolke JG, Naert I, Jansen JA. 2000. A histological evaluation of TiO2-gritblasted and Ca-P magnetron sputter coated implants placed into the trabecular bone of the goat: Parts 1 and 2. *Clin Oral Implants Res* 11(4):305–324.

Wennerberg A, Albrektsson T. 2000. Suggested guidelines for the topographic evaluation of implant surfaces. *Int J Oral Maxillofac Implants* 15(3):331–344.

Wieland M, Textor M, Spencer ND, Brunette DM. 2001. Wavelength-dependent roughness: A quantitative approach to characterizing the topography of rough titanium surfaces. *Int J Oral Maxillofac Implants* 16(2):163–181.

Zalkind, M., Ever-hadani, P. and Hochman, N. 2003. Resin-bonded fixed partial denture retention: A retrospective 13-year follow-up. *J Oral Rehabili* 30:971–977.

Comprehensive Treatment Planning for Complete Arch Restorations

2

Introduction

Treatment of the edentulous patient with dental implants continues to evolve, from the originally described implant-retained fixed prosthesis in the mandible, supported by five to six implants *ad modum* Brånemark, to implant-retained overdentures, to full arch reconstructions using multiple implants in both dental arches.

When dealing with an edentulous jaw or with a terminal dentition patient, the clinician has various prosthetic and surgical treatment alternatives.

Treatment variables include type of restoration (fixed or removable), number and position of implants, loading protocols, interval between tooth extraction and implant insertion, prosthetic design, and, if an overdenture is planned, attachment type.

Since multiple treatment options are available, this chapter will focus only on some aspects involved in the complex pathway of defining a treatment strategy for complete arch implant-supported restorations:

- Indications for overdenture or fixed rehabilitation
- Number of implants and implant positions
- Treatment alternatives for the terminal dentition patient

TREATMENT OF THE EDENTULOUS MAXILLA AND MANDIBLE WITH IMPLANT-RETAINED OVERDENTURES

David A. Felton

Introduction

The treatment of edentulism, whether in one or both dental arches, continues to be a difficult clinical task, and one in which all key predictors (Beltan-Aguilar et al. 2006; Douglas et al. 2002; Marcus et al. 1996; U.S. Census Bureau, Census 2000 2008) suggest that the demand for treatment by the edentulous patient will not decline in the foreseeable future. Although the incidence of complete edentulism is on the decline in the United States (Waldman et al. 2007), current economic conditions in the United States along with a burgeoning population growth will continue to provide an increase in the numbers of edentulous dental arches for the next three to five decades (Douglas et al. 2002). While the curriculum for teaching complete denture therapy has been reduced in U.S. dental schools since the mid-1980s (Rashedi and Petropoulus 2003), there is perhaps no other group of individuals who need access to prosthodontic care more than those patients who have no teeth, or who wear prosthetic replacements that are woefully inadequate. Evidence from the New England Elder Dental Survey (Marcus et al. 1996) and from the U.S. Surgeon General's report (2000), entitled *Oral Health in America*, strongly suggests that many edentulous patients wear removable prostheses that are totally inadequate to meet the basic needs of function, phonetics, and aesthetics. Many of the patients surveyed simply did not (or could not) wear the mandibular prostheses, even for social occasions. The McGill Consensus Conference (Feine et al. 2002) has stated that the *first choice standard of care* for treatment of the edentulous mandible is the use of an overdenture prosthesis retained by two dental implants. Although dental implant therapy has emerged in the last 25 years as one of the fastest growing areas of dentistry, it does not appear that treatment of the edentulous patient (estimated at 27 million adults in the United States alone) with dental implants has reached any significant percentage of the edentulous population. Perhaps access to care, associated costs for implant overdenture therapy and maintenance, and the increasing use of denture adhesives (estimated at over $200 million in the United States alone) are preventing the denture wearer from seeking professional care.

Purpose

The purpose of this section of the chapter is to review the indications for, the biomechanical considerations of, the types of attachment systems used in, and the reported success rates of dental implant-retained overdentures.

Indications for Implant-Retained Overdentures

Dr. Jocelyn Feine has previously reported (2004) that the completely edentulous patient meets the World Health Organization's definition for being handicapped, since patients avoid eating in the company of others due to difficulties in chewing, and the definition of being physically impaired. Additionally, edentulous patients can be defined as having a disability, since they are limited in their ability to perform two of the most essential tasks of life (eating and speaking). Given the recommendations of the McGill Consensus Conference, the indications for implant-retained overdentures, at least in the mandibular arch, are very well defined. What other indications for use of dental implants in the edentulous patient exist? Dental implants used to retain overdenture prostheses should be considered for any patient who has a desire to improve the retention of his or her removable prostheses, regardless of the arch. Additionally, dental implants should be considered for any patient where maintenance of cortical bone is considered essential to providing both stability and retention to a removable prosthesis. Implants should also be considered for patients who wish to improve their ability to masticate food (Boerrigter et al. 1995; Garrett et al. 1998; Geertman et al. 1996). Implants are contraindicated in patients whose manual dexterity is such that they could not remove the prosthesis, and in those individuals whose health is so compromised as to increase the risk of adverse events during the surgical phase.

Biomechanical Considerations in Implant-Retained Overdentures

The most important biomechanical consideration for dental implant therapy is related

Table 2.1. Comparison of different protocols that may be used for the treatment of a terminal dentition patient requiring a complete arch FPD. Loading protocols, definitions, and intervals between extraction and implant placement are according to the ITI consensus (*Int J Oral Maxillofac Implants* 19(Suppl), 2004).

Treatment Strategy	Type of Implant Placement after Extraction	Implant Loading Interval	Timing of Use of Removable Provisional	Timing of Use of Fixed Provisional	Total Treatment Time	Advantages and Indications	Drawbacks and Contraindications
Conventional	After socket healing (16 weeks)	Conventional (3–4 months) or early loading (6–8 weeks)	6–8 months of treatment	Soft tissue conditioning phase (4–8 weeks)	7–10 months	Safe and well-documented protocol. Indicated in case of acute infections of residual teeth and when alveolar reconstruction is required.	Long treatment time. Indirect loading of implants with removable provisional.
Immediate loading	After socket healing (16 weeks)	Immediate loading (within 24 hours after implant insertion)	4 months (to allow socket healing)	2–4 months following implant placement	6–8 months	Reduces the time of denture use, good psychological impact for the patient.	Long and stressful surgical prosthetic phase. Total treatment time is only slightly reduced.
Immediate post-extraction implants	Implants placed in the same surgical session of extractions	Conventional (3–4 months) or early loading (6–8 weeks)	During implant healing (from 6 weeks to 4 months after implant placement)	Soft tissue conditioning phase (4–8 weeks)	4–6 months	Reduces the number of surgical phases and total treatment time.	It is critical to precisely foresee the hard- and soft-tissue response. Indirect loading of implants with removable provisional.
Staged approach	Immediate or after soft-tissue coverage of the sockets (4–8 weeks)	Early or conventional loading	Never	Throughout treatment	4–10 months	Fixed provisional restoration is used throughout the treatment. Minimal risk involved in placement and loading protocols.	Long protocol with simple but multiple surgical and prosthetic steps.
Immediate loading of immediate implants	Implants placed in the same surgical session of extractions	Immediate loading (within 24 hours after implant insertion)	Never	Throughout treatment	4–6 months	Fixed provisional restoration is used throughout the treatment. Reduces the number of surgical phases and total treatment time.	It is critical to precisely foresee the hard- and soft-tissue response. Long and stressful surgical prosthetic phase.

Patients asking for a fixed provisional restoration throughout treatment may benefit from a staged approach or an immediate replacement protocol. The staged approach reduces the aesthetic risk connected to immediate implant placement but increases treatment time and steps. If this approach is chosen, a sufficient number of residual natural abutments should be present in an acceptable position to support the provisional restoration (Figs. 2.1–2.6).

The immediate replacement timetable (immediate loading of implants placed at the time of extractions) reduces overall treatment time and treatment steps. It should be noted that it is difficult to anticipate the final gingival contour when multiple implants are placed in fresh extraction sockets, and this may be critical in the aesthetic zone. If the clinician is planning a hybrid prosthesis with pink acrylic or porcelain and an adequate bone volume is present apically to the remaining roots

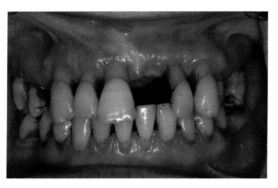

Figure 2.1. Female patient 42 years of age with advanced periodontal disease. Mobility grade III of all upper front teeth.

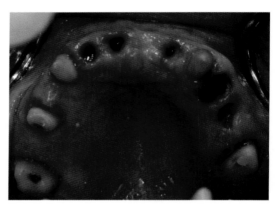

Figure 2.3. The remaining incisors and the first left bicuspid are extracted. The cuspids and second molars are prepared as abutments for a fixed provisional partial denture.

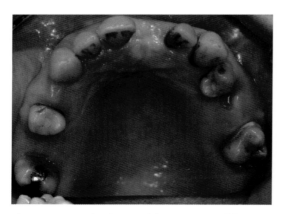

Figure 2.2. Occlusal view of the upper jaw of the same patient: the right first molar and first bicuspid are missing; the left central incisor and the second bicuspid and first molar are missing. It is decided to provide the patient with a fixed implant-supported rehabilitation without the need of a removable provisional prosthesis.

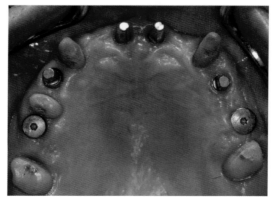

Figure 2.4. The implants were placed in the position of the central incisors, first bicuspid, and first molar bilaterally, and after 8 weeks they can be loaded to support the provisional restoration. At this time the cuspid may be extracted and implants inserted.

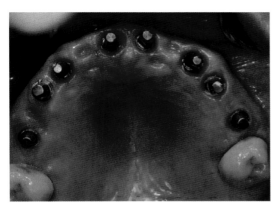

Figure 2.5. Eight weeks after the placement of implants in the cuspid site the case is ready for final impressions. Soft tissue conditioning has been performed throughout the entire provisional phase. Four FPDs will restore the case.

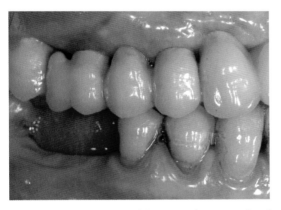

Figure 2.6a. Right view of the case after 20 weeks of active treatment with the final restoration.

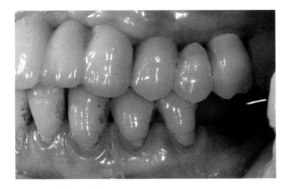

Figure 2.6b. Left view.

(typically in the anterior mandible), the immediate replacement technique may be safely used.

References

Adell R, Eriksson B, Lekholm U, Brånemark PI, Jemt T. 1990. Long-term follow-up study of osseointegrated implants in the treatment of totally edentulous jaws. *Int J Oral Maxillofac Implants* 5:347–359.

Adell R, Lekholm U, Rockler B, et al. 1981. A 15-year study of osseointegrated implants in the treatment of the edentulous jaw. *Int J Oral Surg* 6:387–416.

Allen PF, Thomason JM, Jepson NJ, Nohl F, Smith DG, Ellis J. 2006. A randomized controlled trial of implant-retained mandibular overdentures. *J Dent Res* 85:547–551.

Attard NJ, Zarb GA. 2004. Long-term treatment outcomes in edentulous patients with implant overdentures: The Toronto study. *Int J Prosthodont* 17:425–433.

Awad MA, Locker D, Korner-Bitenshy N, Feine JS. 2000. Measuring the effect of intra-oral implant rehabilitation on health-related quality of life in a randomized controlled clinical trial. *J Dent Res* 79:1659–1663.

Balshi TJ. 1988. Converting patients with periodontally hopeless teeth to osseointegration prostheses. *Int J Periodontics Restorative Dent* 8:8–33.

Beltan-Aguilar ED, Barker LK, Canto MT, Dye BA, Gooch BF, Hyman J, et al. 2006. Surveillance for certain health behaviors among states and selected local areas: Behavioral risk factor surveillance system. United States 2004. *Morb Mortal Wkly Rep* 55(SS-7):1–44.

Bidez MW, Lemons JE, Isenberg BR. 1986. Displacements of precious and nonprecious dental bridges utilizing endosseous implants as distal abutments. *J Biomed Mater Res* 20:785–797.

Bidez MW, Misch CE. 1999. Clinical biomechanics in implant dentistry. In: *Contemporary Implant Dentistry,* 2nd ed. Carl E. Misch (ed.). St. Louis: Mosby. 303–316.

Boerrigter EM, Geertman ME, Van Oort RP, Bouma J, et al. 1995. Patient satisfaction with implant-retained mandibular overdentures. A comparison with new complete dentures not retained by implants—a multicenter randomized clinical trial. *Fr J Oral Maxillofac Surg* 33:282–288.

Bulard RA, Vance JB. 2005. Multi-clinic evaluation using mini-dental implants for long-term denture stabilization: A preliminary biometric evaluation. *Compendium* 26:892–897.

Chiapasco M. 2004. Early and immediate restoration and loading of implants in completely edentulous patients. *Int J Oral Maxillofac Implants* 19(Suppl):76–91.

Cooper LF, Rahman A, Moriarty J, Chaffee N, Sacco D. 2002. Immediate mandibular rehabilitation with endosseous implants: Simultaneous extraction, implant placement, and loading. *Int J Oral Maxillofac Implants* 17:517–525.

Cooper LF, Scurria MS, Lang LA, Guckes AD, Moriarty JD, Felton DA. 1999. Treatment of edentulism using Astra Tech implants and ball abutments to retain mandibular overdentures. *Int J Oral Maxillofac Implants* 14:646–653.

Cordaro L, Torsello F. 2006. Soft tissue conditioning by immediate restoration of immediately placed implants in full-arch rehabilitation: The double provisional technique. *Eur J Esthet Dent* 1:216–229.

Cordaro L, Torsello F, Ercoli C, Gallucci G. 2007. Transition from failing dentition to a fixed implant-supported restoration: A staged approach. *Int J Periodontics Restorative Dent* 27:481–487.

Cordioli G, Majzoub Z, Castagna S. 1997. Mandibular overdentures anchored to single implants: A five-year prospective study. *J Prosthet Dent* 78:159–165.

Douglas CW, Shih A, Ostry L. 2002. Will there be a need for complete dentures in the United States in 2020? *J Prosthet Dent* 87:5–8.

Dudic A, Mericske-Stern R. 2002. Retention mechanisms and prosthetic complications of implant-supported mandibular overdentures: Long-term results. *Clin Implant Dent Relat Res* 4:212–219.

Feine JS. 2004. ADEA pre-doctoral dental implant conference presentation. November 2004.

Feine JS, Carlsson GE, Awad MA, Chehade A, et al. 2002. The McGill consensus statement on overdentures. *Int J Oral Maxillofac Implants* 17:601–602.

Ferrigno N, Laureti M, Fanali S, Grippaudo G. 2002. A long-term follow-up study of non-submerged ITI implants in the treatment of totally edentulous jaws. Part I: Ten-year life table analysis of a prospective multicenter study with 1286 implants. *Clin Oral Implants Res* 13:260–273.

Ganeles J, Rosenberg MM, Holt RL, Reichman LH. 2001. Immediate loading of implants with fixed restorations in the completely edentulous mandible: Report of 27 patients from a private practice. *Int J Oral Maxillofac Implants* 16:418–426.

Garrett NR, Kapur KK, Hamada MO, Roumanas ED, et al. 1998. A randomized clinical trial comparing the efficacy of mandibular implant-supported overdentures and conventional dentures in diabetic patients. Part II: Comparisons of masticatory performance. *J Prosthet Dent* 79:632–640.

Geertman ME, Van Waas MAJ, Van't Hof MA, Kalk W. 1996. Denture satisfaction in a comparative study of implant-retained mandibular overdentures: A randomized clinical trial. *Int J Oral Maxillofac Implants* 11:194–200.

Goodacre CJ, Bernal G, Rungcharassaeng K, Kan JYK. 2003. Clinical complications with implant and implant prostheses. *J Prosthet Dent* 90:121–132.

Gotfredsen K, Holm B. 2000. Implant-supported mandibular overdentures retained with ball or bar attachments: A randomized prospective 5-year study. *Int J Prosthodont* 13:125–130.

Grunder U. 2001. Immediate functional loading of immediate implants in edentulous arches: Two-year results. *Int J Periodontics Restorative Dent* 21:545–551.

Gulizio MP, Agar JR, Kelly JR, and Taylor TD. 2005. Effect of implant angulation upon retention of overdenture attachments. *J Prosthodont* 14:3–11.

Heydecke G, Thomason JM, Lund JP, Feine JS. 2005. The impact of conventional and implant supported prostheses on social and sexual activities in edentulous adults: Results from a randomized trial 2 months after treatment. *J Dent* 33:649–657.

Kawai Y, Taylor JA. 2008. Effect of loading time on the success of complete mandibular titanium implant retained overdentures: A systematic review. *Clin Oral Implants Res* 118:399–408.

Kiener P, Oetterli M, Mericske E, Mericske-Stern R. 2001. Effectiveness of maxillary overdentures supported by implants: Maintenance and prosthetic complications. *Int J Prosthodont* 14:133–140.

Krennmair G, Ulm C. 2001. The symphyseal single-tooth implant for anchorage of a mandibular complete denture in geriatric patients: A clinical report. *Int J Oral Maxillofac Implants* 16:98–104.

Lewis S. 1996. Treatment planning: Teeth versus implants. *Int J Periodontics Restorative Dent* 16:366–377.

Marcus PA, Joshi J, Jones JA, Morgano SM. 1996. Complete edentulism and denture use for elders in New England. *J Prosthet Dent* 76:260–266.

McEntee MI, Walton JN, Glick N. 2005. A clinical trial of patient satisfaction and prosthodontic needs with ball and bar attachments for implant-retained complete overdentures: Three-year results. *J Prosthet Dent* 93:28–37.

Mericske-Stern R, Oetterli M, Kiener P, Mericske E. 2002. A follow-up study of maxillary implants supporting an overdenture: Clinical and radiographic results. *Int J Oral Maxillofac Implants* 17:678–686.

Misch CE. 1997. Prosthodontic considerations. In: *Contemporary Implant Dentistry*. Carl E. Misch (ed.). St. Louis: Mosby. 187–200.

———. 2006. Consideration of biomechanical stress in treatment with dental implants. *Dent Today* 25(5):80–85.

Naert I, Hooghe M, Quirynen M, Van Steenberghe D. 1997. The reliability of implant-retained hinging overdentures for the fully edentulous mandible. An up to 9-year longitudinal study. *Clin Oral Investig* 1:119–124.

Nyman S, Lindhe J. 1976. Prosthetic rehabilitation of patients with advanced periodontal disease. *J Clin Periodontol* 3:135–147.

Raghoebar GM, Meijer HJA, Van't Hof M, Stegenga B, Vissink A. 2003. A randomized prospective clinical trial on the effectiveness of three treatment modalities for patients with lower denture problems: A 10-year follow-up study on patient satisfaction. *Int J Oral Maxillofac Implants* 32:498–503.

Raghoebar GM, Meijer HJA, Stegenga B, Van't Hoff MA, Van Oort RP, Vissink A. 2000. Effectiveness of three treatment modalities for the edentulous mandible: A five-year randomized clinical trial. *Clin Oral Implants Res* 11:195–201.

Randow K, Glantz PO, Zoger B. 1986. Technical failures and some related clinical complications in extensive fixed prosthodontics. An epidemiological study of long-term clinical quality. *Acta Odontol Scand* 44:241–255.

Rashedi B, Petropoulus VC. 2003. Preclinical complete denture curriculum survey. *J Prosthodont* 12:37–46.

Rosenstiel SF, Land MF, Fujimoto J. 1995. Treatment planning. In: *Contemporary Fixed Prosthodontics*, 2nd ed. St. Louis: Mosby. 46–64.

Schnitman PA, Wohrle PS, Rubenstein JE, DaSilva JD, Wang NH. 1997. Ten-year results for Brånemark implants immediately loaded with fixed prostheses at implant placement. *Int J Oral Maxillofac Implants* 12:495–503.

Schwartz-Arad D, Chaushu G. 1997. Placement of implants into fresh extraction sites: 4 to 7 years retrospective evaluation of 95 immediate implants. *J Periodontol* 68:1110–1116.

Schwartz-Arad D, Gulayev N, Chaushu G. 2000. Immediate versus non-immediate implantation for full-arch fixed reconstruction following extraction of all residual teeth: A retrospective comparative study. *J Periodontol* 71:923–928.

Schwartz-Arad D, Kidron N, Dolev E. 2005. A long-term study of implants supporting overdentures as a model for implant success. *J Periodontol* 76:1431–1435.

Shatkin TE, Shatkin S, Oppenheimer BD, Oppenheimer AJ. 2007. Mini dental implants for long-term fixed and removable prosthetics: A retrospective analysis of 2514 implants placed over a five-year period. *Compendium* 28:92–99.

Shillinburg HT, Hobo S, Lowell D, et al. 1997. Treatment planning for the replacement of missing teeth. In: *Fundamentals of Fixed Prosthodontics*, 3rd ed. HT Shillinburg and S Hobo (eds.). Chicago: Quintessence. 85–104.

Smedberg JI, Nilner K, Frykholm A. 1999. A six-year follow-up study of maxillary overdentures on osseointegrated implants. *Eur J Prosthodont Restor Dent* 7:51–56.

Smyd ES. 1952. Mechanics of dental structures: Guide to teaching dental engineering at undergraduate level. *J Prosthet Dent* 2:668–692.

Spiekermann H, Jansen VK, Richter EJ. 1995. A 10-year follow up study of IMZ and TPS implants in the edentulous mandible using bar-retained overdentures. *Int J Oral Maxillofac Implants* 10:231–243.

Stoker GT, Wismeijer D, Van Waas MA. 2007. An eight-year follow-up to a randomized clinical trial of aftercare and cost-analysis with three types of mandibular implant-retained overdentures. *J Dent Res* 86:276–280.

Tylman SD. 1965. *Theory and Practice of Crown and Fixed Partial Prosthodontics*. St. Louis: Mosby.

U.S. Census Bureau, Census 2000. 2008. URL: http://census.gov/population/www/projections/htm. Accessed March 15, 2008.

U.S. Surgeon General's Report. Oral Health in America. Chapter 4. URL: http://www.nidcr.nih.gov/AboutNIDCR/SurgeonGeneral. Accessed March 15, 2008.

Waldman HB, Ferlman SP, Xu L. 2007. Should the teaching of full denture prosthetics be maintained in schools of dentistry? *J Dent Educ* 71:463–466.

Widbom C, Solderfeldt B, Kronstrom M. 2005. A retrospective evaluation of treatments with implant-supported maxillary overdentures. *Clin Implant Dent Relat Res* 7:166–172.

Comprehensive Treatment Planning for the Patient with Complex Treatment Needs

3

THE CHALLENGING PATIENT WITH FACIAL DEFORMITIES, RARE DISORDERS, OR OLD AGE

Birgitta Bergendal, James D. Anderson, and Frauke Müller

Introduction

Treatment with dental implants is now a well-established treatment modality in partial and total edentulousness. The long-term success and survival rates of the implants, as well as improvement in quality of life, are well described in multiple studies of large patient samples. However, meta-analyses, systematic reviews, and statements from consensus conferences reveal that the evidence in many aspects is still limited (Gottfredsen et al. 2008; Swiss Society of Reconstructive Dentistry 2007). Most research on the clinical performance of dental implants is based on studies of healthy individuals, with individuals with chronic diseases, rare disorders, and old age often excluded. In many groups of complex patients, the knowledge base on the use of dental implants is very small and there are few guidelines for treatment with implants in medically compromised patients (Beikler and Flemmig 2003). At the same time individuals with different kinds of developmental malformations, chronic and rare diseases, and disability have an increased risk of early tooth loss and are most in need of oral rehabilitation (Nunn 2000; Storhaug 1989).

The mouth as an organ acts in many vital functions, such as breathing, sucking, chewing, and swallowing (Andersson-Norinder and Sjogreen 2000). The subtle interplay of many different functions increases the vulnerability for damage not only as early as the fetal stage but also later in life. Associated with disease, disability, and aging, these effects can result in compromised orofacial function as well as deterioration of the dental status and early tooth loss.

Present Knowledge Base

A search in PubMed made in January 2008 on the criterion "dental implants" gave just over 10,000 references, and in combination with search terms related to the complex patient the following numbers of references

were found: "rare disorders" and "craniofacial disorders" <10, "geriatric" or "chronic
disease" <50, and "oral cancer" <150. Some
of the references were the same in the different searches, and the majority of the references do not give any information on the
experiences and outcomes of treatment with
implants. This unsophisticated search showed
that roughly 1% of publications on dental
implants refer to complex patients. There is
an apparent need for treatment with dental
implants in people with chronic diseases and
congenital or acquired disabilities compared
to the general population.

However, it seems evident that there is a
substantial lack of information about treatment outcomes, risks for failure, and complications in these segments of the population.
Since the groups are relatively small (and also
for practical and ethical reasons), there are
limited possibilities for designing prospective
studies that would yield a high level of scientific evidence.

The Challenging Patient with Facial Deformity

The use of implants for facial deformities
outside the mouth was contemplated quite
early in the development of the osseointegration technique. The first extraoral implant
was placed by Anders Tjellström in 1977
(Granström 2007) for a bone-anchored
hearing aid, and the first reports of their use
appeared as early as 1980 (Tjellström et al.
1980). Two years later, the same technology
was used to retain the first reported extraoral
prostheses (Tjellström et al. 1981). So by the
time the 1982 Toronto Conference took place,
the use of osseointegration outside the mouth
was already established.

Hardware and Technique

Implants

The implant most commonly used in the
extraoral environment today is a variation of
the original milled commercially pure titanium dental implant. The development of the
surgical protocols for these implants has followed the dental protocols, including the
introduction of single-stage surgery. As a
result of the high success rates, the number of
implants needed at any site for sufficient
retention has diminished over the years
(Abu-Serriah 2001).

Dentists working in the heavily loaded oral
environment are accustomed to the occlusal
forces that dominate our planning decisions.
Implants that are only 3 mm or 4 mm long
therefore appear shockingly short (Fig. 3.1).
They are a reflection not just of the thinness
of the bone where they are used; they hint at
the reduced loads these implants are thought
to support. Whether the reduced loads are so
low as to be clinically insignificant is still an
open question (Del Valle et al. 1997). The
original flange design was thought to prevent
traumatic intrusion into the brain (Granström
2007), as well as to provide some lateral stability at insertion. The value of this feature is
questionable, however. Flangeless designs are
now available.

The implant placement technique is drawn
directly from dental protocols. Arguably,
because of access considerations, extraoral
surgery is substantially easier than intraoral.
As in the intraoral situation, an atraumatic
surgical technique and primary stability are
important conditions for osseointegration.
Similarly, mobility of the soft tissue around

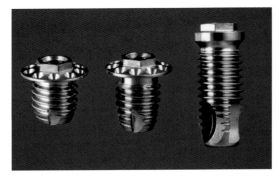

Figure 3.1. Three mm and 4 mm flanged craniofacial
implants compared to a conventional milled 7 mm long
implant.

the abutment compromises the soft tissue attachment to the abutment. Therefore, in the extraoral environment, unlike in the mouth, an aggressive thinning of the skin overlying the implant is necessary to achieve a firm attachment between skin and periosteum, with a minimum of intervening subcutaneous tissue. This is a principle that runs counter to a surgeon's intuition with respect to maintaining a blood supply in the healing site, so it is a new appreciation for surgeons and carries with it a significant learning curve.

Prosthetic Hardware

The prosthetic hardware also is analogous to the intraoral designs. Bar and clip designs are commonly used in the extraoral environment in a way that is no different from the intraoral design. Angulated abutments also are available with much larger angulations ranging from 30 to 110 degrees. These abutments are substantially different from the intraoral designs and are often most useful in the orbit, where there is very little room available for hardware (Fig. 3.2). Given that the loading is thought to be low, retention is placed eccentrically from the axis of the implant in

the expectation of less risk to the bone-implant interface. Magnetic retention also is available.

"Success Rates"

Native Bone

It has been estimated that up to 2007, more than 90,000 craniofacial implants have been placed in more than 45,000 patients (Granström 2007). This widespread use is based on success rates comparable to the intraoral situation. However, as in the mouth, the success rates are not uniform across different bones. In a 10-year follow-up of the earliest craniofacial patients, Granström (2007) reported the percentage of implants lost from the orbit, nasal area, and temporal bone (Table 3.1).

Based on that early experience, implants now are typically placed largely in the superior and lateral orbital rim and the floor of the piriform aperture. Limiting Granström's original data to those areas yields more favorable results that are consistent with the experience in other countries (Abu-Serriah 2001; Parel and Tjellström 1991; Wolfaardt et al. 1993).

Drinias et al. (2007) found that the implant failure rate in the temporal bone correlates with the age of the patient at insertion. Patients over 40 years of age have higher

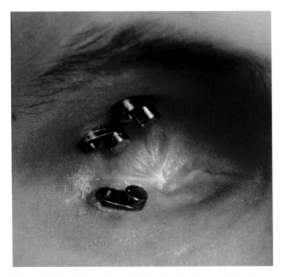

Figure 3.2. Magnetic retention located eccentrically on craniofacial implants where space is confined in the orbit.

Table 3.1. Percentage of craniofacial implants lost from native bone after up to 10 years of follow-up (modified from Granström G, Bergström K, et al. 1994. A detailed analysis of titanium implants lost in irradiated tissues. *Int J Oral Maxillofac Implants* 9:653–662).

Site	% Lost[*]	Modified % Lost[‡]
Orbit	32	14
Nose	20	12.5
Temporal Bone	5	5

[*] As reported.
[‡] Limited to superior and lateral orbital rim and to floor of nose only.

failure rates than patients under 40, and those failures tend to occur later after implant placement. This effect tended to cause the failure rate in the temporal bone to be relatively constant over time, unlike initial loss followed by a successful plateau found in the intraoral situation.

Radiation

In 1988 there was consensus that placement of implants in radiated bone was contraindicated (National Institutes of Health 1988). Since then, however, reports have appeared detailing relatively successful placement of implants in radiated bone (Niimi et al. 1998; Parel and Tjellström 1991; Wolfaardt et al. 1993).

Recent information suggests that the success rate of implants placed in radiated bone is not as high as in bone that has not been radiated. However, the damaging effect of radiation seems to vary in different bones, and unlike the conventional situation, the failures tend to be late. Using pooled data, Granström (2003) calculated that in the radiated mandible, the survival rate does not differ substantially from the non-radiated mandible until about 9 years after placement. At about that time, the survival rate declines sharply to less than 50% at 12 years after placement. In the maxilla, the failures start to occur more frequently at about the 5-year mark, progressing to a survival rate of about 50% as in the mandible. Extraorally, implants placed into the radiated temporal bone are much less affected by radiation, slipping only to about 75% survival at 12 years. The radiated orbital bone, on the other hand, performs much less well, with failures beginning very early and giving survival rates of less than 50% at 12 years (Granström 2003).

Given the higher rates of failure, the question then arises as to whether the use of osseointegrated implants should be offered to patients who have had, or will have, radiation. The question naturally requires a consideration of the consequences of failure. The most serious consequence of implant failure is osteoradionecrosis (ORN). Several reports of follow-ups on implants in radiated patients (Granström and Tjellström 1997; Harrison et al. 2003) suggest the incidence of ORN is remarkably low. With this low risk and given that the benefits of implant-retained prostheses are so great, it seems reasonable to offer implant solutions to selected patients with cautious optimism but fully informed consent.

Hyperbaric Oxygen

Hyperbaric oxygen (HBO) has been used for many years in the treatment of different conditions including ORN. However, the use of HBO in relation to osseointegrated implants is intended to be prophylactic, and this application has been the subject of debate for many years. There are numerous contraindications and complications associated with HBO, and it is an expensive resource. Nevertheless, there is some reason to believe that HBO may have beneficial effects when used with osseointegrated implants. HBO has been shown to improve angiogenesis (Marx et al. 1990) and bone turnover, and on this basis Granström suggests HBO acts as a stimulator of osseointegration (Granström 1998). Granström (2005) has recently offered useful empirical evidence of the benefit of HBO. While the survival rates of implants in all the radiated bones of the skull is significantly worse after radiation, the survival rates are significantly improved with the use of HBO in all these bones to near the levels of non-radiated bone. The exception is the temporoparietal bone. Here the failure rate is only reduced from 33% to 30% after HBO, in contrast to a commonly reported failure rate of less than 5% in non-radiated bone (Tolman and Taylor 1996).

Grafted Bone

The flexibility afforded by osteomyocutaneous-free tissue transfer has made it the surgical reconstructive method of choice following ablative procedures in the maxilla and mandible. Combined with osseointegrated implants, the prospect of near-normal function is possible. Case series and case reports are numerous, all reporting successful use of the combined modality, including implant failure rates similar to that of native bone (Chiapasco et al. 2006; Jaquiery et al. 2004; Vinzenz et al. 1996).

The use of implants in grafted bone outside the mouth, on the other hand, is much less commonly reported than in the intraoral situation. In a series of 28 patients, Gliklich et al. (1998) provided a very useful set of site-specific goals for the use of free-tissue transfers when combined with rehabilitation services, including implant-retained prostheses. In essence, they stated that the main goals of free-tissue transfer are to obtain vascular coverage in addition to a smooth contour of the scalp and a flat temporal platform, while for the orbit additional aims are maintained orbital cavity depth and brow position preservation. Application of these goals increased the successful use of implant-borne prostheses in their series.

Skin Reactions

The most common complication following the placement of extraoral implants is inflammatory skin reaction. However, these complications are not evenly distributed between patients, between age groups, or over time. As many as 60% of patients had a soft tissue complication in the first 2 years, dropping to less than 25% by 5 years in a series reported by Abu-Serriah (2001). On the other hand, Reyes reported that 70% of patients had no reaction over an 8-year follow-up (Reyes et al. 2000). But among the early patients in that series, Tjellström reported that of those experiencing any adverse reactions, only 15% of the patients accounted for over 70% of the skin reactions observed (Tjellström 1989). Similarly, the frequency of skin reactions is higher in the younger age groups (Reyes et al. 2000). In both series, as time from implant placement increased, the incidence of skin reactions decreased, and no reactions

were serious enough to require removal of implants.

Applications

Extraoral Prostheses

The traditional prosthetic solutions in craniofacial prosthetics include replacement of the eye, nose, and ear. The commonest diagnoses leading to ear replacement are syndromic in nature, such as Treacher Collins and Goldenhar's. Loss of the nose is most commonly due to malignancy later in life, while loss of an eye can occur in childhood as a result of retinoblastoma or recurrent rhabdomyosarcoma. Of course, trauma including burns is also an important cause of tissue loss in any of these locations.

Contraindications include unrealistic expectations, alcohol or drug abuse, or any condition that might interfere with skin and prosthesis maintenance. As with the intraoral situation, smoking may limit implant survival but, unlike in the mouth, data directly addressing this question is limited.

Bone-Anchored Hearing Aid

The first extraoral implant was placed in 1977 to support a new type of hearing aid, the bone-anchored hearing aid. Previously, patients who could not wear conventional air-conduction hearing aids used a bone conduction hearing aid that pressed an amplified vibrator against the skin to conduct sound through the bones of the skull to the cochlea. The problem was that the skin attenuated the signal and it became painful with continuous pressure. The bone-anchored aid conducts sound directly to the bone through the implant for better sound transmission with no pressure on the skin (Tjellström and Håkansson 1995). Patients with external otitis, chronic draining ears or canal atresia, and 45 dB average hearing loss or better are candidates for bone-anchored hearing aids (Wazen et al. 1998).

The Autogenous/Prosthetic Choice in Rehabilitation

Early in the planning process (particularly for the nose and ear), the rehabilitation team must decide, together with the patient, between an autogenous and a prosthetic solution. In general, surgical reconstructive procedures take advantage of all remaining tissue. Implant-retained prosthetic solutions, on the other hand, are best carried out with minimal remaining tissue. The decision between autogenous and prosthetic options therefore favors the autogenous as a first option to take advantage of remaining tissue, with the prosthetic option reserved for salvage. If aesthetically acceptable, a surgical reconstruction avoids the maintenance problems of a prosthesis (Wilkes and Wolfaardt 1994). This decision, then, is heavily driven by the availability of sufficiently skilled surgical expertise to undertake the autogenous procedures, and therefore indirectly affects the use of implants in rehabilitation.

On the other hand, in the intraoral environment, where the surgical expertise exists to provide well-designed free flaps, an extremely difficult rehabilitation problem requiring extensive use of implants (Boyes-Varley et al. 2007) can be transformed into an entirely unremarkable dental rehabilitation (Gbara et al. 2007).

The Future

There are numerous areas for future development in extraoral prosthesis construction including new materials (Kiat-amnuay et al. 2008), rapid prototyping (Chen et al. 1997), and robotic prostheses (Klein et al. 1999). However, with regard to osseointegrated implants, skin inflammation around abutments remains a significant problem. Some work has been done on this (Klein et al. 2000), but much more is needed. Finally, given the rapid changes in surgical planning systems and techniques, it is reasonable to look forward to the further transformation of

complex aesthetic and functional dilemmas into simpler rehabilitation solutions.

Challenging Patients with Rare Disorders

When dental implants were recognized as a new treatment alternative in individuals with partial and total edentulousness, the opportunity for habilitation and rehabilitation in rare disorders represented one of many challenging applications. However, it was not until 1988, with a case report on the use of implants in an adult patient with hypohidrotic ectodermal dysplasia (Ekstrand and Thomsson 1988), that a report on the use of implants in a rare disorder was published.

Definitions of Rare Disorders/ Diseases

The concept of rare disorders (diseases) has different definitions in different countries. According to the World Health Organization (WHO Rare Diseases Act of 2002) and the NIH Office of Rare Diseases (http://rarediseases.info.nih.gov), a rare disease is generally considered to have a prevalence of fewer than 200,000 affected individuals in the United States, equivalent to 1 in 1,500 citizens. EURORDIS, the European Organization for Rare Diseases, defines a disorder or disease as rare in Europe when it affects less than 1 in 2,000 citizens (Orphan Drug regulation 141/2000, www.eurordis.org). In Sweden, the definition used in the Swedish Rare Disease Database is disorders or injuries resulting in extensive disability and affecting no more than 100 in 1,000,000 population, equivalent to 1 in 10,000 citizens.

The jaws as well as the teeth are affected in many rare disorders since the mouth and teeth, with their complicated development and sensory and neurological functions, are among the most vulnerable to malformation and malfunction. Therefore, dentists can play

Table 3.2. Number of syndromes matching certain search terms in the Winter-Baraitser Dysmorphology Database* containing nearly 4,000 syndromes.

Search Term	Number of Syndromes
Face	1,591
Oral Region	1,211
Mouth	1,074
Teeth	793
Oligodontia	219
Premature loss of teeth	51
Abnormal salivary glands	11

*London Dysmorphology Database 1.0, www. lmdatabases.com.

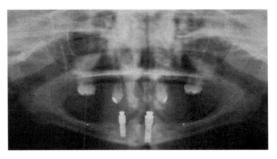

Figure 3.3. Implants replacing teeth missing from tooth agenesis. Seven-year-old boy with hypohidrotic ectodermal dysplasia. In 1986 at age 6 years, two implants were placed in the canine region of the anodontic mandible to support an overdenture.

an important role not only in treatment but also in the diagnosis of rare syndromes. A search of the Winter-Baraitser Dysmorphology Database (www.lmdatabases.com), which has information on nearly 4,000 syndromes, demonstrates that symptoms of the face, mouth, and teeth are common in many hereditary syndromes (Table 3.2).

Rare Disorders and Dental Implants

A search of PubMed using the search terms "rare disease" and "dental implants" in January 2008 found one reference to a publication, which was a case presentation on treatment with bone grafts and implants in a patient with systemic mastocytosis (Thor et al. 2005). This shows that the search criteria and keywords are often unreliable. Ectodermal dysplasia (ED) syndromes were the most well represented among reports on treatment with dental implants with 31 publications (all not cited here). In hypohidrotic ED, the most common of around 200 different ED syndromes, anodontia of the lower jaw is most common in boys with the typical phenotype and several case reports of early treatment with dental implants, from 1.5 to 6 years of age, have been published (Bergendal et al.

1991; Bonin et al. 2001; Guckes et al. 1997; Smith et al. 1993) (Fig. 3.3).

Two retrospective reports on a limited number of patients with ED (6 and 14, respectively) have been published (Kearns et al. 1999; Sweeney et al. 2005). However, there is only one prospective study with a substantial number of patients on habilitation with dental implants in ED (Guckes et al. 2002). Fifty-one patients, aged 8–68 years, had 243 implants placed in the anterior mandible and 21 in the anterior maxilla. The survival rate was 91% in the mandible and 76% in the maxilla. Fourteen individuals (27.5%) had lost an implant and all but two were lost before loading. Recently a compilation of the results of implant treatment in five small Swedish children with hypohidrotic ED showed that all but one had lost implants early after insertion, which was interpreted to be caused by the small size of the jaws rather than ED per se, since those who had lost implants were all successfully re-operated on directly after healing or later in their teens (Bergendal et al. 2008). In osteogenesis imperfecta around half of affected individuals also have dentinogenesis imperfecta or aberrant dentin (Malmgren and Norgren 2002), which can cause early tooth loss, and a few patients are reported who were successfully treated with dental implants (Ambjornsen 2002; Binger et al. 2006; Lee and Ertel 2003; Prabhu et al. 2007; Zola 2000). In cleidocranial dysplasia four cases were reported (Angle and Rebellato 2005; Daskalogiannakis et al. 2006; Lombardas and Toothaker 1997; Petropoulos et al. 2004). In hypophosphatasia, a rare, inherited metabolic disorder of decreased tissue non-specific alkaline phosphatase that results in defective bone mineralization, affected individuals often have a short stature and bowed lower legs. Oral manifestations are aplasia or hypoplasia of cementum, which result in premature loss of primary teeth and early loss of permanent teeth. X-linked hypophosphataemic rickets is another rare bone disorder affecting metabolism, where the oral symptoms are enlarged coronal pulp spaces and grossly defective dentine. Even minor enamel defects like infractions, minor abrasion facets, or superficial enamel caries lead to pulpal necrosis, abscess formation, and osteonecrotic lesions. The infections are difficult to treat and teeth are often lost early (Fig. 3.4).

Individuals with this disorder also have a short stature and bowed lower legs and could easily be mistaken for having hypophosphatasia. Children are nowadays given medication to ameliorate these symptoms. Following the breakthrough of increasing knowledge of genetics, children and young individuals are now diagnosed earlier and are given better information about the name and symptoms of their diagnosis, while the adult population might still be poorly informed. This became evident when a Swedish workshop was arranged in 2001 to evaluate the outcomes of treatment with dental implants in a group of individuals with many failed implants (Bergendal and Ljunggren 2001). Not until the right diagnoses were set—three had hypophosphatasia and three had X-linked hypophosphataemic rickets—was it evident that most of the implants placed in the latter group were lost (Table 3.3).

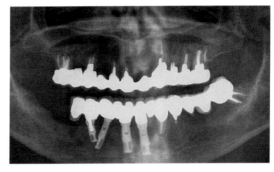

Figure 3.4. Implants replacing teeth lost as a consequence of a rare disorder. Typical dental status of 50-year-old male with X-linked hypophosphataemic rickets. All remaining natural teeth were root-filled, some with apical periodontitis, and a history of failed implants.

Table 3.3.   Outcome of treatment with dental implants in six Swedish individuals with X-linked hypophosphataemic rickets or hypophosphatasia (Bergendal and Ljunggren 2001).

	Patients	Age at Implant Placement	Number of Teeth	Number of Root-Filled Teeth	Number of Implants Placed	Implant Sites				Number of Implants Lost
X-Linked	1	22	26	3	4	43	42	31	33	4
Hypophosphataemic	2	29	19	14	1		45			1
Rickets	3	47	15	14	5	46	44	42	41	3
							31			
Hypophosphatasia	4	30	23	1	4	12	11	21	22	0
	5	34	23	1	1		44			0
	6	51	15	4	8	47	46	45	44	0
						34	35	36	37	

Treatment with dental implants in one patient with X-linked hypophosphataemic rickets (Resnick 1998) and one with hypophosphatasia were reported (Slotte et al. 2006).

Early periodontitis is seen not only in hypophosphatasia but also in Ehlers-Danlos syndrome and Papillon-Lefevre syndrome. Children with Papillon-Lefevre syndrome often lose their primary as well as their permanent teeth early, and there are some experiences from treatment with implants (Adbulwassie et al. 1996; Toygar et al. 2007; Ullbro et al. 2000; Woo et al. 2003). In syndromes affecting the oral mucosa, for example, dystrophic epidermolysis bullosa (EB), where the oral mucosa is very frail, easily bruised, and heals with scarring, there is an increased risk of tooth loss due to the difficulties of maintaining good oral hygiene without damaging the mucosa. Dental implants have been shown to serve well in EB with due caution to the frail oral tissues (Lee et al. 2007; Müller et al. 2006; Penarrocha et al. 2007; Penarrocha-Diago et al. 2000). Low salivary secretion rates and enamel defects have been shown in Prader-Willi syndrome (Young et al. 2001) and 22q11-deletion syndrome (Klingberg et al. 2002). Patients with these conditions may be at risk for dental disease and tooth loss, and in both syndromes oligodontia is also a feature. Hypoplasia of major salivary and lacrimal glands often causes dental erosion, dental caries, and early tooth loss in affected individuals (Entesarian et al. 2005). These are examples of diagnoses where dental implants could be needed in oral rehabilitation, but where there are no publications on outcomes of treatment.

Most tissues and organs in the mouth can be affected in hereditary syndromes. Some typical examples where a need for treatment with dental implants can arise due to tooth agenesis or acquired tooth loss are listed in Table 3.4.

Table 3.5 contains a compilation of publications on implant treatment in rare disorders, searching the diagnosis and "dental implants" where more than one reference was

Table 3.4. Examples of features in syndromes associated with tooth agenesis or acquired tooth loss.

Feature	Examples of Syndromes
Oligodontia	Ectodermal dysplasia syndromes
	Kabuki syndrome
	Prader-Willi syndrome
	22q11-deletion syndrome
	Williams syndrome
Mineralization Disturbancies	Osteogenesis imperfecta
	X-linked hypophosphataemic rickets
Periodontitis	Ehlers-Danlos syndrome
	Hypofosfatasia
	Papillon-Lefevre syndrome
Oral Mucosal Lesions Abnormal	Epidermolysis bullosa
	Pachyonychia congenita
	Hypoplasia of major salivary and lacrimal glands
Salivary Glands	LADD—Lacrimal Auriculo Dental Digital syndrome

found. Also included are published abstracts of posters and presentations at scientific meetings, workshops, and consensus conferences.

Five single case reports were also found covering implant treatment in Erdheim-Chester disease (Brahim et al. 1992), nevoid basal cell carcinoma syndrome (Gorlin syndrome) (Markt 2003), scleroderma (Patel et al. 1998), systemic mastocytosis (Thor et al. 2005), and Williams-Beuren syndrome (Mass et al. 2007). Thus, 57 publications were found: 39 (66%) were single case reports. In all, 151 patients with a rare syndrome treated with dental implants were reported and more than 70% had an ED syndrome.

This is a very weak basis on which to identify risks and complications, and it should be remembered that most publications report favorable outcomes. In addition to the rare disorders with varying degrees of tooth agenesis or an increased risk of early tooth loss, there are also combinations of symptoms that represent rare dental conditions with very challenging treatment needs. Only a few reports were published on treatment with dental implants in case series of individuals

Table 3.5. Publications on treatment with dental implants in rare disorders and syndromes.

Rare Disorder/Syndrome	Treated Patients		No of Case Reports	No of Publications
	No.	%		
Ectodermal Dysplasia Syndromes	110	72.8	19	31
Epidermolysis Bullosa	12	7.9	2	4
Osteogenesis Imperfecta	7	4.6	4	5°
Papillon Lefevre Syndrome	5	3.3	3	4
Cleidocranial Dysplasia	4	2.7	4	4
Hypophosphatasia	4	2.7	1	2*°
X-Linked Hypophosphataemic Rickets	4	2.7	1	2*
Other Syndromes[z]	5	3.3	5	5
	151		39	57

* Abstract.
□ Consensus conference.
[z] Erdheim-Chester disease, nevoid basal cell carcinoma syndrome (Gorlin syndrome), scleroderma, systemic mastocytosis and Williams-Beuren syndrome.

with disabilities and chronic diseases: an evaluation of risk factors in medically compromised patients (Beikler and Flemmig 2003), a prospective study on individuals with neurologic disabilities (Ekfeldt 2005), and a case series of special care patients (Oczakir et al. 2005). In the latter two publications, five of the patients had Down syndrome, and together with one case report (Lustig et al. 2002), there is now information in the literature on six patients with this diagnosis. Down syndrome is not rare but is the most common chromosomal syndrome. Common symptoms in individuals with Down syndrome are not only multiple tooth agenesis but also low salivary secretion and immunological defects. These characteristics increase the risk of early tooth loss, often in combination with skeletal discrepancies and different levels of cognitive impairment.

The Future

Many individuals with rare disorders and rare dental conditions have apparent needs for habilitation and rehabilitation with dental implants. However, reports are still sporadic in the literature, and the lack of knowledge about oral needs and outcomes of treatment with dental implants needs to be addressed urgently in clinical research. The challenges of biological, psychological, cognitive, and technical difficulties associated with the clinical management of individuals with rare disorders make it particularly important to communicate any finding, favorable or—even more important—unfavorable.

Challenging Patients with Old Age

The History of Dental Implants in Gerodontology

When dental implants were first introduced they were applied to healthy individuals with missing teeth. In the very early days the implants were not suitable for fragile individuals or unfavorable anatomical conditions. At the same time, clinical success was not yet backed by long-term scientific evidence. In the 1980s and 1990s the development of sophisticated implant surfaces and bone augmentation techniques allowed for less invasive surgical interventions, and borderline anatomical conditions could be mastered. Encouraged by well-documented success rates and clinical long-term stability, the indication for dental implants was gradually extended to groups of patients who were originally considered at risk, or who were simply at old age. Nowadays, implant-supported reconstructions can undoubtedly be considered a main option in restorative dentistry. However, despite a number of well-conducted useful studies that abnegate an age limit to implant restorations, their use is still scarce in the elderly population (De Baat 2000).

The Geriatric Patient

Demographics indicate an increasing proportion of the elderly in the population. Physiological aging is irreversible, progressive, and general. It starts around the age of 35 years and involves an annual decrease of about 1% of body functions. In principle, nature has provided sufficient physiological spare capacity to enable health and appropriate function throughout life. Nevertheless, healthy aging remains the exception. More often life in old age is characterized by multimorbidity and functional limitations such as reduced mobility and cognitive impairment (Budtz-Jorgensen 1999). Another trend is that elderly subjects tend to retain their natural teeth longer (Hugoson et al. 2005). These developments present a considerable quantitative and qualitative challenge to the dental profession and other health care providers.

Treatment Concepts

Dental treatment planning for geriatric patients deviates from a purely "academic" treatment plan by taking into account the general health and physical and cognitive impairment as well as the autonomy of the

Table 3.6. Treatment planning in gerodontology has to take into account the general health condition and functional limitations as well as the patient's socio-economic context.

Academic treatment plan	Treatment demand Oral examination Complaints/pain Medical reasons for a dental treatment
Clinical treatment plan	General health and functional findings Physical or mental handicap Ratio cost/benefit Autonomy
Practical treatment plan	Subjective treatment demand Wishes of the family Financial aspects Dental preliminary treatment/ invasive diagnostics
Modified treatment	Changes in compliance Changes in general and oral health

patient in handling and maintaining a dental restoration (Table 3.6).

Such a "clinical" treatment plan has to further be modified by the subjective treatment demand, because the ability and motivation to enter invasive and lengthy dental treatments is largely reduced in most elderly patients. Financial aspects and preliminary treatment procedures that assess the patient's resilience might further play a role and lead to a "practical" treatment plan, which in turn has to be modified continuously according to contingent changes in compliance and health (Riesen et al. 2002).

Restorative work in particular has to be planned and designed according to the patient's resilience, manual dexterity, and autonomy. Further functional decline and potential tooth loss in the years to come has to be anticipated. Elderly edentate persons prefer removable dentures for aesthetic reasons and the ease of cleaning (Feine et al. 1994). Indeed, in cases of advanced bone loss it is easier to replace the missing tissues and restore the patient's profile with a removable appliance. Furthermore, removable restorations provide all the flexibility that is necessary to avoid a replacement late in life, when the capacity to adapt to a new prosthesis is largely diminished.

Benefits of Implants in Elderly Patients

Prevention of Bone Atrophy

Numerous studies have shown the beneficial effect of dental implants on the preservation of the peri-implant bony structures. With reference to alveolar ridge atrophy in edentulous persons, as described in the long-term observations of Tallgren (1972), peri-implant bone loss is slowed down seven- to ten-fold when dental implants support a removable denture (Jemt et al. 1996; Lindquist et al. 1988; Naert et al. 1991). However, occlusal load distribution needs to be carefully balanced; implant support in the lower interforaminal region increases the chewing forces and might consequently lead to pronounced bone resorption in the lower posterior and upper anterior edentulous regions (Jacobs et al. 1992; Kreisler et al. 2003).

Muscle Coordination

Motor control loses its precision with age due to the loss of individual motor units and the recruitment of the remaining muscle fibers by neighboring units. These changes are also observed in the chewing muscles, which renders motor control of complete dentures difficult. With an increasing prevalence of dysphagia in geriatric patients, dentures become at risk in aspiration (Arora et al. 2005; Chapman 2006). In these situations, dental implants provide a substantial advantage in retaining a removable denture independent of muscle control.

Chewing Efficiency and Bite Force

Chewing efficiency with complete dentures is limited by three factors: physical retention,

stability, and pain in the denture-bearing tissues. All these limitations are abolished in implant-supported overdentures, resulting in a significantly improved masticatory efficiency (Van der Bilt et al. 2006; Van Kampen et al. 2004). However, the muscle bulk diminishes with age and bite force is largely reduced. This atrophy is even more pronounced after tooth loss, probably due to the lack of physiological stimulation (Newton et al. 1993). It is likely, but not yet proven, that the stabilization of complete dentures by means of dental implants counteracts this atrophy with an increased utilization of the chewing muscles.

Nutritional State

Undernutrition has a prevalence of 5–8% in community-dwelling elderly adults, but it rises to 30–60% in the institutionalized population (Guigoz et al. 1994). Nutritional intake depends on a variety of very different factors such as appetite, cognitive state, general health, education, mobility, financial resources, and cultural and religious habits, as well as cooking skills. Despite a confirmed correlation between the number of teeth and the nutritional intake, it has to be borne in mind that chewing efficiency is only one among many factors contributing to an adequate nutritional intake (Sheiham et al. 2001). The stabilization of complete dentures by means of osseointegrated implants might improve the nutritional state (Morais et al. 2003), but it is nevertheless recommended that any dental restoration is complemented by professional nutritional advice (Moynihan et al. 2000).

Psychosocial Aspects

Tooth loss and denture-wearing can have a substantial impact on self-esteem and psychosocial well-being. Among the most feared incidents of complete denture wearers is the loss of retention in a social context, which reveals immediately the presence of a removable prosthesis. The inability to finish a meal within the habitual time is no less feared and might lead to social isolation, even in an institutionalized context. Wismeijer and his group (1997) reported an almost complete psychosocial rehabilitation of 104 complete denture wearers, 16 months after stabilization of their lower prostheses by ITI implants. After having been restored, the patients felt more comfortable visiting their families, entertaining friends at their homes, and eating out in restaurants.

Risks of Implant Restorations

While the general health and local anatomical risk of surgical intervention can be handled by careful preoperative anamnesis and diagnostics, there is an unforeseeable risk in elderly persons concerning their future health and functional impairment. Once autonomy is lost, oral hygiene measures and denture manipulation rely on carers who generally have little experience with sophisticated implant restorations. It should further be considered that with declining health and cognitive impairment, the use of dentures becomes less frequent (Taji et al. 2005). Even with sore spots a patient might be tempted to eat without the prosthesis when a dental appointment is not easily available. Implant attachments that have the female part in the mouth might then fill up with food debris (Fig. 3.5).

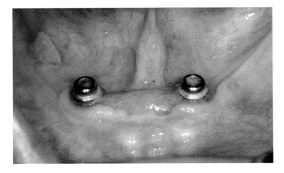

Figure 3.5. This 92-year-old institutionalized female patient ate without her dentures because she had sore spots and did not dare ask the nurse for a dental appointment. The locators filled with food debris and the denture did not fit anymore.

When reduced vision and dexterity preclude cleaning the attachments, the denture can no longer be worn. Treatment concepts should therefore avoid attachments that can fill up with food or calculus. Attachments should also not be cemented permanently. Terminally ill patients who prefer not to wear their dentures, for example when chemotherapy renders the mucosa sensitive, might want to have their implant attachments replaced by less disturbing healing caps.

Survival Rates and Peri-implant Bone Loss

Only very few comparative studies looked into the effect of age on the osseointegration process and clinical success rates. Among the first was a Swedish paper by Köndell and co-workers (1988), who reported on equal survival rates of dental implants in a group of 18- to 54-year-old patients and one with an age range of 65–84 years. Later, a Dutch group conducted a prospective study to determine the influence of age on implant survival rates in patients treated with mandibular overdentures supported by two implants (Meijer et al. 2001). Long-term data are also available from a cohort study by Bryant and Zarb (2003), while Engfors et al. (2004) examined in a retrospective study the outcomes in patients 80 years of age and over and compared the results with a matched younger control group. The studies suggest no relationship between age and bone loss or implant survival rates. Thus, the placement of dental implants in elderly patients should not be discouraged.

Apprehensions of Elderly Persons

Besides the known barriers to oral health care for elderly adults such as access to care and financial limitations, implant treatment options might furthermore be confined by their poor general health condition. In addition to those "objective" barriers, there are a number of subjective apprehensions that preclude the acceptance of an implant treatment (Table 3.7).

Table 3.7. Apprehensions concerning a potential implant treatment in 92 volunteers with an average age of 81.2 ± 8.0 years judged on a 100 mm VAS scale (modified from Salem 2008).

I would not like to benefit from dental implants because . . .

	Women (n = 61)		Men (n = 31)		p
	Mean	SD	Mean	SD	
I find implants too expensive	65.1	±32.8	74.5	±25.0	n.s
I don't see the necessity	54.5	±43.9	64.2	±46.0	n.s
I consider myself too old	52.0	±42.4	47.7	±43.9	n.s
It is not worthwhile	38.5	±43.0	58.4	±46.4	n.s
I am afraid of the operation	52.7	±36.6	9.7	±13.0	<0.0001
My bone is of bad quality	31.5	±34.7	3.2	±6.5	<0.0001
I fear implant rejection	27.9	±30.1	6.1	±14.8	<0.0001
I fear a foreign body feeling	25.7	±30.8	9.0	±20.1	0.0004
The integration time is too long	17.9	±27.1	6.5	±12.5	0.0247
I know persons with bad experience	12.3	±23.7	5.5	±18.0	0.0203
Total	37.8	±17.4	28.5	±12.8	0.0229

Even when cost was removed as a factor, 36% of elderly and edentulous subjects refused implants within the context of a clinical trial (Walton and MacEntee 2005). In a semi-structured interview of 92 volunteers, Salem investigated the attitude toward and knowledge of dental implants, as well as the hypothetical acceptance of an implant treatment. A step-wise backward multiple linear regression analysis revealed that it is not age as such that predicts possible apprehensions of an implant treatment but limited knowledge of implants, poor oral health, and being a woman, as well as institutionalized living, that are the predominant factors (Salem 2008).

Future Perspective

To increase the number of old and very old patients who benefit late in life from the proven advantages of implant-supported restorations, implants should be placed when the patient is still independent and resilient.

Also, less invasive surgical techniques should be developed. The dissemination of objective knowledge on dental implants would help to reduce existing apprehensions in the elderly population.

Concluding Remarks

Methods for Health Care Improvement and Quality Evaluation

Many clinical achievements in complex patients fall more appropriately in the category of health care improvement than of high-level evidence-based research (Bergendal 2006). Publications of results in small groups of patients and in single cases can contribute to the gradual building of knowledge of methods and outcomes in oral rehabilitation for complex patients. However, data can be gathered faster by using new information techniques, cooperation between centers, and networks of professionals.

The establishment of easy access databases for evaluation of outcomes of treatment with dental implants could be an optimal method for continuously adding new information on treatment results. Ideally, each patient could be given a classification of their medical diagnosis. It would then be possible to search for patients with a certain disease or syndrome, medication, or other characteristics and learn the outcome of treatment with dental implants. When widely used by clinicians, this type of database could supply the information that today is scattered and unsystematic. Another strategy is to create fora and networks and establish multicenter cooperation in order to increase study sample size in specific projects. Consensus conferences can also be an effective way to gather current knowledge and to present statements based on the best available evidence (Gottfredsen et al. 2008; Koch et al. 1996; Swiss Society of Reconstructive Dentistry 2007).

Similarly, the establishment of care programs and research strategies for certain groups of patients, like the conferences on ectodermal dysplasia (Bergendal et al. 1998) and osteogenesis imperfecta (Storhaug 2002), would add focused information.

References

Abu-Serriah MM. 2001. Outcome of extra-oral craniofacial endosseous implants. *Brit J Oral Maxillofac Surg* 39(4):269.

Abu-Serriah MM, McGowan DA, Moos KF, Bagg J. 2003. Extra-oral craniofacial endosseous implants and radiotherapy. *Int J Oral Maxillofac Surg* 32(6):585–592.

Adbulwassie H, Dhanrajani PJ, et al. 1996. Papillon-Lefevre syndrome. Reappraisal of etiology, clinical features and treatment. II: Oral rehabilitation using osseointegrated implants. *Indian J Dent Res* 7(2):63–70.

Ambjornsen E. 2002. Maintenance and rehabilitation of the dentition in osteogenesis imperfecta. Challenges for the dental profession? OI-Consensus Conference. Oslo, Norway: Norwegian Directorate for Health and Social Welfare.

Andersson-Norinder J, Sjogreen L. 2000. Orofacial dysfunction. In: *Disability and Oral Care*. J Nunn (ed.). London: FDI World Dental Press Ltd. 82–92.

Angle AD, Rebellato J. 2005. Dental team management for a patient with cleidocranial dysostosis. *Am J Orthod Dentofacial Orthop* 128(1):110–117.

Arora A, Arora M, et al. 2005. Mystery of the missing denture: An unusual cause of respiratory arrest in a nonagenarian. *Age and Ageing* 34(5):519–520.

Beikler T, Flemmig TF. 2003. Implants in the medically compromised patient. *Crit Rev Oral Biol Med* 14(4):305–316.

Bergendal B. 2006. Evidence and clinical improvement: Current experiences with dental implants in individuals with rare disorders. *Int J Prosthodont* 19(2):132–134.

Bergendal T, Eckerdal O, et al. 1991. Osseointegrated implants in the oral habilitation of a boy with ectodermal dysplasia: A case report. *Int Dent J* 41(3):149–156.

Bergendal B, Ekman A, Nilsson P. 2008. Implant failure in young children with ectodermal dysplasia. A retrospective evaluation of use and outcome of dental implant treatment in children in Sweden. *Int J Oral Maxillofac Implants* 23(3):520–524.

Bergendal B, Koch G, et al. 1998. Consensus Conference on Ectodermal Dysplasia with Special Reference to Dental Treatment. Stockholm: Förlagshuset Gothia Ltd.

Bergendal B, Ljunggren Ö. 2001. Treatment with oral implants in X-linked hypophosphataemic rickets and hypophosphatasia—report from a workshop. Abstract *Swedish Dent J* 25:165.

Binger T, Rucker M, et al. 2006. Dentofacial rehabilitation by osteodistraction, augmentation and implantation despite osteogenesis imperfecta. *Int J Oral Maxillofac Surg* 35(6):559–562.

Bonin B, Saffarzadeh A, et al. 2001. Early implant treatment of a child with anhidrotic ectodermal dysplasia. Apropos of a case. *Rev Stomatol Chir Maxillofac* 102(6): 313–318.

Boyes-Varley JG, Howes DG, Davidge-Pitts KD, Brånemark I, McAlpine JA. 2007. A protocol for maxillary reconstruction following oncology resection using zygomatic implants. *Int J Prosthodont* 20(5):521–531.

Brahim JS, Guckes AD, et al. 1992. Implant rehabilitation in Erdheim-Chester disease: A clinical report. *J Prosthet Dent* 68(3): 399–401.

Bryant SR, Zarb GA. 2003. Crestal bone loss proximal to oral implants in older and younger adults. *J Prosthet Dent* 89(6): 589–597.

Budtz-Jorgensen E. 1999. *Prosthodontics for the Elderly: Diagnosis and Treatment.* Chicago: Quintessence Publishing Co, Inc.

Chapman L. 2006. Another case of missing dentures. *Age and Ageing* 35(2):205.

Chen LH, Tsutsumi S, Iizuka T. 1997. A CAD/CAM technique for fabricating facial prostheses: A preliminary report. *Int J Prosthodont* 10(5):467–472.

Chiapasco M, Biglioli F, Autelitano L, Romeo E, Brusati R. 2006. Clinical outcome of dental implants placed in fibula-free flaps used for the reconstruction of maxillo-mandibular defects following ablation for tumors or osteoradionecrosis. *Clin Oral Implants Res* 17(2):220–228.

Daskalogiannakis J, Piedade L, et al. 2006. Cleidocranial dysplasia: 2 generations of management. *J Can Dent Assoc* 72(4): 337–342.

De Baat C. 2000. Success of dental implants in elderly people—a literature review. *Gerodontology* 17(1):45–48.

Del Valle V, Faulkner G, Wolfaardt JF. 1997. Craniofacial osseointegrated implant-induced strain distribution: A numerical study. *Int J Oral Maxillofac Implants* 12(2): 200–210.

Drinias V, Granström G, Tjellström A. 2007. High age at the time of implant installation is correlated with increased loss of osseointe-grated implants in the temporal bone. *Clin Implant Dent Relat Res* 9(2):94–99.

Ekfeldt A. 2005. Early experience of implant-supported prostheses in patients with neurologic disabilities. *Int J Prosthodont* 18(2):132–138.

Ekstrand K, Thomsson M. 1988. Ectodermal dysplasia with partial anodontia: Prosthetic treatment with implant fixed prosthesis. *ASDC J Dent Child* 55(4):282–284.

Engfors I, Ortorp A, et al. 2004. Fixed implant-supported prostheses in elderly patients: A 5-year retrospective study of 133 edentulous patients older than 79 years. *Clin Implant Dent Relat Res* 6(4):190–198.

Entesarian M, Matsson H, et al. 2005. Mutations in the gene encoding fibroblast growth factor 10 are associated with aplasia of lacrimal and salivary glands. *Nat Genet* 37(2):125–127.

Feine JS, De Grandmont P, et al. 1994. Within-subject comparisons of implant-supported mandibular prostheses: Choice of prosthesis. *J Dent Res* 73(5):1105–1111.

Gbara A, Darwich K, Li L, Schmelzle R, Blake F. 2007. Long-term results of jaw reconstruction with microsurgical fibula grafts and dental implants. *J Oral Maxillofac Surg* 65(5):1005–1009.

Gliklich RE, Rounds MF, Cheney ML, Varvares MA. 1998. Combining free flap reconstruction and craniofacial prosthetic technique for orbit, scalp, and temporal defects. *Laryngoscope* 108(4):482–487.

Gottfredsen K, Carlsson G, et al. 2008. Implants and/or teeth. Consensus statements and recommendations. *J Oral Rehabil* 35(Suppl 1):2–8.

Granström G. 1998. Hyperbaric oxygen therapy as a stimulator of osseointegration. *Advances in Oto-Rhino-Laryngology* 54:33–49.

———. 2003. Radiotherapy, osseointegration and hyperbaric oxygen therapy. *Periodontology 2000* 33:145–162.

———. 2005. Osseointegration in irradiated cancer patients: An analysis with respect to implant failures. *J Oral Maxillofac Surg* 63(5):579–585.

———. 2007. Craniofacial osseointegration. *Oral Dis* 13(3):261–269.

Granström G, Tjellström A. 1997. Effects of irradiation on osseointegration before and after implant placement: A report of three cases. *Int J Oral Maxillofac Implants* 12(4):547–551.

Guckes AD, McCarthy GR, et al. 1997. Use of endosseous implants in a 3-year-old child with ectodermal dysplasia: Case report and 5-year follow-up. *Pediatr Dent* 19(4):282–285.

Guckes, AD, Scurria MS, et al. 2002. Prospective clinical trial of dental implants in persons with ectodermal dysplasia. *J Prosthet Dent* 88(1):21–25.

Guigoz Y, Vellas B, et al. 1994. Mini nutritional assessment: A practical assessment tool for grading the nutritional state of elderly patients. *The Mini Nutritional Assessment, Facts and Research in Gerontology* (Suppl I). Paris: Serdi.

Harrison JS, Stratemann S, Redding SW. 2003. Dental implants for patients who have had radiation treatment for head and neck cancer. *Spec Care Dentist* 23(6): 223–229.

Hugoson A, Koch G, et al. 2005. Oral health of individuals aged 3–80 years in Jonkoping, Sweden during 30 years (1973–2003). I: Review of findings on dental care habits and knowledge of oral health. *Swedish Dent J* 29(4):125–138.

Jacobs R, Schotte A, et al. 1992. Posterior jaw bone resorption in osseointegrated implant-supported overdentures. *Clin Oral Implants Res* 3(2):63–70.

Jaquiery C, Rohner D, Kunz C, Bucher P, Peters F, Schenk RK, Hammer B. 2004. Reconstruction of maxillary and mandibular defects using prefabricated microvascular fibular grafts and osseointegrated dental implants—a prospective study. *Clin Oral Implants Res* 15(5):598–606.

Jemt T, Chai J, et al. 1996. A 5-year prospective multicenter follow-up report on overdentures supported by osseointegrated implants. *Int J Oral Maxillofac Implants* 11(3):291–298.

Kearns G, Sharma A, et al. 1999. Placement of endosseous implants in children and adolescents with hereditary ectodermal dysplasia. *Oral Surg Oral Med Oral Pathol Oral Radiol Endod* 88(1):5–10.

Kiat-amnuay S, Chambers MS, Jacob RF, Anderson JD, Sheppard RA, Johnson DA, Haugh GS, Gettleman L. 2008. Clinical trial of chlorinated polyethylene for facial prostheses. In preparation.

Klein M, Hohlfeld T, Moormann P, Menneking H. 2000. Improvement of epidermal adhesion by surface modification of craniofacial abutments. *Int J Oral Maxillofac Implants* 15(2):247–251.

Klein M, Menneking H, Schmitz H, Locke HG, Bier J. 1999. A new generation of facial prostheses with myoelectrically driven moveable upper lid. *Lancet* 353(9163):1493.

Klingberg G, Oskarsdottir S, et al. 2002. Oral manifestations in 22q11 deletion syndrome. *Int J Paediatr Dent* 12(1):14–23.

Koch G, Bergendal T, et al. 1996. Consensus Conference on Oral Implants in Young Patients. Stockholm: Förlagshuset Gothia Ltd.

Köndell PA, Nordenram A, et al. 1988. Titanium implants in the treatment of edentulousness: Influence of patient's age on prognosis. *Gerodontics* 4(6): 280–284.

Kreisler M, Behneke N, et al. 2003. Residual ridge resorption in the edentulous maxilla in patients with implant-supported mandibular overdentures: An 8-year retrospective study. *Int J Prosthodont* 16(3): 295–300.

Lee CY, Ertel SK. 2003. Bone graft augmentation and dental implant treatment in a patient with osteogenesis imperfecta: Review of the literature with a case report. *Implant Dent* 12(4):291–295.

Lee H, Al Mardini M, et al. 2007. Oral rehabilitation of a completely edentulous epidermolysis bullosa patient with an implant-supported prosthesis: A clinical report. *J Prosthet Dent* 97(2):65–69.

Lindquist LW, Rockler B, et al. 1988. Bone resorption around fixtures in edentulous patients treated with mandibular fixed tissue-integrated prostheses. *J Prosthet Dent* 59(1):59–63.

Lombardas P, Toothaker RW. 1997. Bone grafting and osseointegrated implants in the treatment of cleidocranial dysplasia. *Compend Contin Educ Dent* 18(5):509–512, 514.

Lustig JP, Yanko R, et al. 2002. Use of dental implants in patients with Down syndrome: A case report. *Spec Care Dentist* 22(5):201–204.

Malmgren B, Norgren S. 2002. Dental aberrations in children and adolescents with osteogenesis imperfecta. *Acta Odontol Scand* 60(2):65–71.

Markt JC. 2003. Implant prosthodontic rehabilitation of a patient with nevoid basal cell carcinoma syndrome: A clinical report. *J Prosthet Dent* 89(5):436–442.

Marx RE, Ehler WJ, Tayapongsak P, Pierce LW. 1990. Relationship of oxygen dose to angiogenesis induction in irradiated tissue. *Am J Surg* 160(5):519–524.

Mass E, Oelgiesser D, et al. 2007. Transitional implants in a patient with Williams-Beuren syndrome: A four-year follow-up. *Spec Care Dentist* 27(3):112–116.

Meijer HJ, Batenburg RH, et al. 2001. Influence of patient age on the success rate of dental implants supporting an overdenture in an edentulous mandible: A 3-year prospective study. *Int J Oral Maxillofac Implants* 16(4):522–526.

Morais JA, Heydecke G, et al. 2003. The effects of mandibular two-implant overdentures on nutrition in elderly edentulous individuals. *J Dent Res* 82(1):53–58.

Moynihan PJ, Butler TJ, et al. 2000. Nutrient intake in partially dentate patients: The effect of prosthetic rehabilitation. *J Dent* 28(8):557–563.

Müller F, Bergendal B, et al. 2006. Implant-supported FPDs in a patient with dystrophic epidermolysis bullosa. *Int J Oral Maxillofac Implants*. Submitted.

Naert I, Quirynen M, et al. 1991. Prosthetic aspects of osseointegrated fixtures supporting overdentures. A 4-year report. *J Prosthet Dent* 65(5):671–680.

National Institutes of Health. 1988. Consensus development conference statement. NIH Consensus Development Conference: Dental Implants. National Institutes of Health. U.S. Department of Health and Human Services.

Newton J, Yemm R, et al. 1993. Changes in human jaw muscles with age and dental state. *Gerodontology* 10(1):16–22.

Niimi A, Ueda M, Keller EE, Worthington P. 1998. Experience with osseointegrated implants placed in irradiated tissues in Japan and the United States. *Int J Oral Maxillofac Implants* 13(3):407–411.

Nunn J. 2000. *Disability and Oral Care.* London: FDI World Dental Press Ltd.

Oczakir C, Balmer S, et al. 2005. Implant-prosthodontic treatment for special care patients: A case series study. *Int J Prosthodont* 18(5):383–389.

Parel SM, Tjellström A. 1991. The United States and Swedish experience with osseointegration and facial prostheses. *Int J Oral Maxillofac Implants* 6(1):75–79.

Patel K, Welfare R, et al. 1998. The provision of dental implants and a fixed prosthesis in the treatment of a patient with scleroderma: A clinical report. *J Prosthet Dent* 79(6): 611–612.

Penarrocha M, Larrazabal C, et al. 2007. Restoration with implants in patients with recessive dystrophic epidermolysis bullosa and patient satisfaction with the implant-supported superstructure. *Int J Oral Maxillofac Implants* 22(4):651–655.

Penarrocha-Diago M, Serrano C, et al. 2000. Placement of endosseous implants in patients with oral epidermolysis bullosa. *Oral Surg Oral Med Oral Pathol Oral Radiol Endod* 90(5):587–590.

Petropoulos VC, Balshi TJ, et al. 2004. Treatment of a patient with cleidocranial dysplasia using osseointegrated implants: A patient report. *Int J Oral Maxillofac Implants* 19(2):282–287.

Prabhu N, Duckmanton N, et al. 2007. The placement of osseointegrated dental implants in a patient with type IV B osteogenesis imperfecta: A 9-year follow-up.

Oral Surg Oral Med Oral Pathol Oral Radiol Endod 103(3):349–354.

Resnick, D. 1998. Implant placement and guided tissue regeneration in a patient with congenital vitamin D-resistant rickets. *J Oral Implantol* 24(4):214–218.

Reyes RA, Tjellström A, Granström G. 2000. Evaluation of implant losses and skin reactions around extraoral bone-anchored implants: A 0- to 8-year follow-up. *Otolaryngology—Head & Neck Surgery* 122(2):272–276.

Riesen M, Chung JP, et al. 2002. Interventions bucco-dentaires chez les personnes âgées. *Médecine & Hygiène* 2414:2178–2188.

Salem K. 2008. Attitude, connaissance et acceptation du traitement implantaire chez la personne âgée. Division of Gerodontology and Removable Prosthodontics. Geneva, University of Geneva. Doctoral thesis.

Sheiham A, Steele JG, et al. 2001. The relationship among dental status, nutrient intake, and nutritional status in older people. *J Dental Res* 80(2):408–413.

Slotte C, Thorstensson B, et al. 2006. A case of hypophosphatasia followed from childhood to adulthood over a period of more than thirty years. *J Oral Disabil Oral Health* 7:126.

Smith RA, Vargervik K, et al. 1993. Placement of an endosseous implant in a growing child with ectodermal dysplasia. *Oral Surg Oral Med Oral Pathol* 75(6):669–673.

Storhaug K. 1989. Disability and oral health. A study of living conditions, oral health and consumption of social and dental services in a group of disabled Norwegians. Institute of Community Dentistry, University of Oslo. Thesis.

———. 2002. OI-Consensus Conference (Osteogenesis Imperfecta). Oslo: TAKO-centre, Resource Centre for Oral Health in Rare Medical Conditions.

Sweeney IP, Ferguson JW, et al. 2005. Treatment outcomes for adolescent ectodermal dysplasia patients treated with dental implants. *Int J Paediatr Dent* 15(4):241–248.

Swiss Society of Reconstructive Dentistry. 2007. First European Workshop on Evidence-Based Reconstructive Dentistry. *Clin Oral Implants Res* 18:1–261.

Taji T, Yoshida M, et al. 2005. Influence of mental status on removable prosthesis compliance in institutionalized elderly persons. *Int J Prosthodont* 18(2):146–149.

Tallgren A. 1972. The continuing reduction of the residual alveolar ridges in complete denture wearers: A mixed-longitudinal study covering 25 years. *J Prosthet Dent* 27(2):120–132.

Thor A, Stenport VF, et al. 2005. Bone graft and implants in a patient with systemic mastocytosis. *Clin Implant Dent Relat Res* 7(2):79–86.

Tjellström A. 1989. Osseointegrated systems and their applications in the head and neck. *Adv Otolaryngol Head Neck Surg* 3:39–70.

Tjellström A, Håkansson B. 1995. The bone-anchored hearing aid. design, principles, indications and long term results. *Otolaryngol Clin North Am* 28:53–72.

Tjellström A, Håkansson B, Lindstrom J, Brånemark PI, Hallen O, Rosenhall U, Leijon A. 1980. Analysis of the mechanical impedance of bone-anchored hearing aids. *Acta Otolaryngol (Stockh)* 89(1–2):85–92.

Tjellström A, Lindstrom J, Nylen O, Albrektsson T, Brånemark PI, Birgersson B, Nero H, Sylven C. 1981. The bone-anchored auricular episthesis. *Laryngoscope* 91(5):811–815.

Tjellström A, Yontchev E, Lindstrom J, Brånemark PI. 1985. Five years' experience with bone-anchored auricular prostheses. *Otolaryngology—Head and Neck Surgery* 93(3):366–372.

Tolman DE, Taylor PF. 1996. Bone-anchored craniofacial prosthesis study. *Int J Oral Maxillofac Implants* 11(2):159–168.

Toygar HU, Kircelli C, et al. 2007. Combined therapy in a patient with Papillon-Lefevre syndrome: A 13-year follow-up. *J Periodontol* 78(9):1819–1824.

Ullbro C, Crossner CG, et al. 2000. Osseointegrated implants in a patient with Papillon-Lefevre syndrome. A 4 1/2-year follow up. *J Clin Periodontol* 27(12):951–954.

Van der Bilt A, Van Kampen FM, et al. 2006. Masticatory function with mandibular implant-supported overdentures fitted with different attachment types. *Eur J Oral Sci* 114(3):191–196.

Van Kampen FM, Van der Bilt A, et al. 2004. Masticatory function with implant-supported overdentures. *J Dent Res* 83(9): 708–711.

Vinzenz KG, Holle J, Wuringer E, Kulenkampff KJ. 1996. Prefabrication of combined scapula flaps for microsurgical reconstruction in oro-maxillofacial defects: A new method. *J Craniomaxillofac Surg* 24(4):214–223.

Walton JN, MacEntee MI. 2005. Choosing or refusing oral implants: A prospective study of edentulous volunteers for a clinical trial. *Int J Prosthodont* 18(6):483–488.

Wazen JJ, Caruso M, Tjellström A. 1998. Long-term results with the titanium bone-anchored hearing aid: The U.S. experience. *Am J Otol* 19(6):737–741.

Wilkes GH, Wolfaardt JF. 1994. Osseointegrated alloplastic versus autogenous ear reconstruction: Criteria for treatment selection. *Plast Reconstr Surg* 93(5): 967–979.

Wismeijer D, Van Waas MA, et al. 1997. Patient satisfaction with implant-supported mandibular overdentures. A comparison of three treatment strategies with ITI-dental implants. *Int J Oral Maxillofac Surg* 26(4):263–267.

Wolfaardt JF, Wilkes GH, Parel SM, Tjellström A. 1993. Craniofacial osseointegration: The Canadian experience. *Int J Oral Maxillofac Implants* 8(2):197–204.

Woo I, Brunner DP, et al. 2003. Dental implants in a young patient with Papillon-Lefevre syndrome: A case report. *Implant Dent* 12(2):140–144.

Young W, Khan F, et al. 2001. Syndromes with salivary dysfunction predispose to tooth wear: Case reports of congenital dysfunction of major salivary glands, Prader-Willi, congenital rubella, and Sjogren's syndromes. *Oral Surg Oral Med Oral Pathol Oral Radiol Endod* 92(1): 38–48.

Zola MB. 2000. Staged sinus augmentation and implant placement in a patient with osteogenesis imperfecta. *J Oral Maxillofac Surg* 58(4):443–447.

Comprehensive Treatment Planning for the Patient with Oral or Systemic Inflammation

4

THE EFFICACY OF OSSEOINTEGRATED DENTAL IMPLANTS FOR PERIODONTALLY COMPROMISED PATIENTS

Myron Nevins and David M. Kim

Twenty-five years have elapsed since the North American continent was graced by the presentation from P.I. Brånemark and his breakthrough research on osseointegrated implants at the 1982 Toronto Conference on Osseointegration in Clinical Dentistry. His team's treatment regime to reverse edentulism and restore the dignity and mastication of dentally disadvantaged patients has revolutionized dental treatment planning and significantly upgraded the prognosis both of edentulous patients and partially dentate patients (Adell et al. 1981, 1990; Brånemark et al. 1977; Buser et al. 1990; Jemt et al. 1989; Lekholm et al. 1999; van Steenberghe et al. 1990).

Since the introduction, the patient population who would benefit from safe and efficacious prostheses anchored by titanium implants has continually expanded. However, the debate continues on whether similar success and survival rates can be anticipated in partially edentulous, periodontally compromised patients. These patients demonstrated damage in quality and dimension of the remaining alveolar ridge due to a history of periodontal disease and consequential loss of teeth (Ellegaard et al. 1997). It may be reasonable to anticipate that the risk of peri-implant infections is higher if the periodontal disease is not definitely treated before the implant placement. A 10-year prospective study comparing the clinical and radiographic changes in periodontal and peri-implant conditions revealed a correlation between these conditions (Karoussis et al. 2004).

Before a pessimistic argument can be made for implant treatment in periodontally compromised patients, it is necessary to evaluate available evidence and collate this with an awareness of current treatment trends and clinical judgment (Nevins 2001). There have been numerous studies documenting a high degree of success in implant therapy in properly treated and well-maintained periodontitis-susceptible subjects (Ellegaard et al. 1997; Mengel et al. 2001; Nevins and Langer 1995; Sbordone et al. 1999) (Figs. 4.1a–4.1d).

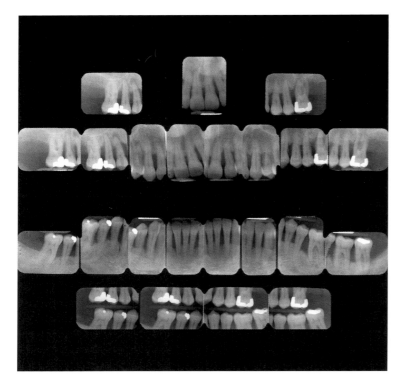

Figure 4.1a. Patient was diagnosed with generalized aggressive periodontitis in 1991.

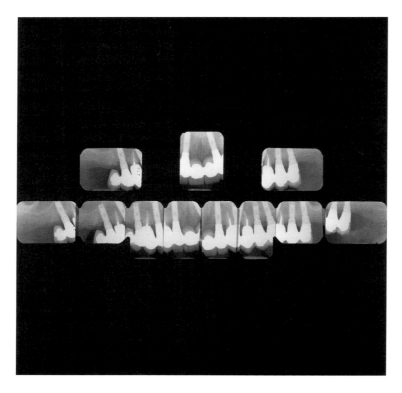

Figure 4.1b. In 1994, majority of maxillary teeth were extracted and replaced with dental implants.

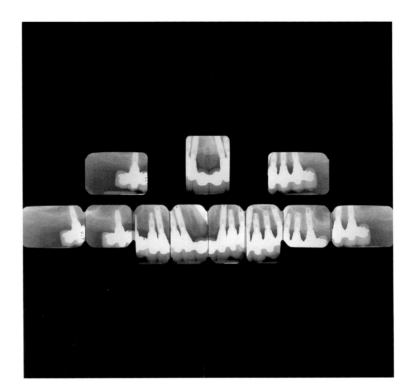

Figure 4.1c. In 2000, two remaining cuspids required extraction and were replaced with dental implants.

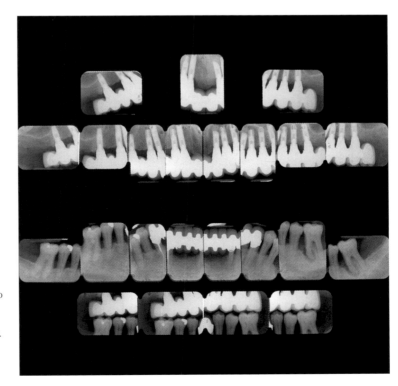

Figure 4.1d. Twelve years following initial placement of maxillary implants (2006) revealed that the bone level around implants remained very stable. Interestingly, apical portion of the left later incisor implant had to be resected due to inflammatory disease. This patient is on a strict 3-month periodontal maintenance therapy. Note the advancement of periodontal disease on mandibular left molar.

The results of these studies pointed out that implant therapy in periodontally compromised patients has a 3- to 5-year prognosis, similar to the well-documented long-term prognosis of implant treatment in non-periodontally compromised patients. For example, the 5-year survival rates of 258 dental implants in patients with a history of periodontitis who had previously undergone periodontal surgery and maintained a high standard of oral hygiene were 97% (two-stage implants) and 94% (one-stage implants) (Baelum and Ellegaard 2004). For this same group, the 10-year survival rates were 97% (two-stage implants) and 78% (one-stage implants) (Baelum and Ellegaard 2004). The higher failure rate with one-stage implants can be explained by lower reported survival rates for hollow screw implants when compared to solid screw implants (Baelum and Ellegaard 2004; Buser et al. 1997). A randomized, controlled clinical trial of partially edentulous periodontitis-susceptible subjects demonstrated that bone loss during the first year of function was minor, as well as annually thereafter (Wennström et al. 2004). Thus, to date there is no consensus or evidence to support an unfavorable prognosis for implants in periodontally compromised patients.

Early Loss and Late Loss of Dental Implants

The decisive factors in implant success rates depend on the thresholds chosen to distinguish between success and failure. Even though the consensus on success varies considerably, current criteria for success includes both radiographic and clinical confirmations (Albrektsson et al. 1986). They are as follows:

1. The individual implant should be clinically immobile.
2. There should be no radiographic peri-implant radiolucency.
3. There should be an absence of persistent pain, infections, neuropathies, and paresthesia.

4. There should be 85% success at the end of a 5-year period of observation and 80% at the end of a 10-year period of observation.
5. There should be less than 0.2 mm of bone loss annually following the implant's first year of loading.

Longitudinal studies have reported implant survival rates of around 90–95% over periods of 5–10 years (Berglundh et al. 2002; Esposito et al. 1998). Implant failure can be classified as "early implant loss" (before functional loading) or "late implant loss" (following functional loading) (Berglundh et al. 2002). An early loss is not synonymous with peri-implantitis because peri-implantitis is considered an inflammatory process affecting the tissues around an osseointegrated implant that is in function, which ultimately results in loss of supporting bone and eventually in late implant loss (Albrektsson and Isidor 1994). A variety of factors may be responsible for early failure, such as surgical trauma, overheating during the implant site preparation, delayed wound healing, lack of implant stability, bacterial contamination, or premature overloading. Factors associated with late loss are less well understood, but may include infection and overloading.

Critical Reviews

A systematic approach to reviewing articles on the efficacy of osseointegrated implants for periodontally compromised patients is a reliable method for understanding current knowledge and consensus. In their systematic approach to evaluate the long-term (≥5 years) success of implants placed in partially edentulous patients with a history of periodontitis (evidenced by loss of supporting bone and implant loss), Van der Weijden et al. in 2005 concluded that the outcome of implant therapy in periodontitis patients may be different from that of individuals without such a history. In contrast to this article, a thorough MEDLINE search of the relationship between susceptibility to periodontitis and peri-implantitis with implant outcome up to 2006 indicated differing results. For example, periodontally compromised patients were successfully treated with minimally or moderately rough implants, in the presence of maintenance therapy (Quirynen et al. 2007). Other systematic reviews conclude that in the presence of maintenance therapy, associated with minimally rough implants, the rate of late implant failure did not differ between patients with or without a history of periodontitis (Mengel and Flores-de-Jacoby 2005; Rosenberg et al. 2004).

Chronic and Aggressive Periodontitis

Karoussis conducted a comprehensive and critical review of dental implant prognosis in periodontally compromised partially edentulous patients (Karoussis et al. 2007). Implant survival rates in patients with a history of chronic periodontitis were well above 90% for both short-term (<5 years) and long-term (≥5 years) studies. These results were comparable to the mean implant survival rates reported for the general population. This raises the question, why do we expect implants to be successful when other periodontal treatment regimes have failed?

While the short-term implant survival rates for patients treated for aggressive periodontitis were above 95%, the long-term survival rates of implants in those patients were uncertain. These patients will probably have more inflammatory episodes than patients with chronic periodontitis. The above finding is in agreement with the results of other studies (Mengel et al. 2001; Nevins and Langer 1995).

Confounding Variables to Consider

Microorganisms

The peri-implant microbiota in well-maintained implant patients resembles that found around healthy dentitions (Leonhardt et al. 1999; Mombelli et al. 1987). However, a past history of periodontitis may represent a significant risk factor for complications around implants (Van der Weijden et al. 2005). In partially edentulous patients, microorganisms in periodontal pockets may act as a reservoir for colonization of the subgingival area around implants (Mombelli 2002; Quirynen et al. 2002). Thus, periodontal pathogens may be transmitted from residual pockets at teeth to implant sites, elevating the risk of peri-implant infection (Apse et al. 1989; Lee et al. 1999; Leonhardt et al. 1993; Mombelli et al. 1995; Quirynen and Listgarten 1990). However, a 10-year follow-up of osseointegrated implants in individuals treated for advanced periodontal disease prior to their implant treatment revealed that the mere presence of these putative periodontal pathogens within implant sites may not influence the long-term outcome of the implant treatment (Leonhardt et al. 2002). Sbordone and Quirynen also reported similar findings (Sbordone et al. 1999; Quirynen et al. 2001). These species were likely a part of the normal resident microbiota, and therefore may be randomly presented at both stable and progressing peri-implant sites (Leonhardt et al. 2002).

It is reasonable to anticipate that neglected or poorly treated periodontal disease would increase the risk for development of peri-implant infections (Leonhardt et al. 2002). Therefore the state of periodontal health reached following successful periodontal therapy is of utmost importance for the success of implant treatment. Nonetheless, the presence of periodontal pathogens around dental implant sites alone should not be considered as a prediction of implant failure (Nevins 2001; Quirynen et al. 2001; Sbordone et al. 1999).

Smoking

Smoking is a risk factor for periodontitis, and it may also be a significant risk factor for the development of peri-implantitis (Leonhardt et al. 2003). Wilson and Nunn (1999) found an increased risk for implant failure by a factor of almost 2.5 among smokers. Wallace also reported failure rates of 16.6% in smokers versus 6.9% in non-smokers (Wallace 2000). Smoking has also been associated as a major risk factor for multiple implant failure in retrospective analysis (Ekfeldt et al. 2001). Smoking cessation in periodontally compromised patients should therefore be recommended and instituted before considering implant therapy.

Maintenance Therapy

It has been suggested that patients should not be considered for dental implant therapy if they present with local inflammation or inadequate oral hygiene (Buser et al. 1997). It is important to diagnose existing periodontal disease and finite end point goal of therapy before introducing dental implants. It is assumed that red flags such as diabetes, steroid treatment, bisphosphonate treatment, and oncologic-related treatment regimes including radiation therapy will be recognized before implant treatment is initiated. Individually designed maintenance therapy following oral hygiene instruction, debridement procedure, and definitive periodontal therapy forms the basis of long-term success, as it is effective in preventing recurrence of periodontitis (Becker et al. 1984). Patients with untreated periodontal disease and refractory periodontitis are at risk for complications, and a regular maintenance program is essential to maintain the health of the periodontium and periodontal tissue (Leonhardt et al. 1993). Patients complying with a periodontal maintenance program have historically outperformed their counterparts. Hardt and Wennström both reported a significant marginal bone loss with no maintenance program compared to almost no bone loss in compliant patients (Hardt et al. 2002; Wennström et al. 2004). In addition, a 3-year prospective longitudinal study of implants in patients treated for generalized aggressive

and chronic periodontitis reported positive findings when they underwent periodontal surgery and a strict 3-month periodontal recall system (Mengel and Flores-de-Jacoby 2005).

Conclusion (Paradigm Shift Since 1982)

Since the 1982 Toronto Conference we have witnessed many changes, including implants being placed into immediate extraction sites and bone enhancement surgeries using a variety of osteopromotive materials such as autografts, allografts, xenografts, and alloplasts with and without barrier membrane. These products are also used at the time of tooth extraction in order to preserve the ridge. This procedure can be done in conjunction with immediate implant placement or as a staged event with later return for implant placement. Horizontal and vertical ridge augmentation has been accomplished, and bone is now routinely developed on the floor of the maxillary sinus to provide implant delivery to replace maxillary molars. Perhaps the most exciting additions to this field have been the emergence of recombinant proteins such as recombinant bone morphogenic protein 2 (rhBMP-2) and recombinant platelet derived growth factor (rhPDGF-BB) that potentiate the ability to manage bone deficiencies that ultimately save teeth and enhance placement of dental implants (Figs. 4.2a–4.2d). Both products have passed regulatory scrutiny and are available for patient use.

After considerable review of available evidence and clinical evaluation, it is the authors' belief that implant placement and restoration can be performed in periodontally compromised patients who are definitely treated and enrolled in periodontal maintenance therapy. With success and survival rates similar to those observed among periodontally healthy patients, there is no substantial evidence to exclude implant treatment options for patients with a past history of chronic periodontitis.

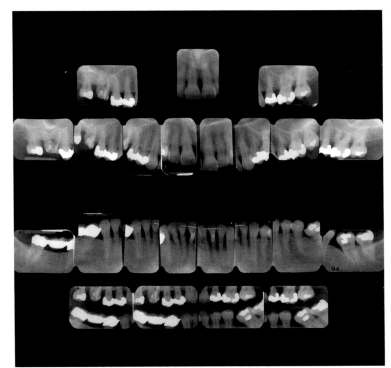

Figure 4.2a. Patient was diagnosed with generalized chronic periodontitis in 1994. Previously, the right maxillary first molar was treated with distal root resection. However, the tooth was not salvageable due to severe bone loss and furcation involvement. After the extraction, the patient was placed on strict 3-month periodontal maintenance therapy.

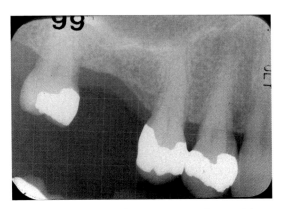

Figure 4.2b. In 1999, this patient agreed to participate in a clinical trial that would provide a novel method to restore the edentulous region of the first molar.

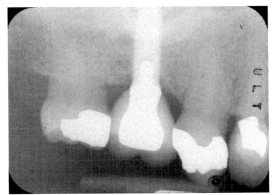

Figure 4.2c. It was determined that this patient was eligible to participate in a sinus lift study (clinical trial on rhBMP-2) and ultimately treated with sinus lift surgery, implant placement surgery, and an implant crown by 2002.

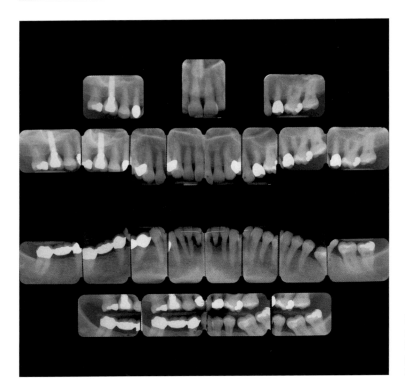

Figure 4.2d. Full mouth radiographs at the 6-year follow-up (2008) revealed very good implant stability with no noticeable bone loss.

PROFILES AND TREATMENT OPTIONS FOR REFRACTORY PATIENTS IN A PERIODONTAL PRACTICE

Øystein Fardal and Gerard James Linden

The term "refractory periodontal disease" has been used to describe individuals who are characterized by continued degeneration of the periodontium despite ongoing sanative, surgical, and/or pharmacological therapy (American Academy of Periodontology 2000). Haffajee et al. (2004) have suggested that refractory periodontitis may represent a state in which the clinician and the patient are unable to lower the infectious bacterial burden to a level that can be tolerated by the host's innate and acquired resistance. Other data have suggested that patients suffering from refractory periodontitis may also be hyperimmune so that they mount destructive inflammatory reactions even against normal oral flora (Bhide et al. 2006)

It is not known what proportion of long-term maintenance patients are unresponsive to treatment to the extent that they lose multiple teeth. Tooth loss is ultimately the major problem facing both the affected patients and their dentists. But limited information exists on periodontal maintenance patients who continue to lose teeth to such an extent that major prosthetic replacements are required. Similarly, there is not much information regarding the distribution of tooth loss, predisposing factors, or the outcomes of tooth replacements. A number of studies have reported complications when implants were used in patients with a history of progressive periodontal disease (Fardal et al. 1999; Hardt et al. 2002; Karoussis et al. 2003; Roos-Jansåker et al. 2006).

All periodontal maintenance patients treated initially by the same periodontist in a specialist practice in Norway between 1986 and 2006 were screened to identify and characterize refractory patients (Fardal and Linden 2008). The refractory cases were identified as patients who received initial periodontal therapy followed by at least 8 years of maintenance treatment in the specialist practice, and who lost multiple teeth during the maintenance period such that they were classified as downhill or extreme downhill as defined by Hirschfeld and Wasserman (1978). In addition, the loss of teeth was not part of an initial treatment plan to extract hopeless teeth. The maintenance therapy in the specialist practice was shared between three hygienists and the investigator (øF). A control group was selected from age- and gender-matched patients who attended the specialist practice for treatment and maintenance over the same period. For each case two controls were chosen as a representative convenience sample from the practice database.

Gender, date of birth, date of initial assessment, and medical history including drug history at the time of the initial assessment were obtained from the clinical records for all participants. Participants were questioned at the initial assessment regarding whether they thought they were under stress and whether they were currently taking, or had taken, antidepressants. Each participant was questioned in detail about whether close relatives (parents, children, brothers or sisters) had a history of periodontal disease. The diagnosis of periodontal disease and the type of definitive periodontal therapy (non-surgical and/or surgical) were recorded. Smoking habits were recorded in terms of the numbers of cigarettes smoked per day. Patients who only smoked on social occasions were not classified as smokers. Also noted were the average levels of plaque control during maintenance (good, moderate, poor) as outlined by Fardal and Linden (2005) and compliance with maintenance therapy (complete, erratic).

At the final assessment, the type of prosthetic treatment carried out to replace lost teeth was recorded. The use of implants and any complications relating to implant treatment such as non-integration, peri-implantitis, or loss of implants were recorded from the clinical notes.

In addition, patients were asked how satisfied they were with the prosthetic therapy they received to replace their lost teeth.

It was found that a total of 27 (17 female, 10 male) out of 1,251 patients (2.2%) who received initial periodontal treatment between 1986 and 1998 met the criteria for inclusion in the downhill/extreme downhill refractory group. The average age of these patients at their initial examination was 48.5 years (SD 10.0, range 21–71) and they had on average 20.6 (SD 4.6, range 13–28) teeth. Twenty-five (93%) of the refractory group and 42 (78%) of the control group were diagnosed with uncertain to poor initial prognosis. Twenty-three (85%) of the refractory group were compliant with the maintenance regimens prescribed, while 4 (15%) showed erratic compliance. The average period of monitoring of the refractory group was 13.4 years (SD 3.3, range 8–19).

On average, each downhill subject lost 10.4 (range 4–16) teeth during the monitoring period, which represented 50% of the teeth present at the start of the study. The rate of tooth loss in the refractory group was 0.78 teeth per year, which was 35 times greater than that in the control group. The distribution of tooth loss by tooth type and arch in the refractory group is shown in Table 4.1.

The distribution of tooth loss in the present study is different from previous tooth loss studies (Fardal et al. 2004; Hirschfeld and Wassermann 1978). These studies reported that the predominant tooth loss was mainly in the first and second molar regions. The present study shows a more even distribution between the teeth, with a slight predominance for the anterior and premolar teeth in the upper jaw and the second molars in the lower jaw. Table 4.2 shows tooth loss distribution from a previous study (Fardal et al. 2004) of 100 regular maintenance patients.

Multivariate analysis indicated that being in the refractory group was predicted by heavy smoking ($p = 0.026$), being under stress ($p = 0.016$), or having a family history of periodontitis ($p = 0.002$). A comparison between the variables of the refractory and control groups is summarized in Table 4.3.

Table 4.1. Distribution of tooth loss in the downhill group by tooth type and arch: 280 teeth were lost in total (27 patients, observation period 13.6 years).

Upper		9	12	11	13	11	19	15	13	16	16	16	10	13	6	1
	8	7	6	5	4	3	2	1	1	2	3	4	5	6	7	8
Lower	1	11	7	7	6	3	7	8	7	7	5	4	4	9	13	

Table 4.2. Distribution of tooth loss in a "normal" maintenance population of 100 patients observed over 10 years, 36 teeth lost in total (Fardal et al. 2004).

Upper		5	3	3	1				1			2	2	2	3	
	8	7	6	5	4	3	2	1	1	2	3	4	5	6	7	8
Lower		5	2	1	1	1								1	3	

Table 4.3. Comparison between refractory and control subjects.

	Refractory	Control	*p*
Age initial assessment Mean (SD)	48.5 (10.0)	48.1 (10.2)	0.86
Years in maintenance since treatment started Mean (SD)	13.4 (3.3)	13.9 (3.2)	0.50
Teeth present at start of treatment Mean (SD)	20.6 (4.6)	25.8 (2.6)	<0.0001
Number of teeth lost during treatment Mean (SD)	10.4 (3.75)	0.3 (0.57)	<0.0001
Smoking			
Non	11 (40.7)	39 (72.2)	
Light	5 (18.5)	10 (18.5)	
Heavy	11 (40.7)	5 (9.3)	0.0026
n (%)			
Systemic disease n (%)	8 (29.6)	17 (31.5)	0.86
Hygiene			
Good	11 (40.7)	22 (40.7)	0.02
Moderate	11 (40.7)	31 (57.4)	
Poor	5 (18.5)	1 (1.9)	
n (%)			
Stress n (%)	11 (40.7)	1 (1.9)	<0.0001
Family history of periodontitis n (%)	19 (70.4)	13 (24.1)	<0.0001

Implant Therapy in Refractory Cases

Implants were placed in 14 (52%) of the refractory group compared with 2 (4%) of the control group, $p < 0.0001$. Those who received implants lost 8.8 (SD 3.7) teeth, which was less than those who were not treated with implants (12.0, SD 3.2), $p = 0.027$. Those treated with implants in the refractory group received an average of 4.9 (SD 2.1) implants. Within the refractory group there was little difference in age at assessment of those who were eventually treated with implants compared to those who were not: 50.2 (SD 10.6) compared with 46.7 (SD 9.4) years, $p = 0.37$. Within the refractory group the period of supportive periodontal treatment for those who received implants was virtually the same as for non-implant cases: 13.2 (3.9) compared with 13.6 (SD 2.6) years, $p = 0.76$. The implants were followed up for on average 5.4 years (range 2–9). A total of 14 implants in 7 refractory patients did not integrate. A further 5 implants in 4 patients developed peri-implantitis (1 after 3 years, 1 after 5 years, 1 after 6 years, and 2 after 8 years), and 3 of these implants were finally lost. In total, 17 (25%) of the implants placed in the refractory group were lost during the study period and 9 (64%) of the refractory group lost at least one implant. For the patients in the control group none of the implants placed were lost. Table 4.4 shows a summary of implant therapy for the refractory group of patients.

The type of restorations used to replace the lost teeth, with arch distribution, is given in Table 4.5.

The patients gave the highest satisfaction scores for fixed restorations. In addition, the combination of a complete or partial upper denture with a tooth- or implant-supported bridge in the lower jaw scored equally high in patients' satisfaction.

The remaining removable restorations scored as only moderately satisfactory except for the combination of complete upper and lower dentures, which were scored as being unsatisfactory.

Table 4.4. Results of implant placement for the refractory patient group.

		Number of Patients
Number of patients receiving implants	24	27
Average number of implants placed for each patient	4.9 (SD 2.1)	24
Average observation period (years and range)	5.4 (2–9)	24
Number of non-integrated implants	14	7
Peri-implantitis	5	4
Implants lost due to peri-implantitis	3	2
Total number of implants lost (%)	17 (25)	9

Table 4.5. Distribution of tooth replacements by restoration type and arch.

Upper Restorations	7 Complete dentures	6 Partial dentures	3 Tooth-supported fixed bridges	7 Combination tooth/ implant fixed bridges	4 Implant-supported fixed bridges
Lower	3	3	8	3	0

Conclusion

In conclusion, a small number of periodontal maintenance patients seem to be refractory to treatment and go on to experience continued and significant tooth loss. These subjects also have a high level of implant complications and failure. Smoking, stress, and a family history of periodontal disease were identified as factors associated with a refractory outcome, and these variables remained significant after multivariate analysis. In the context of the current study it is possible that these factors were not only associated with an increased risk of progressive periodontitis and tooth loss but also with an increased likelihood of implant failure.

SYSTEMIC IMPLICATIONS OF PERI-IMPLANT INFLAMMATION: MIMICRY OF THE PERIODONTITIS-SYSTEMIC DISEASE MODEL?

Howard C. Tenenbaum, Michael Glogauer, Michael Landzberg, and Michael Goldberg

Background

Inflammation around endosseous implants, or peri-implantitis as it is often referred to, is a condition associated both with ailing and/or failing implants (Mombelli and Lang 1998). An upsurge of clinical and animal studies in the last two decades has addressed the prevention and management of peri-implantitis (Chen and Darby 2003), the goal being to avert the loss of a failing implant; however, little attention has been paid to the possibility that this condition could increase the risk for development of systemic illnesses similar to that which has been reported in patients with gingivitis and periodontitis (Seymour et al. 2007). As alluded to above, there is clear evidence of an epidemiological association between periodontal inflammation and/or infection and certain systemic conditions like cardiovascular disease (CVD) (Janket et al. 2003; Khader et al. 2004). Similarly and as addressed below, there appears to be a bidirectional relationship between periodontal disease and control of diabetes. That being said, it is unknown whether a similar risk of systemic disease exists insofar as dental implants are concerned.

Brief Review of Periodontal Disease/ Systemic Disease Evidence

There is a groundswell of data showing significant, albeit modest, positive associations between CVD and periodontitis, including findings from two recent meta-analyses that investigated periodontal diseases and the risk of coronary heart disease, stroke, and cerebrovascular diseases (Janket et al. 2003; Khader et al. 2004; Seymour et al. 2007). For instance, it has been shown that patients who suffer from severe chronic periodontitis have a significantly increased risk for the development of CVD including stroke, atherosclerosis, and myocardial infarction. These findings appear to hold even after adjusting for the traditional risk factors such as smoking and serum lipid concentration (Beck et al. 1996; DeStefano et al. 1993; Desvarieux et al. 2003; Grau et al. 1997; Hung et al. 2003; Jansson et al. 2001; Valtonen 1999). Most extraordinary, however, have been the findings showing that poor oral health is a significant risk indicator of death due to CVD (Jansson et al. 2001). Although current opinion on the association between periodontal disease and CVD is divided, there are several hypotheses to account for this relationship, including the notion of a common genetic predisposition and pathophysiological mechanisms of seemingly disparate disorders, direct bacterial damage to the endothelium, molecular mimicry between bacterial and self-antigens, and finally a role for systemic inflammation concerning increased levels of circulating cytokines and other inflammatory mediators (Seymour et al. 2007).

Further in this regard, there is a significant amount of evidence to suggest that diabetes is associated with increased prevalence, extent, and severity of gingivitis and periodontitis (Mealey and Oates 2006). In fact, severe periodontitis has been characterized as the "sixth complication of diabetes" (Loe 1993). Patients with type 2 diabetes mellitus have an almost three-fold increase in their risks for development of destructive periodontal disease over those without diabetes (Emrich et al. 1991) and are four times more likely to have alveolar bone loss progression than healthy controls (Taylor et al. 1998a). Increased gingival pocket depth and loss of dentition are other indicators of periodontal disease that are seen more frequently in patients with diabetes (Emrich et al. 1991). Evidence suggests that poor glycemic control is a major contributor to poorer periodontal health as measured by increased levels of glycated hemoglobin (HbA1c) (Ainamo et al. 1990; Taylor et al. 1998a, 1998b). A large U.S. study showed that patients with poorly controlled diabetes, and who had an HbA1c level greater than 9, were three times more likely to have severe periodontitis than controls (Tsai et al. 2002).

The mechanisms for the association between periodontal disease and diabetes include decreased collagen production, reduced polymorphonuclear neutrophil (PMN) function, and the accumulation of advanced glycation end products (AGEs) in tissues, including the periodontium (Perrino 2007). Interactions between AGEs and their cognate receptors (RAGE) on inflammatory cells induce increased expression of proinflammatory cytokines responsible for tissue destruction (Schmidt et al. 1996). It is this interaction that is central to diabetic complications and that may contribute to the increased prevalence and severity of periodontal diseases among individuals with diabetes (Kinane and Marshall 2001; Perrino 2007). Hence insofar as diabetes and periodontitis is concerned, there is good evidence for the existence of a bidirectional relationship between the two, such that exacerbation of one disease can lead to exacerbation of the other (Grossi and Genco 1998; Mealey and Oates 2006). It has been hypothesized that the inflammatory process in periodontal disease leads to increased levels of TNF alpha, which in turn is known to promote insulin resistance (Nishimura et al. 2003). This relationship has also been demonstrated in interventional studies showing that when periodontitis is treated in patients who have diabetes, significant reductions in glycated hemoglobin occur, thus indicating that periodontal treatment affects glycemic control in a positive manner (Janket et al. 2005). A randomized controlled trial of 44 patients with type 2 diabetes mellitus showed that patients who received mechanical treatment for periodontal disease had an 11% reduction in HbA1c levels at 3 months follow-up compared with a 4% increase in HbA1c levels in the control group (Kiran et al. 2005). Similarly, when diabetes is brought under better control, parameters of periodontal disease also improve (Mealey and Klokkevold 2002).

There is also new evidence that appears to confirm a possible causal relationship between periodontitis in mothers and the delivery of pre-term low-birthweight infants. Treatment of maternal periodontitis led to significant reductions in the incidence of pre-term birth and increases in birthweight, as well as combinations of the two (Tarannum and Faizuddin 2007).

What Is Peri-implantitis?

Dental implants are an effective treatment for replacing missing teeth; however, their long-term success is dependent on whether the inflammatory and regenerative processes at work are in proper balance. Peri-implantitis is arguably one of the most significant risk factors associated with implant failures and can be best described as an inflammatory reaction with loss of bone in the tissues surrounding an osseointegrated implant in function (Albrektsson et al. 1994). Symptoms of peri-implantitis may include but not be limited to bleeding on probing, increased probing "pocket" depth, mobility, suppuration, and pain.

The incidence data for peri-implantitis show that in general it occurs relatively rarely ranging from 2% to 10% (Berglundh et al. 2002). However, a higher incidence of peri-implantitis has been reported in individuals with a history of chronic periodontitis (28.6%) compared with individuals with good periodontal health (Karoussis et al. 2003). Nevertheless, an estimation of the prevalence of peri-implantitis is very difficult to make and depends on the criteria used to differentiate between health and disease (Chen and Darby 2003; Karoussis et al. 2003).

The microbiota associated with successful implants are similar to the flora seen in people with good periodontal health, whereas the organisms associated with failing implants resemble those isolated from individuals with periodontitis (Chen and Darby 2003). It follows that factors that influence the supragingival and subgingival microflora may contribute to peri-implantitis. The clinical implication of this could be that patients with a history of chronic periodontitis may be at increased risk of peri-implantitis should the need for implantation arise, ideas that are discussed elsewhere in this section in relation to patients receiving implants who had either extremely severe periodontitis or refractory periodontitis prior to treatment with implants. Successful implants are typically colonized, albeit sparsely, by Gram positive cocci, while failing implants harbor large numbers of Gram negative anaerobes (Mombelli and Lang 1992; Mombelli et al. 1987, 1995). Traditional periodontal pathogens such as Actinobacillus actinomycetemcomitans, Prevotella intermedia, Porphyromonas gingivalis, Fusobacterium species, and Campylobacter rectus have all been associated with failing implants (Chen and Darby 2003). The relationship between the surface roughness of implants and bacterial colonization has also been assessed clinically (Quirynen et al. 1993). As shown in Figures 4.3 and 4.4 (original photos

courtesy of Dr. Asbjorn Jokstad, Faculty of Dentistry, University of Toronto), plaque/biofilm accumulation does occur around endosseous implants leading to soft tissue inflammation (Fig. 4.3) as well as peri-implant bone loss (Fig. 4.4)—similar to what is observed in teeth affected by periodontitis.

It has also been shown that smoking habits represent an increased risk for impaired bone healing and implant failure and, in parallel, smoking also brings an increased risk for chronic periodontitis (Albandar et al. 2000; Bergstrom 1989). A review of 56 patients with a total of 187 endosseous dental implants over 4 years demonstrated a significant association between increased implant failure rates and cigarette smoking, with failure rates of 16.6% in smokers compared to 6.9% in non-smokers (Wallace 2000). More recently, a retrospective analysis over a 5-year period

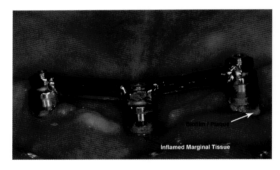

Figure 4.3.   Clinical image of failing/ailing implant.

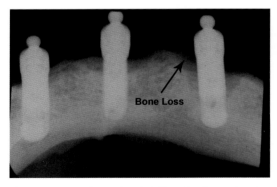

Figure 4.4.   Radiograph of failing implants showing bone loss.

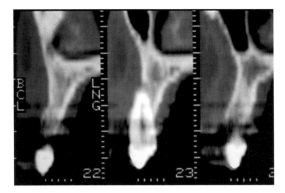

Figure 5.2. CT scan film circa 1989, showing 3 mm slice cross-sectional images.

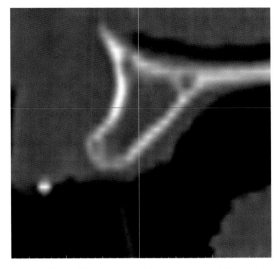

Figure 5.3a. Cross-sectional image revealed the height and width of available bone.

(Materialise Dental, Glen Burnie, Maryland) became available in 1994 on the Windows 3.1 platform. This innovative software program provided the clinician with the tools to easily and quickly visualize and manipulate axial, cross-sectional, and panoramic images while adding treatment planning capabilities and bone density assessment necessary for dental implant planning. Clinicians were able to use their own computers and monitors equipped with the proper software to "scroll" through distortion-free slices to assess all relevant CT images without the need for a roomful of large chest X-ray-size lightboxes. Virtual implant simulation allowed clinicians to plan receptor sites with an improved understanding of the receptor site anatomy.

The cross-sectional view revealed the width and height of available bone (Fig. 5.3a). A virtual schematic implant replica could then be placed in a position to maximize the available bone volume (Fig. 5.3b). The length, width, and angulation of the implant could be determined within this 2-D slice. An important addition to the planning process was the ability to simulate the abutment projection from the implant to aid in linking the surgical plan to the desired restoration (Fig. 5.3c). These new views allowed for the "Triangle of Bone™" concept by the GANZ in 1995 to be visualized as a "zone" that would help define the bone volume within a potential implant receptor site to determine a decision tree for

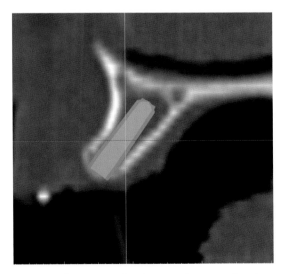

Figure 5.3b. A virtual schematic implant placed to maximize bone volume.

the proper course of treatment (Fig. 5.3d). Additionally, in the mandible the path of the inferior alveolar nerve could be identified and traced as an aid to implant placement to avoid potential complications. In the maxilla,

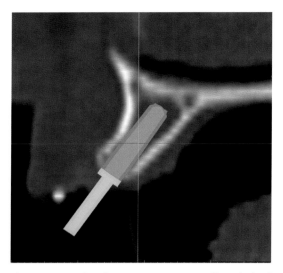

Figure 5.3c. The abutment projection (yellow) helped link the implant to the desired restoration.

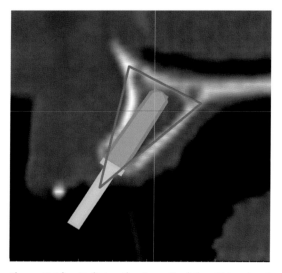

Figure 5.3d. Defining the "zone" of the "Triangle of Bone™" for identifying available bone volume.

the topography of the bilateral sinuses could be clearly seen in the axial, cross-sectional, and panoramic views to be assessed for pathology, thickening of the membrane, and as a receptor for augmentation procedures.

The continued maturation of SIM/Plant™ included direct manipulation of the 3-D reconstructed images and interactive implant placement. This was followed by other similar software applications introduced to the dental implant marketplace for the purposes of making CT scan technology available to clinicians around the world. Advances in 3-D reformatting technologies provided highly refined, accurate assessment of the CT scan data in a manner that exceeded information gleaned from film alone. The evolution of the software capabilities was then expanded to link the virtual plan to a surgical template or guide. During this period from the late 1990s and early into the new millennium, the technology was available through links with SIM/Plant and other software applications, but not widely utilized.

As the implant industry developed new and improved implants there was a paradigm shift from Brånemark's original two-stage surgical protocol to early and immediate loading. Immediate loading protocols should obligate a better understanding of the underlying bone anatomy to achieve long-term success. Despite these new modalities, published anecdotal papers, consensus position papers, and research reporting immediate placement and restorations were being accomplished largely without the use of advanced diagnostic imaging technology or CT-guided surgery. It was not until the advent, and the subsequent introduction, of new smaller in-office CBCT scanning machines such as the NewTom (AFP Imaging, Elmsford, New York) and the i-CAT (Imaging Sciences, Hatfield, Pennsylvania) that one major barrier was removed—patients no longer needed to leave the office for a scan. The second major event that served as a potent catalyst to promote the use of CT/CBCT and guided surgery was when the largest dental implant company, Nobel BioCare (Göteborg, Sweden), embraced this technology with the introduction of their NobelGuide™ "total solution" combining treatment planning software with data from the CT scan and the clinical hardware for placing implants with special templates.

Barium Sulfate Scanning Appliance

Prior to the scan itself, a protocol of pre-surgical prosthetic planning should include the fabrication of a scanning or scanographic appliance. The use of radiopaque templates of the desired tooth position can help maximize the technology and facilitate true restorative-driven implant dentistry. Duplicating a patient's ideal denture or a diagnostic wax-up with a mixture of barium sulfate and acrylic will result in an appliance that can be worn by the patient during the scanning process (Fig. 5.4a). The completely opaque template will then be visualized in all of the CT scan images, but most significantly in the 3-D reconstruction, as the ultimate planning aid (Fig. 5.4b).

The next evolution of interactive treatment planning software was the incorporation of realistic implants. The use of realistic implants has greatly expanded the application of this technology. A Tapered Internal Implant of two different diameters is visualized in Figures 5.5a and 5.5b.

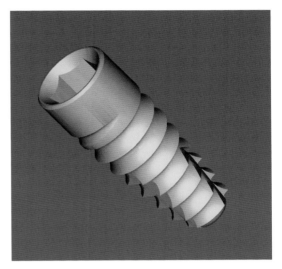

Figure 5.5a. A Tapered Internal Implant of two different diameters, color-coded (yellow and green) to the manufacturer's specifications (BioHorizons, Birmingham, Alabama).

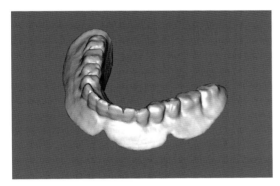

Figure 5.4a. Barium sulfate radiopaque scanning appliance worn during the scan is virtually revealed on the interactive software application.

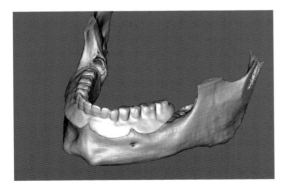

Figure 5.4b. The completely opaque template visualized on the 3-D reconstructed mandible.

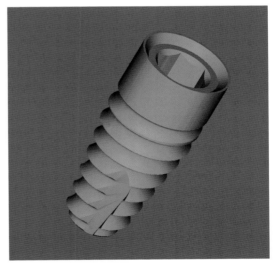

Figure 5.5b. Note that all aspects of the implant can be appreciated, including thread design and internal hexagonal connection.

Note that all aspects of the implant can be appreciated, including the thread design and internal hexagonal connection (Bio-Horizons, Birmingham, Alabama). The 2-D cross-sectional image reveals the radiopaque scanning appliance and helps the clinician evaluate the relationship of the tooth and flange position to the underlying bone (Fig. 5.6).

A realistic implant (Astra Tech, Inc., Waltham, Massachusetts) was positioned, and a realistic virtual Locator attachment/abutment (Zest Anchors, Inc., Escondido, California) was placed in anticipation of an implant-supported overdenture restoration. With the scanning prosthesis removed, four implants can be visualized and assessed for proper placement using the 3-D reconstruction (Fig. 5.7).

Proper use of this technology is greatly enhanced when the available software tools are fully appreciated and utilized. For this example, the implant-to-implant distance can be measured, the proximity to the adjacent mental foramina can be visualized, and a thorough assessment of the mandibular bone

can be understood before the scalpel ever touches the patient. From this dataset, a CT-derived template can be fabricated. A bone-borne stereolithographic template is seen in Figure 5.8.

A dual-scan technique was adopted by the NobelGuide™ system for soft tissue–borne templates as another method for combining pre-surgical planning with the CT scan and guided surgical intervention. In this method, a scanning appliance is fabricated with the incorporation of gutta percha markers to act as future reference points. The patient wears the template when the scan is taken. Different from the method previously described, the scanning appliance is then placed back in to

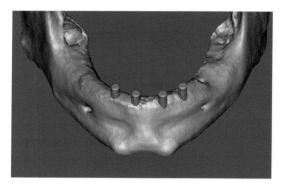

Figure 5.7. Four Locator attachments placed on realistic implants (Astra Tech, Inc. Waltham, Massachusetts) in anticipation of an implant-supported overdenture prosthesis.

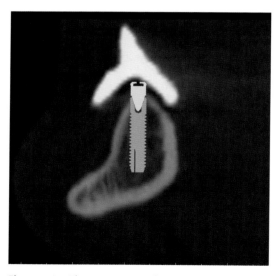

Figure 5.6. The cross-sectional image reveals the scanning appliance, the underlying bone, and a realistic Locator attachment (Zest Anchors, Inc., Escondido, California) placed on a realistic implant.

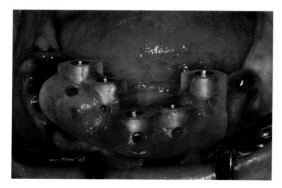

Figure 5.8. Bone-borne stereolithographic surgical guide seated on the exposed mandibular symphysis.

the CT/CBCT machine to be scanned separately from the patient. The two datasets are then combined with the proprietary Procera Planning Software™ (Nobel BioCare, Göteborg, Sweden) and the planning can be accomplished (Figs. 5.9a, 5.9b).

Presently, this software differs from others on the market in that only manufacturer-specific implants can be used with the companion surgical armamentarium. CT-derived templates are then created from the virtual plan with stainless steel cylinders that allow for both osteotomy drilling and placement of the implants through the templates to maximize accuracy.

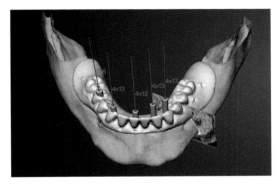

Figure 5.9a. The dual-scan technique soft-tissue template adopted by the NobelGuide™ system.

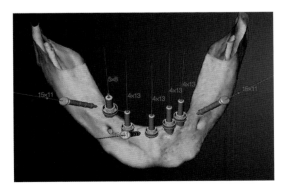

Figure 5.9b. With the scanning template removed, the implants and fixation screws can be clearly visualized on the mandible.

Virtual Teeth and Realistic Abutments

Using CT/CBCT scan technology has forced clinicians to re-evaluate previous conventions. The axial section of the maxilla reveals the root morphology of the teeth as they emerge from the bone (Fig. 5.10).

This view alone signifies a new paradigm in diagnosis and treatment planning for dental implants, as it illustrates the "restorative dilemma" as described by GANZ. After inspection, it is clear that the root morphology of the maxillary teeth is varied in size and shape. The implants that we utilize are all round in shape. Therefore the "restorative dilemma" refers to how we must emerge from a round implant platform to re-establish correct tooth morphology for the definitive restoration. In addition, the lamina dura surrounding the individual teeth can be clearly visualized, which helps define a new method to measure tooth-to-implant proximity—identification of the periodontal ligament space.

The posterior mandible is difficult to assess for dental implant placement due to the proximity of the inferior alveolar nerve, the mental foramen, the lingual concavity, the size of the teeth and number of missing roots, and the desired scheme of occlusion. With the advent

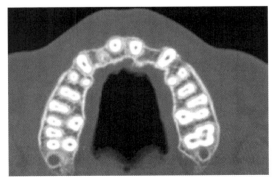

Figure 5.10. An axial slice of the maxilla illustrating the "restorative dilemma" referring to the actual root morphology compared with the round shape of dental implants.

of 3-D interactive planning, when all of the 2-D images have been utilized the final plan can be assessed with the 3-D model. Three implants placed in the posterior mandible are visualized with schematic abutment projections in Figure 5.11.

To properly evaluate implant positioning, embrasure design, and the restorative requirements of this area, a virtual occlusion can be established (Fig. 5.12).

The abutment projections can be visualized above the occlusal plane of the virtual teeth (Fig. 5.13a). Using an interactive transparency tool, realistic stock, pre-machined abutments can be chosen to fit within the envelope of each tooth at the proper soft tissue level (Fig. 5.13b).

Through software manipulation the mandibular bone can be "removed," and use of the "zoom" feature allows for close inspection of the relationship of the implant, the abutment, and the virtual tooth position (Fig. 5.14a). Additionally the proximity to the adjacent teeth and the neighboring mandibular nerve can be viewed and measured to ensure safe placement of the proposed implant(s). When the virtual teeth are removed, the realistic stock abutments can be visualized and examined for soft tissue cuff height and accuracy of placement (Fig. 5.14b).

Using all of the available views and software tools, the final position of each implant is examined for accuracy and verified in the

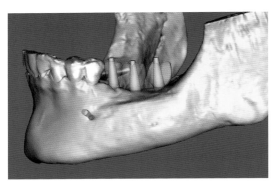

Figure 5.11. Side view of three implants and schematic abutment projections placed in a partially edentate posterior mandible.

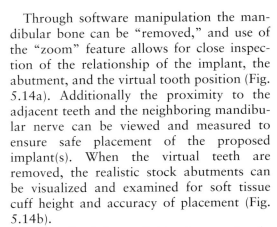

Figure 5.13a. Abutment projections extend above the occlusal surface of the virtual teeth.

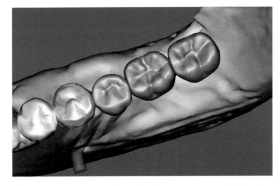

Figure 5.12. A virtual occlusion can be established to properly evaluate implant position, embrasure design, and the restorative requirements of this area.

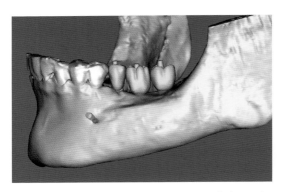

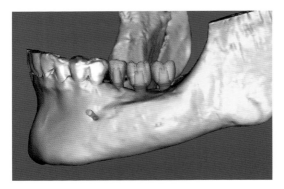

Figure 5.13b. The interactive transparency tool reveals the realistic stock, pre-machined abutments that fit within the envelope of each tooth.

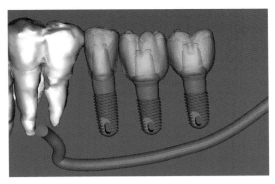

Figure 5.14a. "Removing" the mandibular bone, and zooming in, allows for close inspection of the implant-restorative complex.

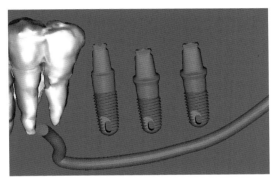

Figure 5.14b. Removing the virtual teeth reveals the pre-contoured abutments, which can then be evaluated for proper tissue cuff heights and accuracy of placement.

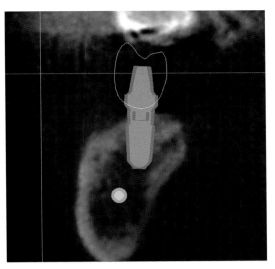

Figure 5.15a. The final position of the implant within the envelope of the virtual tooth is examined for accuracy in the cross-sectional image.

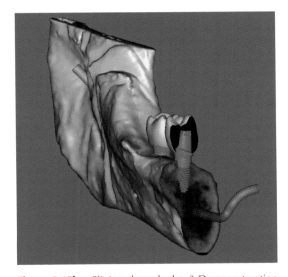

Figure 5.15b. Slicing through the 3-D reconstruction allows for further assessment of the position of the implant in relation to the inferior alveolar nerve.

cross-sectional image (Fig. 5.15a). Avoiding the path of the inferior alveolar nerve is most important, and further assessment can be accomplished by slicing through the 3-D reconstructed view containing the implant, the realistic abutment, and the virtual tooth (Fig. 5.15b).

Once the plan is finalized, the clinician can then send it via e-mail for the fabrication of a tooth-borne stereolithographic surgical template, and in select cases a stereolithographic model (SurgiGuide, Materialise, Lueven, Belgium) (Fig. 5.16a). The original and basic SurgiGuide consisted of stainless steel cylinders, 5 mm in height and embedded into the acrylate material. Three guides were

to be used for this example, one for each drill diameter specific to the implant manufacturer's drilling protocol (Fig. 5.16b).

The CT-scan fabricated stereolithographic model can be utilized to further link the plan to the restoration by utilizing replica implants

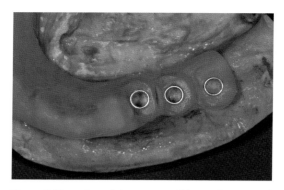

Figure 5.16a. A tooth-borne stereolithographic surgical guide with stainless steel cylinders.

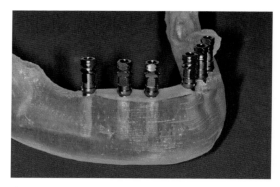

Figure 5.17a. The stereolithographic model of the patient's mandible provides a valuable tool to link the plan to the restoration by inserting replica implants into the acrylate.

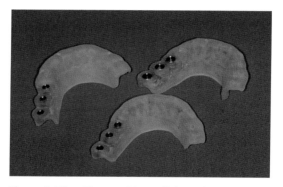

Figure 5.16b. Three guides will be utilized, one for each drill diameter specific to the implant manufacturer's drilling protocol.

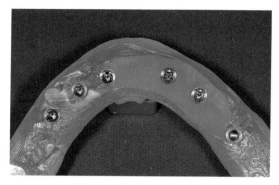

Figure 5.17b. The clinician can have an actual reproduction of the patient's mandible on hand to evaluate the plan and the implant placement and to aid in the fabrication of a transitional prosthesis.

placed within the acrylate (Fig. 5.17a). Using the SIM/Plant plan, six implants were placed in parallel on the stereolithographic model (Zimmer Dental, Carlsbad, California). In this manner, the clinician can have the actual reproduction of the patient's mandible or maxilla on hand to evaluate the plan, inter-implant distance, implant angulation, and proximity to the mental foramina (Fig. 5.17b).

In addition, these models can be mounted with proper articulation to aid in the fabrication of a transitional prosthesis to be delivered at time of surgery.

Conclusion

CT and CBCT scans allow for an unparalleled view of the patient's anatomy that when properly utilized removes the guesswork associated with placing implants, empowers clinicians with enhanced diagnostic information aiding the process of making informed decisions for their patients, and provides an improved foundation for communication between all members of the implant team. CT/CBCT scan technology allows for precise measurements of height, width, and depth of

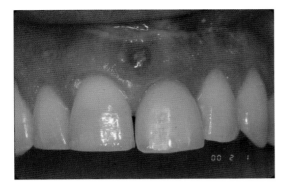

Figure 5.18. Clinically, the appearance of a fistula is often present.

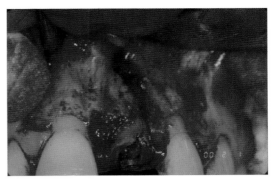

Figure 5.20. Following administration of local anesthesia, a 15 blade is used to create a simplified papilla preservation flap as described by Cortellini and Tonetti (2001). A full thickness flap is elevated along the buccal, gaining access to the planned implant site and the associated periapical pathology.

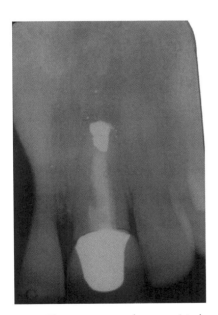

Figure 5.19. The appearance of an associated periapical radiolucency is common.

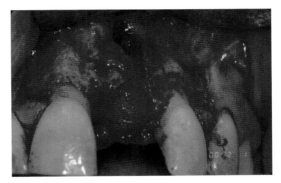

Figure 5.21. Following thorough degranulation, the tooth is extracted.

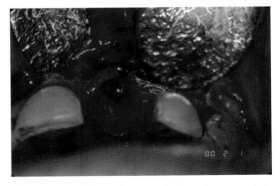

Figure 5.22. The socket morphology is assessed to determine if primary implant stability will be possible.

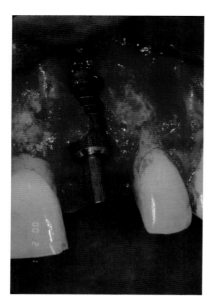

Figure 5.23. The implant bed preparation follows standard procedures, ensuring that the implant shoulder is 2–3 mm apical to the mid-buccal soft tissue height of adjacent teeth and the rough-smooth border of the implant surface is placed in an infra-osseous location relative to the interdental bone.

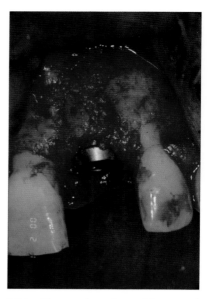

Figure 5.25. Closure of any bone dehiscence/fenestration defect is accomplished using an autogenous and deproteinized bovine bone veneer graft.

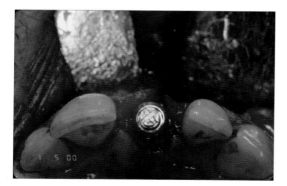

Figure 5.24. The implant shoulder is 1–2 mm lingual to the buccal aspects of the adjacent teeth.

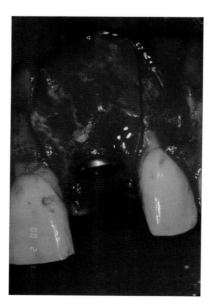

Figure 5.26. The bone veneer graft is protected by a resorbable collagen membrane that extends beyond the borders of the defect and tightly surrounds the neck of the implant.

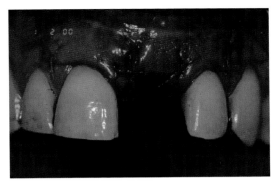

Figure 5.27. Tension-free flap closure with a semi-submerged covering of the healing cap is beneficial, especially when treating sites with a thick, scalloped periodontium. Buccal view.

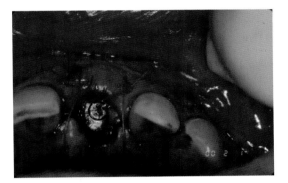

Figure 5.28. Tension-free flap closure with a semi-submerged covering of the healing cap is beneficial, especially when treating sites with a thick, scalloped periodontium. Occlusal view.

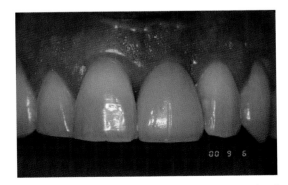

Figure 5.29. Final restorative care can be completed with the implant fulfilling the clinical criteria for success. Clinical view.

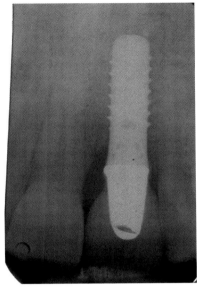

Figure 5.30. Final restorative care can be completed with the implant fulfilling the radiological criteria for success. Radiographical view.

or along the lateral walls of the extraction site. The use of CT radiographs may offer the clinician greater insight to treatment planning in these cases for immediate versus delayed placement.

IMAGE-BASED IMPLANT THERAPY: CURRENT STATUS AND FUTURE PERSPECTIVES

Homah Zadeh

The objective of successful implant therapy is to achieve predictable replacement of teeth with enduring implant-supported prostheses, mimicking natural dentition in form and function. In the initial stages of the clinical application of osseointegration in the early 1980s, the protocol emphasized the surgical aspects of implant therapy. The next stage in the progression of concepts recognized the significance of implant prosthetics for overall treatment success. Current concepts reflect more advanced understanding of the biology of implant-prosthesis interactions with host tissues. Presently, concurrent consideration of surgical, prosthetic, aesthetic, and biomechanical principles is advocated in planning implant therapy. This necessitates a carefully devised plan, constructed by all members of the treatment team including the surgeon, restorative dentist, laboratory technician, and patient. It is also important to execute the plan with a great deal of precision to achieve optimal aesthetics and function. Recent advances have provided the enabling tools to assist with collaborative virtual planning and implementation of that plan during surgery and prosthetic implant. Innovations in imaging, computer software development, and rapid prototyping have provided the tools for a new approach in implant therapy, referred to as "image-based implant therapy." Image-based implant therapy is the utilization of data obtained by diagnostic imaging in the planning and implementation phases of treatment. There are three components to image-based therapy: (1) 3-D diagnostic imaging of the relevant anatomical region(s); (2) application of interactive image manipulation software and its associated tools in pre-surgical planning; and (3) transfer of the virtual plan to the surgical field.

Diagnostic Imaging

In the past, the evaluation of implant sites was limited to 2-D imaging, including periapical radiographs, panoramic radiographs, and lateral cephalograms. Two-dimensional imaging has a number of shortcomings that limits its utility in implant site planning. Firstly, 2-D imaging superimposes multiple anatomical structures, limiting true assessment of implant sites. Secondly, 2-D imaging is more useful for evaluation of bone height and anterior-posterior dimensions and will not provide width measurement. Thirdly, a number of studies have demonstrated significant distortion of conventional dental radiographic imaging, such as panoramic images. Though the manufacturers provide the mag-

nification factor of their units, different values have been obtained in research studies for horizontal and vertical distortions (Laster et al. 2005). Therefore these studies have suggested that panoramic radiographs should be used with caution in making absolute measurements. On the other hand, other investigators have used a large patient base, patients who have safely undergone implant surgery to argue for the safety of panoramic examination. Vazquez et al. (2008) have suggested that panoramic examinations are an appropriate preoperative evaluation procedure for routine posterior mandibular implant placement, when a safety margin of at least 2 mm above the mandibular canal is respected.

The accuracy of image acquisition by CT imaging depends on a number of factors, including slice thickness, voxel size, movement, and metallic artifact. Both CT and CBCT have been determined to yield submillimeter accuracy for linear measurements (Loubele et al. 2008).

In a position paper, the American Academy of Oral and Maxillofacial Radiology (AAOMR) has recommended that cross-sectional tomography should be the method of choice for most patients receiving implants (Tyndall and Brooks 2000).

The guidelines of the European Association of Osseointegration have also suggested that cross-sectional imaging should be the method of choice for most dental implants. It has been suggested that 2-D imaging only be used in minor and/or established low-risk surgery (Harris et al. 2002).

Three-dimensional imaging is now performed by a variety of techniques. In the 1970s computed tomography was developed and was initially referred to as computed axial tomography (CAT or CT scan) and body section roentgenography. The first CT scanner was developed by Sir Godfrey Hounsfield at EMI Central Research Laboratories in England and independently by Allan Cormack at Tufts University. Hounsfield and Cormack shared the 1979 Nobel Prize in Medicine. The first patient brain-scan was made in England in 1972. More recently, CBCT has been developed. CBCT utilizes flat-panel technology to provide volumetric imaging.

In order to capture prosthetic landmarks, a scanning prosthesis is fabricated and worn by the patient during image acquisition. A variety of techniques are currently utilized, incorporating an array of radiopaque material into the scanning of the prosthesis in an attempt to provide landmarks that will be visible in the diagnostic imaging. The utilization of a scanning prosthesis will allow the assessment of the concordance of anatomical and prosthetic landmarks.

Interactive Image Manipulation Software

In order to take full advantage of digital diagnostic imaging data, a number of interactive image manipulation software programs have been developed. By virtue of its digital nature, 3-D imaging allows a number of manipulations to aid with pre-surgical planning. It is possible to scan through various views to trace the path of the inferior alveolar nerve. It is also possible to reconstruct the images into 3-D objects and segment various anatomic structures such as teeth, maxilla, mandible, scanning prosthesis, and so forth so that these objects can be toggled on or off. It is also possible to digitally add objects, such as implants, abutments, and teeth in order to construct a virtual treatment plan. These tools are extremely useful in providing a digital platform for collaboration among the various members of the treatment team. It allows the clinician to test a treatment plan in the digital phase and anticipate any pitfalls prior to surgery.

Bone quality has traditionally been classified by a variety of indices, most prominently by Lekholm and Zarb (1985). Though this classification system is widely used and has been extremely useful clinically, it is relatively subjective. A more objective measurement of bone density can be obtained by the imaging software. Bone density is measured in Houns-

field units (HU). Type 1 bone measures over 1,250 HU, type 2 measures in the 850–1,250 HU range; type 3 bone is 350–850 HU; and type 4 bone is less than 150 HU. Quantitative measurements of bone density in planned osteotomy sites have been positively correlated with the cutting torque values observed during implant placement (Ikumi and Tsutsumi 2005). This observation suggests that quantitative measurement of bone density may be possible on pre-surgical CT data analyzed by image manipulation software. These values provide a predictive measure of bone quality and initial implant stability. Digital bone density measurement can aid in site selection, as well as in determination of the implant loading protocol that will best fit the planned implant's stability.

Transfer of Virtual Plan to the Surgical Field

There are three general methods for transfer of a 3-D plan to the patient. These are: (1) stereolithographic drill guides; (2) intraoperative navigation; and (3) robotics. The latter two technologies are currently utilized in neurosurgery and orthopedic surgery as well as in other areas of medical surgery where precision is of the utmost importance. Intraoperative navigation and robotics are not currently widely available for clinical application in dental implant surgery. The present discussion will therefore be limited to the application of stereolithographic drill guides. Stereolithography, also known as rapid prototyping, is the process for construction of physical models. It utilizes a laser beam to selectively polymerize a light-sensitive resin. It also incorporates rigid sleeves that will assist in guiding drills into pre-defined positions. There are two basic approaches for utilizing stereolithographic drill guides for aiding in osteotomy. In the first approach, the osteotomy is performed through a series of typically three drill guides with increasing sleeve diameter. These drill guides control the axial orientation of the osteotomy. In the second method (Fig. 5.31a), a singular drill guide is used and the osteotomy is performed through a series of drill keys (Van Steenberghe et al. 2003).

These drill keys (Fig. 5.31b) serve as adaptors for drills with a diameter matching the internal diameters of the drill keys.

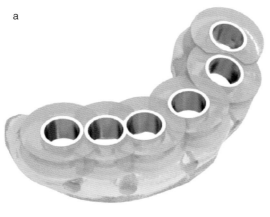

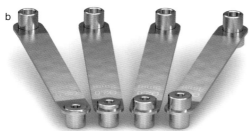

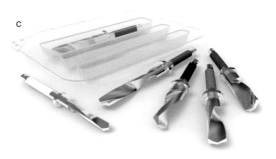

The drill guides control the axial orientation of osteotomy as well as the depth of insertion. The osteotomy depth is controlled by utilizing stops in the drill shanks to limit the entrance of the drill at a pre-determined position inside the key depth (Fig. 5.31c).

There are three forms of support for stereolithographic drill guides: (1) tooth-supported (Figs. 5.31d, 5.31e); (2) bone-supported (Figs. 5.31f, 5.31g); and (3) mucosa-supported (Figs. 5.31h, 5.31i).

Tooth-supported and mucosa-supported guides both provide an opportunity for flapless surgery. These will be indicated when an adequate volume of bone is available (Figs. 5.31j–5.31l).

Bone-supported guides allow implant placement in conjunction with other osseous manipulations. For example, in situations

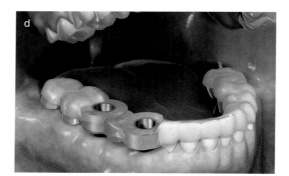

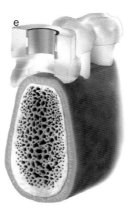

Figures 5.31a–c. The application of a stereolithographic guide in implant surgery. Stereolithographic guide (a) is used to control implant positioning. Drill adaptors (b) are used along with corresponding drills with depth stops (c) to control the depth of placement.

Figures 5.31d and e. Tooth-supported stereolithographic drill guide.

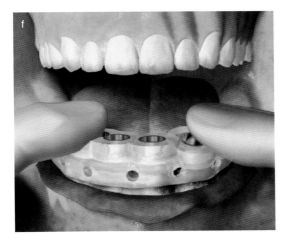

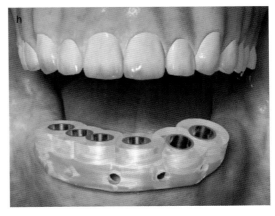

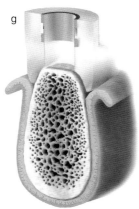

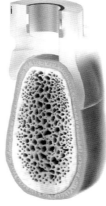

Figures 5.31h and i. Mucosa-supported stereolithographic drill guide.

Figures 5.31f and g. Bone-supported stereolithographic drill guide.

where a narrow crestal bone is present, it will be desirable to perform alveoplasty in the crestal area to provide for a wider crestal ridge. In addition, bone augmentation may be required in conjunction with implant placement, which is only possible if a surgical flap is reflected.

The Accuracy of Implant Placement Using Image-Based Approaches

The precision of implant positioning is an important predictor of implant outcome. It is therefore prudent to embrace technologies that assist in improving precision. The precision of implant placement is a potential predictor of treatment outcome for a number of reasons. Firstly, the position of the implant can determine the volume of bone and soft tissue around the implant. Malpositioning can potentially lead to bone dehiscence and soft tissue recession. Secondly, correct positioning of implants is important in order to avoid impingement on adjacent anatomic structures such as the inferior alveolar nerve, the maxillary sinus, or neighboring teeth. Thirdly, correct positioning of implants is required for concordance of the anatomic

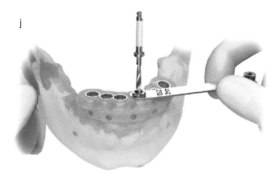

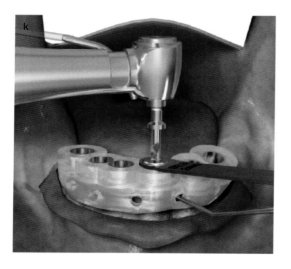

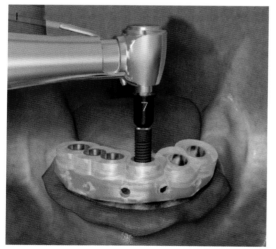

position of the implant with the desired prosthetic position. Lastly, to ensure favorable biomechanical performance, implant position determines the direction of forces.

The accuracy of transfer of the preoperative plan from the 3-D images to the surgical field by stereolithographic drill guides has been addressed in a number of in vitro, ex vivo, and in vivo studies. In an in vitro study, Sarment et al. (2003a, 2003b) compared the traditional surgical guide with the stereolithographic drill guide. The mean discrepancy between the planned implant position and the actual osteotomy was 1.5 mm at the entrance and 2.1 mm at the apex when traditional surgical guides were used. The same measurements were significantly reduced to 0.9 mm and 1.0 mm when stereolithographic guides were used.

Ex vivo and in vivo studies using CT as well as CBCT and stereolithographic drill guides have validated improved accuracy of this method over conventional surgical templates.

Adjunctive Applications of Stereolithography

Stereolithography provides an accurate three-dimensionally printed rigid appliance with a variety of adjunctive applications in addition to implant placement. Guides may be fabricated for assistance with the removal of bone fixation screws. Bone reduction templates may be fabricated for assistance with alveoloplasty. Surgical templates may be fabricated

Figures 5.31 j–l. In the application of the stereolithographic guide, the guide is first tested on the stereolithographic model of the jaw (j) to ensure appropriateness of the plan. Next, the guide is positioned in vivo (k), depending on the form of support for the guide. During this phase, care must be taken to apply external irrigation to ensure adequate irrigation. Following completion of osteotomy, the implant is also placed through the guide (l).

for aiding in precise positioning of a lateral window over the maxillary sinus. Engelke and Capobianco (2005) have reported on the endoscopic subantroscopic laterobasal sinus floor augmentation (SALSA) technique in the atrophic maxilla. As a refinement of the SALSA technique, these investigators have utilized stereolithographic templates to aid in flapless subantral augmentation and implant placement.

Clinical Applications of Image-Based Implant Therapy

Clinical Case 1

The patient illustrated in Figure 5.32a was a 27-year-old female who presented with periodontitis with severe bone loss in the maxillary incisors.

Following extraction of the incisors and some initial soft tissue healing, a tunneling access was elevated utilizing an incision through the frenum to expose the maxillary anterior area (Fig. 5.32b).

The rationale for this novel incision and tunnel approach was to preserve the vascularity of the overlying mucosa and to prevent wound dehiscence during healing. Bone augmentation surgery was performed utilizing autogenous bone blocks (Fig. 5.32c) in conjunction with a mixture of autogenous particulate bone mixed with bovine anorganic bone, covered with a collagen membrane, and sutured (Fig. 5.32d).

Following a 6-month healing period, a CT scan was taken (Fig. 5.32e) illustrating significant volume of bone augmentation. Virtual teeth were added digitally and implant positions and virtual abutments were planned, taking into account their optimal position relative to both the

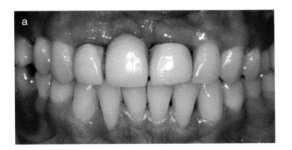
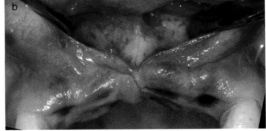
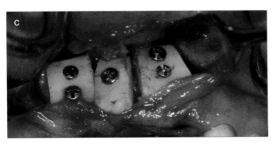
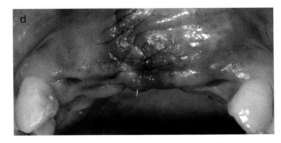

Figures 5.32a–d.   This patient presented with severe bone loss due to aggressive periodontitis in the maxillary incisors (a). Following extraction of the incisors and initial soft-tissue healing, an incision was made through the frenum and a tunnel was elevated to expose the maxillary anterior region (b). Bone augmentation surgery was performed utilizing autogenous bone blocks (c) in conjunction with a mixture of autogenous particulate bone mixed with bovine anorganic bone, covered with a collagen membrane (not shown), and sutured (d).

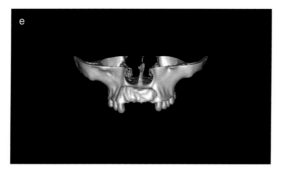 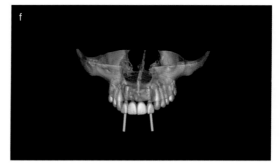

Figures 5.32e and f. Following a 6-month healing period, a CT scan was taken (e), illustrating significant volume of bone augmentation. Virtual teeth were added digitally and implant positions were planned (f).

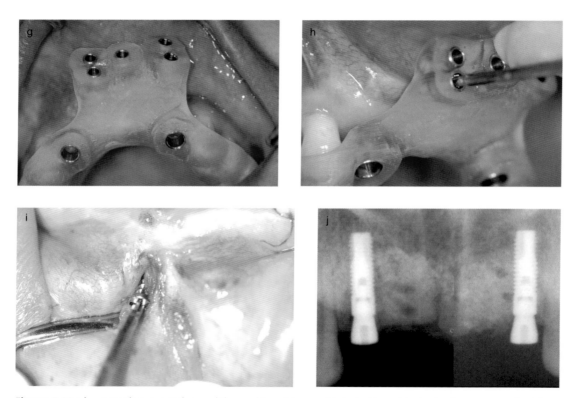

Figures 5.32g–j. A tooth-supported stereolithographic guide was fabricated to guide the implant osteotomies (g), as well as to guide the driver to the head of the fixation screws (h) in order that they could be removed with minimal incision over the screw heads (i). Radiograph of two implants placed in the position of lateral incisors (j).

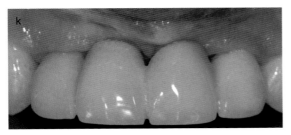

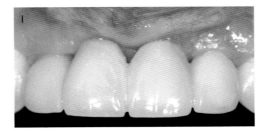

Figures 5.32k and l.   Provisional restoration following a 6-week healing (k). Final metal ceramic restoration was fabricated and cemented (l).

alveolar ridge as well as the planned prosthesis (Fig. 5.32f).

A tooth-supported stereolithographic guide was fabricated to guide the osteotomy for placement of the implants (Fig. 5.32g). In addition, a stereolithographic guide was devised with sleeves to guide the driver to the head of the fixation screws (Fig. 5.32h) in order that they could be removed with minimal incision over the screw heads (Fig. 5.32i).

To devise a guide that can aid in screw removal, in the planning software virtual implants with the same dimensions as the fixation screws were positioned superimposed over the fixation screws. Guide sleeves with the same diameter as the driver were requested from the stereolithographic guide manufacturer (Materialise, Glenbernie, Maryland). Two implants (Astratech, Molndal, Sweden) in the precise position planned were placed (Fig. 5.32j). Following a 6-week healing period, custom zirconium abutments and provisional restoration were fabricated and delivered (Fig. 5.32k). A final metaloceramic restoration was fabricated and cemented (Fig. 5.32l).

Clinical Case 2

The patient illustrated in Figure 5.33a was a 65-year-old female who has worn a removable prosthesis for the past 30 years. A pre-surgical 3-D image by CBCT was performed, which revealed severe atrophy of the poste-

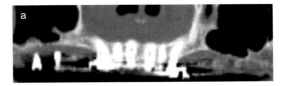

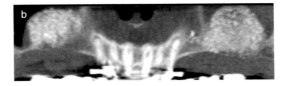

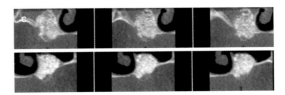

Figures 5.33a–c.   This patient presented with a 30-year history of wearing a removable prosthesis. Pre-surgical three-dimensional CBCT image demonstrated severe atrophy of the posterior maxilla with pneumatization of the maxillary sinus (a). Panoramic (b) and cross-sectional (c) reconstruction of a CBCT scan taken 9 months post–sinus augmentation surgery.

rior maxilla with pneumatization of the maxillary sinus (Fig. 5.33a).

Sinus augmentation surgery was performed with anorganic bovine bone graft. After a 9-month healing period, a follow-up 3-D CBCT image was taken, which revealed adequate volume of bone in the planned sites (Figs. 5.33b, 5.33c).

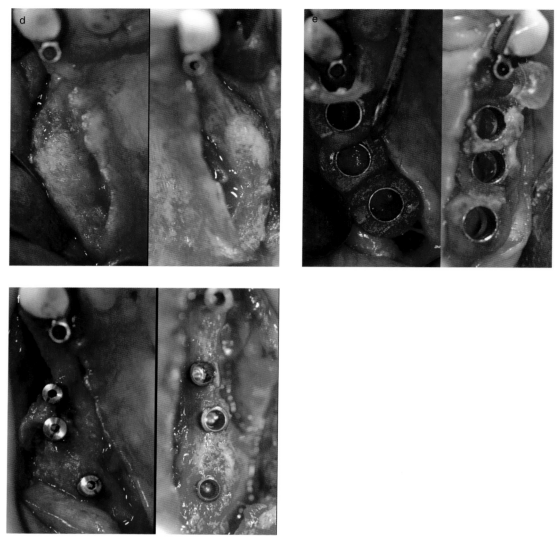

Figures 5.33d–f. A mucoperiosteal flap was elevated (d) and a bone-supported stereolithographic guide was placed on the alveolar ridge (e). The implants were placed, using the guide (f).

A mucoperiosteal flap was elevated (Fig. 5.33d) and a bone-supported stereolithographic guide was placed on the alveolar ridge (Fig. 5.33e).

The implants were placed, using the guide (Fig. 5.33f). Guided bone regeneration was performed utilizing tenting screws (Fig. 5.33g), bovine anorganic bone (Fig. 5.33h), and collagen membrane (not shown).

The purpose of this augmentation was to support the soft tissues horizontally, especially in the area of the first premolar pontics. This allowed correction of the preoperative horizontal atrophy (Fig. 5.33i) by fabrication of a final metaloceramic restoration that restored ridge form (Fig. 5.33j).

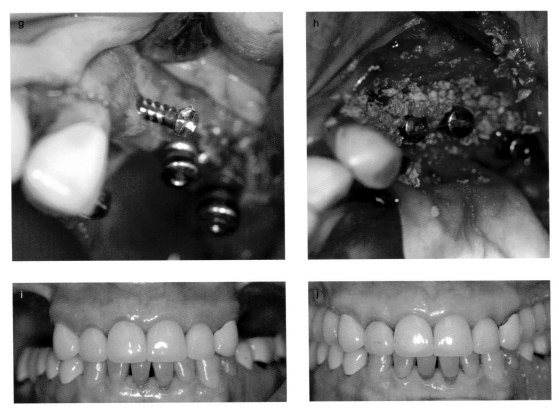

Figures 5.33g–j. Guided bone regeneration was performed utilizing tenting screws (g), bovine anorganic bone (h), and collagen membrane (not shown). Preoperative clinical photograph demonstrating horizontal atrophy of the posterior maxilla (i). Final metal ceramic restoration illustrating the restoration of posterior maxilla arch form (j).

Limitations of Image-Based Implant Therapy

Despite advancements there are a number of limitations for image-based implant surgery. Three-dimensional imaging necessitates radiographic modalities that require increased radiation dosage. The advent of CBCT has provided a 3-D modality with significantly reduced radiation dosage. Another limitation of current imaging technologies is the lack of an ability to image soft tissue volumes. Metal scatter artifacts also remain a problem (Sukovic 2003).

Stereolithographic guides have the limitation that they lack prosthetic landmarks. It is therefore critical to utilize a scanning prosthesis in order to acquire prosthetic landmarks. These landmarks will then be considered in constructing the virtual plan. However, the surgeon cannot modify the osteotomy during surgery.

There is limited documentation of the safety and efficacy of implant surgery performed with stereolithographic guides. Stereolithographic guides for applications using rigid support (tooth and bone-supported) have been well investigated. Mucosa-supported guides have a more limited documentation.

References

Adell R, Lekholm U, Rockler B, Brånemark PI. 1981. A 15-year study of osseointegrated implants in the treatment of the edentulous jaw. *Int J Oral Surg* 10(6): 387–415.

Araujo MG, Lindhe J. 2005. Dimensional ridge alterations following tooth extraction. An experimental study in the dog. *J Clin Periodontol* 32(2):212–218.

Araujo MG, Sukekava F, Wennstrom JL, Lindhe J. 2005. Ridge alterations following implant placement in fresh extraction sockets: An experimental study in the dog. *J Clin Periodontol* 32(6):645–652.

Atwood DA, Coy WA. 1971. Clinical, cephalometric, and densitometric study of reduction of residual ridges. *J Prosthet Dent* 26(3):280–295.

Barzilay I. 1993. Immediate implants: Their current status. *Int J Prosthodont* 6(2): 169–175.

Basten CH. 1995. The use of radiopaque templates for predictable implant placement. *Quintessence Int* 26:609–612.

Basten CH, Kois JC. 1995. The use of barium sulfate for implant templates. *J Prosthet Dent* 76(4):451–454.

Botticelli D, Berglundh T, Lindhe J. 2004. Hard-tissue alterations following immediate implant placement in extraction sites. *J Clin Periodontol* 31(10):820–828.

Brånemark PI, Adell R, Breine U, Hansson BO, Lindstrom J, Ohlsson A. 1969. Intraosseous anchorage of dental prostheses. I: Experimental studies. *Scand J Plast Reconstr Surg* 3(2):81–100.

Brånemark PI, Zarb GA, Albrektsson T (eds.). 1985. *Tissue-Integrated Prostheses: Osseointegration in Clinical Dentistry.* Chicago: Quintessence.

Buser D, Mericske-Stern R, Bernard JP, et al. 1997. Long-term evaluation of non-submerged ITI implants. Part 1: 8-year life table analysis of a prospective multi-center study with 2359 implants. *Clin Oral Implants Res* 8(3):161–172.

Buser DA, Tonetti M. 1997. Clinical trials on implants in regenerated bone. *Ann Periodontol* 2(1):329–342.

Camargo PM, Lekovic V, Weinlaender M, et al. 2000. Influence of bioactive glass on changes in alveolar process dimensions after exodontia. *Oral Surg Oral Med Oral Pathol Oral Radiol Endod* 90(5): 581–585.

Casap N, Tarazi E, Wexler A, Sonnenfeld U, Lustmann J. 2005. Intraoperative computerized navigation for flapless implant surgery and immediate loading in the edentulous mandible. *Int J Oral Maxillofac Implants* 20(1):92–98.

Chen ST, Wilson TG, Jr., Hammerle CH. 2004. Immediate or early placement of implants following tooth extraction: Review of biologic basis, clinical procedures, and outcomes. *Int J Oral Maxillofac Implants* 19(Suppl):12–25.

Chiapasco M. 2004. Early and immediate restoration and loading of implants in completely edentulous patients. *Int J Oral Maxillofac Implants* 19(Suppl):76–91.

Cornelini R. 2000. Immediate transmucosal implant placement: A report of 2 cases. *Int J Periodontics Restorative Dent* 20(2): 199–205.

Cortellini P, Tonetti MS. 2001. Microsurgical approach to periodontal regeneration. Initial evaluation in a case cohort. *J Periodontol* 72(4):559–569.

Covani U, Cornelini R, Barone A. 2003. Bucco-lingual bone remodeling around implants placed into immediate extraction sockets: A case series. *J Periodontol* 74(2): 268–273.

Denissen HW, Kalk W, Veldhuis HA, Van Waas MA. 1993. Anatomic consideration for preventive implantation. *Int J Oral Maxillofac Implants* 8(2):191–195.

Di Giacomo GA, Cury PR, de Araujo NS, Sendyk WR, Sendyk CL. 2005. Clinical application of stereolithographic surgical guides for implant placement: Preliminary results. *J Periodontol* 76(4):503–507.

Engelke W, Capobianco M. 2005. Flapless sinus floor augmentation using endoscopy combined with CT scan-designed surgical templates: Method and report of 6 consecutive cases. *Int J Oral Maxillofac Implants* 20(6):891–897.

Espinosa Marino J, Alvarez Arenal A, Pardo Ceballos A, Fernandez Vazquez JP, Ibaseta Diaz G. 1995. Fabrication on an implant radiological-surgical stent for the partially edentulous patient. *Quintessence Int* 26(2):111–114.

Fortin T, Champleboux G, Lormee J, Coudert JL. 2000. Precise dental implant placement in bone using surgical guides in conjunction with medical imaging techniques. *J Oral Implantol* 26(4):300–303.

Ganeles J, Wismeijer D. 2004. Early and immediately restored and loaded dental implants for single-tooth and partial-arch applications. *Int J Oral Maxillofac Implants* 19(Suppl):92–102.

Ganz SD. 1995. The Triangle of Bone—a formula for successful implant placement and restoration. *Implant Society* 5(5): 2–5.

———. 2001. CT scan technology: An evolving tool for predictable implant placement and restoration. *Int Mag Oral Implantol* 1:6–13.

———. 2003. Use of stereolithographic models as diagnostic and restorative aids for predictable immediate loading of implants. *Pract Proced Aesthet Dent* 15(10):763–771.

———. 2005a. Presurgical planning with CT-derived fabrication of surgical guides. *J Oral Maxillofac Surg* 63(9 Suppl 2):59–71.

———. 2005b. Techniques for the use of CT imaging for the fabrication of surgical guides. *Atlas Oral Maxillofac Surg Clin North Am* 14(1):75–97.

———. 2007. CT-derived model-based surgery for immediate loading of maxillary anterior implants. *Pract Proced Aesthet Dent* 19(5):311–318.

Grunder U, Polizzi G, Goene R, et al. 1999. A 3-year prospective multicenter follow-up report on the immediate and delayed-immediate placement of implants. *Int J Oral Maxillofac Implants* 14(2):210–215.

Harris D, Buser D, Dula K, Grondahl K, Jacobs R, Lekholm U, Nakielny R, Van Steenberghe D, Van der Stelt P. 2002. E.A.O. guidelines for the use of diagnostic imaging in implant dentistry. A consensus workshop organized by the European Association for Osseointegration in Trinity College Dublin. *Clin Oral Implants Res* 13(5):566–570.

Iasella JM, Greenwell H, Miller RL, et al. 2003. Ridge preservation with freeze-dried bone allograft and a collagen membrane compared to extraction alone for implant site development: A clinical and histologic study in humans. *J Periodontol* 74(7): 990–999.

Ikumi N, Tsutsumi S. 2005. Assessment of correlation between computerized tomography values of the bone and cutting torque values at implant placement: A clinical study. *Int J Oral Maxillofac Implants* 20(2):253–260.

Israelson H, Plemons JM, Watkins P, Sory C. 1992. Barium-coated surgical stents and computer-assisted tomography in the preoperative assessment of dental implant patients. *Int J Periodont Rest Dent* 12(1): 52–61.

Jacobs R, Adriansens A, Verstreken K, Suetens P, Van Steenberghe D. 1999. Predictability of a three-dimensional planning system for oral implant surgery. *Dentomaxillofacial Radiol* 28:105–111.

Johnson K. 1963. A study of the dimensional changes occuring in the maxilla after tooth extraction. Part 1: Normal healing. *Aust Dent J* 8:428–434.

———. 1969. A study of the dimensional changes occurring in the maxilla following closed face immediate denture treatment. *Aust Dent J* 14(6):370–375.

Klein M. 2002. Implant surgery using customized surgical templates: The Compu-Guide Surgical Template System. *Dent Implantol Update* 13(6):41–45.

Klein M, Abrams M. 2001. Computer-guided surgery utilizing a computer-milled surgical template. *Pract Proced Aesthet Dent* 13(2):165–169.

Klein M, Cranin AN, Sirakian A. 1993. A computerized tomographic (CT) scan appliance for optimal presurgical and preprosthetic planning of the implant patient. *Pract Periodont Aesthet Dent* 5(6):33–39.

Lam R. 1969. Contour changes of the alveolar process following extraction. *Aust Dent J* 14:241–244.

Laster WS, Ludlow JB, Bailey LJ, Hershey HG. 2005. Accuracy of measurements of mandibular anatomy and prediction of asymmetry in panoramic radiographic images. *Dentomaxillofac Radiol* 34(6): 343–349.

Lazzara RJ. 1989. Immediate implant placement into extraction sites: Surgical and restorative advantages. *Int J Periodontics Restorative Dent* 9(5):332–343.

Lekholm U, Zarb GA. 1985. Patient selection and preparation. In: *Tissue-Integrated Prostheses: Osseointegration in Clinical Dentistry*. PI Brånemark, GA Zarb, and T Albrektsson (eds.). Chicago: Quintessence. 199–209.

Lekovic V, Kenney EB, Weinlaender M, et al. 1997. A bone regenerative approach to alveolar ridge maintenance following tooth extraction. Report of 10 cases. *J Periodontol* 68(6):563–570.

Loubele M, Van Assche N, Carpentier K, Maes F, Jacobs R, Van Steenberghe D, Suetens P. 2008. Comparative localized linear accuracy of small-field cone-beam CT and multislice CT for alveolar bone measurements. *Oral Surg Oral Med Oral Pathol Oral Radiol Endod* 105(4):512–518.

Lundgren D, Nyman S. 1991. Bone regeneration in 2 stages for retention of dental implant. A case report. *Clin Oral Implants Res* 2(4):203–207.

Marcaccini AM, Novaes AB, Jr., Souza SL, Taba M, Jr., Grisi MF. 2003. Immediate placement of implants into periodontally infected sites in dogs. Part 2: A fluorescence microscopy study. *Int J Oral Maxillofac Implants* 18(6):812–819.

Mayfield L. 1999. *Immediate, Delayed, and Late Submerged and Transmucosal Implants*. Berlin: Quintessence.

Misch KA, Yi ES, Sarment DP. 2006. Accuracy of cone beam computed tomography for periodontal defect measurements. *J Periodontol* 77(7):1261–1266.

Missika P, Abbou M, Rahal B. 1997. Osseous regeneration in immediate postextraction implant placement: A literature review and clinical evaluation. *Pract Periodont Aesthet Dent* 9(2):165–175; quiz 175.

Morton DM, Martin WC, Buser D. 2008. General principles for the pre-treatment assessment of and planning for partially dentate patients receiving dental implants. In: *ITI Treatment Guide*, Vol 2. D. Wismeijer, D. Buser, and U Belser (eds.). Berlin: Quintessence. 19–27.

Novaes AB, Jr., Novaes AB. 1995. Immediate implants placed into infected sites: A clinical report. *Int J Oral Maxillofac Implants* 10(5):609–613.

Novaes AB, Jr., Papalexiou V, Grisi MF, Souza SS, Taba M, Jr., Kajiwara JK. 2004. Influence of implant microstructure on the osseointegration of immediate implants placed in periodontally infected sites: A histomorphometric study in dogs. *Clin Oral Implants Res* 15(1):34–43.

Novaes AB, Jr., Marcaccini AM, Souza SL, Taba M, Jr., Grisi MF. 2003. Immediate placement of implants into periodontally infected sites in dogs: A histomorphometric study of bone-implant contact. *Int J Oral Maxillofac Implants* 18(3):391–398.

Novaes AB, Jr., Vidigal GM, Jr., Novaes AB, Grisi MF, Polloni S, Rosa A. 1998. Immediate implants placed into infected sites: A histomorphometric study in dogs. *Int J Oral Maxillofac Implants* 13(3): 422–427.

Paolantonio M, Dolci M, Scarano A, et al. 2001. Immediate implantation in fresh extraction sockets: A controlled clinical and histological study in man. *J Periodontol* 72(11):1560–1571.

Papalexiou V, Novaes AB, Jr., Grisi MF, Souza SS, Taba M, Jr., Kajiwara JK. 2004. Influence of implant microstructure on the dynamics of bone healing around immediate implants placed into periodontally infected sites: A confocal laser scanning microscopic study. *Clin Oral Implants Res* 15(1):44–53.

Parel SM, Triplett RG. 1990. Immediate fixture placement: A treatment planning alternative. *Int J Oral Maxillofac Implants* 5(4):337–345.

Pontual MAB, Freire JNO, Souza DC, et al. 2004. A newly designed template device for use with the insertion of immediately loaded implants. *J Oral Implantol* 30(5): 325–329.

Rosenberg ES, Cho SC, Elian N, Jalbout ZN, Froum S, Evian CI. 2004. A comparison of characteristics of implant failure and survival in periodontally compromised and periodontally healthy patients: A clinical report. *Int J Oral Maxillofac Implants* 19(6):873–879.

Rosenfeld A, Mandelaris G, Tardieu P. 2006. Prosthetically directed placement using computer software to insure precise placement and predictable prosthetic outcomes. Part 1: Diagnostics, imaging, and collaborative accountability. *Int J Periodontics Restorative Dent* 26:215–221.

Rosenfeld AL, Mecall RA. 1996. Use of interactive computed tomography to predict the esthetic and functional demands of implant-supported prostheses. *Compend Contin Educ Dent* 17(12):1125–1146.

Rosenfeld AL, Mecall RA. 1998. Use of prosthesis-generated computed tomographic information for diagnostic and surgical treatment planning. *J Esthet Dent* 10(3): 132–148.

Rosenquist B, Grenthe B. 1996. Immediate placement of implants into extraction sockets: Implant survival. *Int J Oral Maxillofac Implants* 11(2):205–209.

Sammartino G, Della Valle A, Marenzi G, Gerbino S, Martorelli M, di Lauro AE, di Lauro F. 2004. Stereolithography in oral implantology: A comparison of surgical guides. *Implant Dent* 13(2):133–139.

Sarment DP, Al-Shammari K, Kazor CE. 2003a. Stereolithographic surgical templates for placement of dental implants in complex cases. *Int J Periodont Rest Dent* 23(3):287–295.

Sarment DP, Misch CE. 2002. Scannographic templates for novel pre-implant planning methods. *Int Mag Oral Implantol* 3:16–22.

Sarment DP, Sukovic P, Clinthorne N. 2003b. Accuracy of implant placement with a stereolithographic surgical guide. *Int J Oral Maxillofac Implants* 18(4):571–577.

Schropp L, Wenzel A, Kostopoulos L, Karring T. 2003. Bone healing and soft tissue contour changes following single-tooth extraction: A clinical and radiographic 12-month prospective study. *Int J Periodontics Restorative Dent* 23(4):313–323.

Schultz AJ. 1993. Guided tissue regeneration (GTR) of nonsubmerged implants in immediate extraction sites. *Pract Periodontics Aesthet Dent* 5(2):59–65; quiz 65.

Schwartz-Arad D, Chaushu G. 1997. Placement of implants into fresh extraction sites: 4 to 7 years retrospective evaluation of 95 immediate implants. *J Periodontol* 68(11): 1110–1115.

Shanaman RH. 1992. The use of guided tissue regeneration to facilitate ideal prosthetic placement of implants. *Int J Periodontics Restorative Dent* 12(4):256–265.

Siegenthaler DW, Jung RE, Holderegger C, Roos M, Hammerle CH. 2007. Replacement of teeth exhibiting periapical pathology by immediate implants: A prospective, controlled clinical trial. *Clin Oral Implants Res* 18(6):727–737.

Sonic M, Abrahams J, Faiella R. 1994. A comparison of the accuracy of periapical, panoramic, and computerized tomographic radiographs in locating the mandibular canal. *Int J Oral Maxillofac Implants* 9:455–460.

Sukovic P. 2003. Cone beam computed tomography in craniofacial imaging. *Orthod Craniofac Res* 6(Suppl 1):31–36.

Tardieu PB, Vrielinck L, Escolano E. 2003. Computer-assisted implant placement. A case report: Treatment of the mandible. *Int J Oral Maxillofac Implants* 18(4): 599–604.

Tolman DE, Keller EE. 1991. Endosseous implant placement immediately following dental extraction and alveoloplasty: Preliminary report with 6-year follow-up. *Int J Oral Maxillofac Implants* 6(1):24–28.

Tyndall AA, Brooks SL. 2000. Selection criteria for dental implant site imaging: A position paper of the American Academy of Oral and Maxillofacial Radiology. *Oral Surg Oral Med Oral Pathol Oral Radiol Endod* 89:630–637.

Van Assche N, Van Steenberghe D, Guerrero ME, Hirsch E, Schutyser F, Quirynen M, Jacobs R. 2007. Accuracy of implant placement based on pre-surgical planning of three-dimensional cone-beam images: A pilot study. *J Clin Periodontol* 34:816–821.

Van Steenberghe D, Glauser R, Blombäck U, Andersson M, Schutyser F, Pettersson A, Wendelhag I. 2005. A computed tomographic scan-derived customized surgical template and fixed prosthesis for flapless surgery and immediate loading of implants in fully edentulous maxillae: A prospective multicenter study. *Clin Implant Dent Relat Res* 7(Suppl 1):S111–120.

Van Steenberghe D, Malevez C, Van Cleynenbreugel J, Serhal CB, Dhoore E, Schutyser F, Suetens P, Jacobs R. 2003. Accuracy of drilling guides for transfer from three-dimensional CT-based planning to placement of zygoma implants in human cadavers. *Clin Oral Implants Res* 14(1):131–135.

Vazquez L, Saulacic N, Belser U, Bernard J-P. 2008. Efficacy of panoramic radiographs in the preoperative planning of posterior mandibular implants: A prospective clinical study of 1527 consecutively treated patients. *Clinical Oral Implants Res* 19(1): 81–85.

Wagenberg B, Froum SJ. 2006. A retrospective study of 1925 consecutively placed immediate implants from 1988 to 2004. *Int J Oral Maxillofac Implants* 21(1):71–80.

Watzek G, Haider R, Mensdorff-Pouilly N, Haas R. 1995. Immediate and delayed implantation for complete restoration of the jaw following extraction of all residual teeth: A retrospective study comparing different types of serial immediate implantation. *Int J Oral Maxillofac Implants* 10(5): 561–567.

Werbitt MJ, Goldberg PV. 1992. The immediate implant: Bone preservation and bone regeneration. *Int J Periodontics Restorative Dent* 12(3):206–217.

Wilson TG, Jr. 1992. Guided tissue regeneration around dental implants in immediate and recent extraction sites: Initial observations. *Int J Periodontics Restorative Dent* 12(3):185–193.

Wilson TG, Jr., Schenk R, Buser D, Cochran D. 1998. Implants placed in immediate extraction sites: A report of histologic and histometric analyses of human biopsies. *Int J Oral Maxillofac Implants* 13(3): 333–341.

Pre-implant Surgical Interventions

6

HORIZONTAL AND VERTICAL BONE REGENERATION IN THE MAXILLA AND MANDIBLE

Burton Langer

At the time of the original 1982 Osseointegration Conference in Toronto, the major emphasis of implant therapy was on rescuing edentulous patients who could not wear full denture prostheses with any degree of comfort. While most cases of mandibular edentulism could be treated without bone grafting, many maxillary patients required autologous grafts harvested from remote sites. Partial edentulism and anterior cosmetics were not a priority.

As the indications for implant therapy evolved, more people became interested in replacing removable partial dentures or missing or diseased anterior teeth. The use of implants to treat cases of partial edentulism and single-tooth replacement became more commonplace. As this occurred, augmenting bone became one of the most sought-after goals.

The late 1980s saw the development of many procedures for improving the height of the bone inferior to the maxillary sinus. Some were aggressive and required major autologous grafts taken from remote sites. Since patients were reluctant to accept these regimes, and the results were not always predictable, more conservative techniques also were developed.

The most conservative of these was mentioned by Professor P I Brånemark in his text on osseointegration (Brånemark et al. 1985). In it he described a technique for lifting the sinus membrane superiorly in order to increase the height of bone (Fig. 6.1).

However, many clinicians did not succeed with this approach unless they added bone or a synthetic material into the osteotomy site (Davarpanah et al. 2001; Summers 1994a, 1994b) to induce bone formation at the most apical portion. The use of allografts, xenografts, and alloplasts has all yielded impressive results. Another approach is to elevate the apical bone in the osteotomy site and the sinus membrane as a unit (Fig. 6.2). This gives the tissue an inductor from which to form new bone at the apex of the implant site.

With the development of the lateral window approach to sinus elevation (Boyne and James 1980; Tatum 1986), clinicians filled the sinus

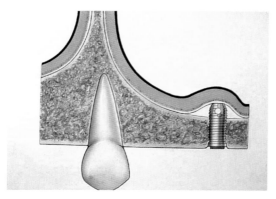

Figure 6.1. Internal sinus elevation. Schneiderian membrane elevated to allow bone to grow over the apical area of the implant.

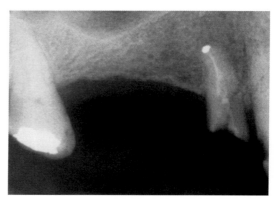

Figure 6.3a. Preoperative radiograph showing an insufficient amount of bone to place an implant.

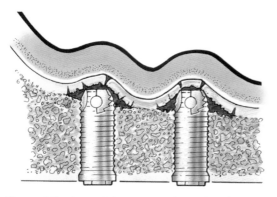

Figure 6.2. Internal bone core sinus elevation performed in such a manner as to retain the apical bone attached to the Schneiderian membrane to assist in bone-forming capacity over the apical end of the implant.

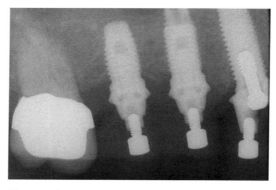

Figure 6.3b. Postoperative radiograph with implant in place after the internal bone core sinus elevation showing an increase in the amount of bone at the apex of the implant.

cavity not only with autogenous bone grafts but also with other bone-grafting materials (Langer and Langer 1999; Wallace and Froum 2003) (Figs. 6.3a, 6.3b).

Most were not bone inducers but rather acted as scaffolds on and through which new bone could grow. These techniques also yielded results that in some cases were as favorable as those obtained when using autogenous bone (Figs. 6.4a–6.4c).

These procedures made it possible to replace missing maxillary posterior teeth in almost all cases, regardless of how little bone was present at the outset of treatment.

As these techniques evolved, implant macrotopography and surface morphology also underwent changes (Buser et al. 1991; Wennerberg et al. 1995). Since it was postulated that the augmented bone was of lesser quality than the native osseous structures, it was felt that a rougher surface on the implants would allow for denser apposition of the newly grafted bone. Over the years, most implant manufacturers gravitated to this concept, and dental professionals embraced it. Implants also generally became more tapered in order to achieve better stabilization in the denser alveolar crest of cortical bone. The use of

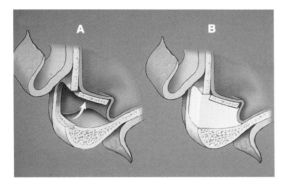

Figure 6.4a. Diagram showing the technique of the lateral window sinus elevation.

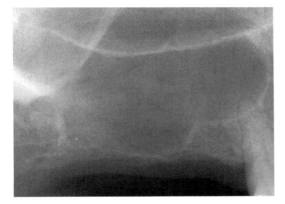

Figure 6.4b. Preoperative radiograph showing less than 2 mm of bone between the crest of the alveolar ridge and the maxillary sinus.

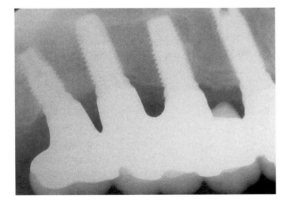

Figure 6.4c. Postoperative radiograph showing three 10 mm implants in place after the lateral window sinus elevation and demineralized bone allograft procedure.

membranes over the lateral sinus window was also introduced to enhance the formation of viable bone in the grafted site (Froum et al. 1998; Tarnow et al. 2000). This approach gained popularity with some clinicians, but others reported comparably successful results without using membranes.

At approximately the same time, the concept of extracting teeth and placing implants simultaneously was introduced (Becker and Becker 1990; Gelb 1993; Lazzara 1989). This shortened by many months the waiting time between extraction and optimal dental aesthetics and function. It also introduced many innovative techniques for rejuvenating, at the time of implant placement, bone that had been lost as a result of periodontal disease or reoccurring apical pathology (Figs. 6.5a–6.5e).

Many different types of bone grafting materials were used—autografts, allografts, alloplasts, and xenografts, alone or in combination. These were further combined in some cases with various types of occlusive membranes. Initially, the membranes were non-resorbable, but resorbable versions soon proved suitable for some indications. Some clinicians advocated guided bone regeneration as the only viable way to accomplish extraction followed immediately by implant placement. Yet others showed comparable results by placing bone grafts around the implants without the membrane.

Assisting in the quest to build bone both horizontally and vertically was the use of subepithelial connective-tissue grafts used over the bone-graft material in an attempt to restore the normal architecture over the newly placed implant (Langer and Calagna 1980, 1982) (Figs. 6.6a–6.6d).

Often large 3-D deficiencies could be rejuvenated so that the implant matched the aesthetic profile of the adjacent teeth. This approach was particularly suitable when the surrounding bone could support the implant and bone graft, as when the buccal plate of bone was resorbed but the surrounding proximal and lingual or palatal bone were still intact.

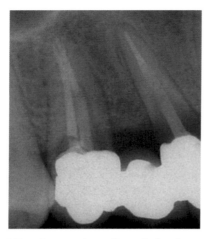

Figure 6.5a. Preoperative radiograph showing two fractured premolars.

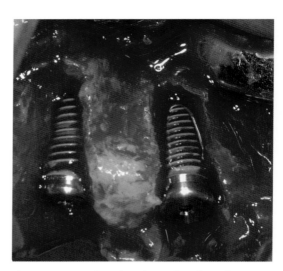

Figure 6.5c. Implants have been placed into the extraction sites.

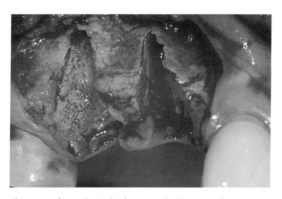

Figure 6.5b. Clinical photograph showing the extraction sites in which the buccal plates of bone of both premolars have been lost.

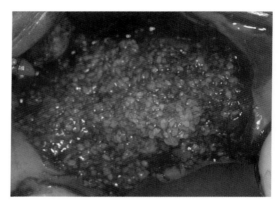

Figure 6.5d. Demineralized bone allograft has been placed over the implants to cover the deficient buccal plates of bone.

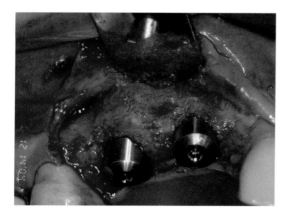

Figure 6.5e. Re-entry showing the horizontal regenerated buccal bone.

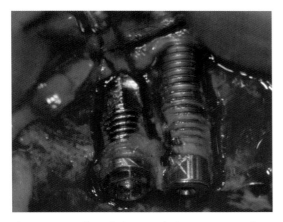

Figure 6.6a.   Clinical photograph showing two implants with loss of three-quarters of the surrounding bone.

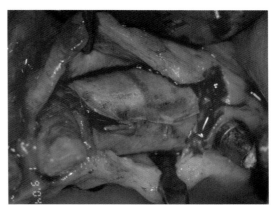

Figure 6.6c.   Bone graft and membrane uncovered.

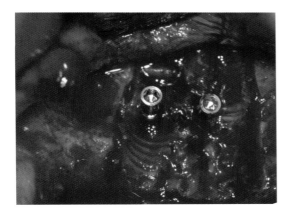

Figure 6.6b.   Two miniscrews are placed to act as tenting screws for a bone graft and titanium membrane placement.

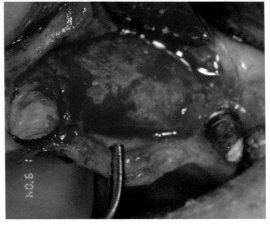

Figure 6.6d.   Bone regenerated horizontally at the 6-month re-entry.

When the amount of bone loss resulting from infection, trauma, or previous implant failure was so significant that bone grafts could not be contained, it became necessary to use accessory tenting screws and titanium membranes to hold the graft material in the desired position (Buser et al. 1990; Schenk et al. 1994; Simion et al. 1998) (Figs. 6.7a–6.7e).

Some authors used the implants to hold the bone grafts and placed titanium membranes over the implants to augment the bone in a vertical direction. The result of these innova-tions was that clinicians were able to place implants in the most compromised locations imaginable. With the advent of new bone additives such as growth factors, this capabil-ity will certainly improve. The same technique is often useful in horizontal augmentation.

The development of the split-ridge tech-nique (Simion et al. 1992) has also enabled clinicians to widen thin areas of bone without having to harvest bone from remote sites. In most cases, grafting material is inserted into the spaces created by the separation of the buccal and lingual bone plates. Often implants

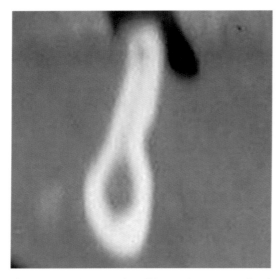

Figure 6.7a. Preoperative CT scan in cross-sectional view showing a narrow bucco-lingual alveolar ridge. Insufficient width to place implants.

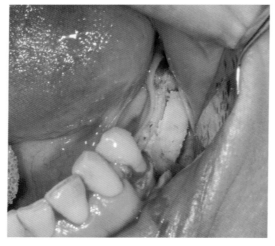

Figure 6.7b. Clinical photograph showing the osteotomy at the crest of the ridge, lateral, and apical borders of the intended ridge expansion.

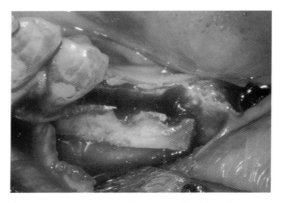

Figure 6.7c. Bone spread apart to allow the placement of bone.

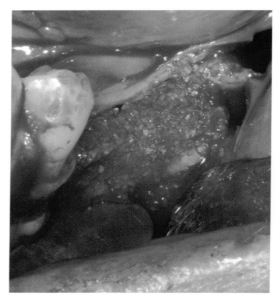

Figure 6.7d. Bone allograft inserted into the trough created when the buccal and lingual plates of bone have been displaced.

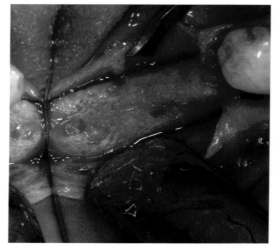

Figure 6.7e. Re-entry into the area and note the increase in width so that 4 mm wide implants could be installed.

can be inserted into the center of the displaced plates of bone, eliminating the need for an additional surgical visit (Figs. 6.8a–6.8e).

Onlay and veneer grafts harvested from remote sites (Bell 1980) are still needed in some situations. This is especially true when there is insufficient bone in the premaxilla to anchor implants.

The final development to enhance vertical bone growth was the introduction of distraction osteogenesis (Chin 1998) and the down

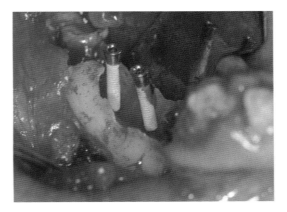

Figure 6.8c. Minipins inserted into the bone defect and extending occlusally to act as a support for a bone allograft and titanium membrane placement.

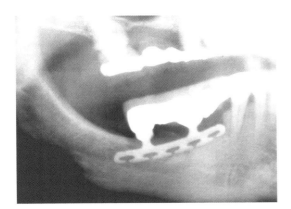

Figure 6.8a. Radiograph showing the bone resorption around a blade implant.

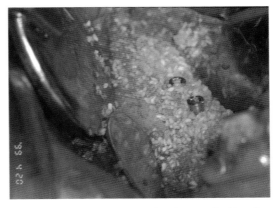

Figure 6.8d. Bone graft placed and covered with a titanium membrane.

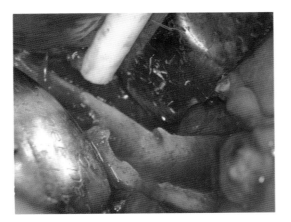

Figure 6.8b. Clinical photograph showing the wide resorption of bone after the blade implant was removed. The extent of the bone loss is encroaching upon the mandibular canal.

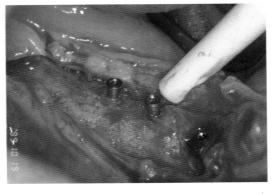

Figure 6.8e. Re-entry showing vertical bone growth almost to the top of the miniscrews.

fracture (Bell 1975; Blomqvist et al. 1997; Cawood et al. 1994) (Figs. 6.9a–6.9e).

This approach relies on the ability of the body and its circulation to regenerate bone that has been moved away from its original position and been brought down in the maxilla or occlusally in the mandible.

While these innovations have revolutionized ossseointegration, many of the original doctrines set forth by the pioneers of the field still serve as the basic framework of implant therapy.

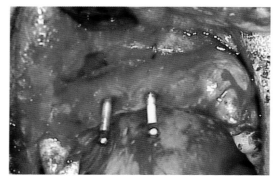

Figure 6.9c.   After both lateral and central incisor extractions, the bone inferior to the nasal spine is distracted in one visit and stabilized in that position. The void that was created by bringing the bone inferiorly was filled with an allograft.

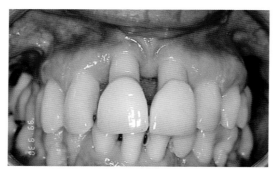

Figure 6.9a.   Clinical photograph showing severe recession and bone loss around anterior teeth resulting in a cosmetic problem.

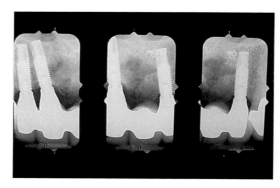

Figure 6.9d.   After 3 months of stabilization, the stabilizing implants were removed and three 15 mm implants were installed.

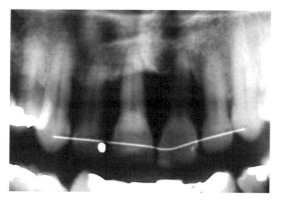

Figure 6.9b.   Radiograph showing advanced bone loss around central and lateral incisors.

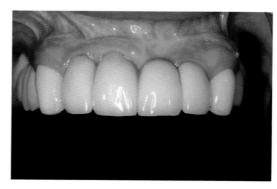

Figure 6.9e.   Final photograph showing a significant decrease in the vertical length of the anterior incisors.

PRE-IMPLANT SURGICAL INTERVENTIONS TISSUE-ENGINEERING SOLUTIONS

E. Todd Scheyer

Surgical methods for the reconstruction of hard- and soft-tissue defects that are predictable, yet without the morbidity associated with the autogenous donor site, are a valuable tool in reconstructive periodontal and implant procedures. Patient preference for procedures that bypass the need for a donor site has impelled surgeons to search for predictable, efficient strategies that use engineered tissue, growth factors, and biomimetic therapies. Tissue engineering has been applied to many areas of medicine. Tissue-engineered skin products have been used in wound healing centers for treating burns, venus statis, pressure, and diabetic ulcers and because of this, applications have come into dentistry to see if the same technology can be utilized to treat oral deficiencies and pathology.

The collection of evidence in the literature for guided tissue regeneration is vast and growing, while the success of dental implants has intensified the need for predictable tissue regenerative procedures. For years dental surgeons have been using, with high levels of predictability, resorbable and non-resorbable barrier membranes with techniques that are a form of *passive* tissue engineering around teeth and dental implant dehiscence and fenestrations (Dahlin et al. 1995; McGuire and Scheyer 2008b; Mellonig and Nevins 1995). By employing *active* tissue engineering new levels of predictability and success can be reached to resolve hard- and soft-tissue defects. With the addition of growth factors, extracellular matrices, and/or live cell therapies to procedures already using barrier membranes or bone replacement grafts, we can make our treatment more predictable in the most challenging situations.

Before proceeding, it is necessary to differentiate between small and large volume defect classifications of periodontal versus alveolar ridge deficiencies. Small volume defects are the intrabony and furcation periodontal defects along with gingival recession defects. This is a simplification of very complex wound healing categories, but should help translate the benefits of using tissue-engineering procedures in all oral defect reconstructive therapies. It is in the small volume defects in which periodontal regeneration has occurred, and the periodontal literature documenting this clinical regeneration has become the foundation for our clinical decision-making tree (Scheyer et al. 2002). True periodontal regeneration with histological evidence of new cementum, periodontal ligament, and alveolar bone has been shown in the human model (Camelo et al. 2003; Nevins et al. 2003; Yukna and Mellonig 2000). The large volume defects are considered the alveolar ridge and maxillary sinus defects needing reconstruction for implant restorations.

The ability to reconstruct these tissues in an area that was previously infected with periodontal disease serves as the ultimate regenerative test. Human recombinant PDGF BB plus beta tricalcium phosphate was shown to accelerate clinical attachment level gains and significantly increase bone growth in severe periodontal defects (Nevins et al. 2005). Materials such as rhPDGF and enamel matrix derivative have met the proof of principle that true regeneration can be obtained when used adjacent to a previously diseased root surface (Camelo et al. 2003; Nevins et al. 2003; Yukna and Mellonig 2000). Furthermore, new histologic evidence from a current study shows proof of principle that true regeneration can be achieved with rhPDGF + β-TCP + collagen in gingival recession-type defects (McGuire and Scheyer 2008a) (Fig. 6.11). Because these materials have been through such comprehensive evaluation in periodontics, we begin to see the advantages of using biosurgical techniques in both periodontics and implant dentistry. When evaluating the more challenging aesthetic concerns such as open interproximal spaces and other severe soft-tissue deficiencies in implant dentistry, there exist no augmentation techniques that can predictably correct these defects. With the application of cell-based therapies, there may be opportunities to repair challenging defects that in the past have remained unpredictable to treat with only clinical reports as published evidence for success. In summary, it is small volume defects that have allowed us to support clinical decisions for material selection when a challenging defect presents to our clinical practice. We then are encouraged to graft the large alveolar ridge and maxillary sinus deficiencies with materials that have strong evidence for success in the acid test models of periodontal hard- and soft-tissue regeneration.

Based on the findings in the periodontal defect model, McGuire and Scheyer (2006) have used rhPDGF + β-TCP with a collagen membrane to treat recession defects in the oral cavity (Fig. 6.10).

This was compared to a subepithelial connective tissue graft within a case series (McGuire and Scheyer 2006) and more recently in a controlled clinical trial showing comparable root coverage outcomes between test and control (McGuire and Scheyer 2008a, 2008c) (Fig. 6.10). This study also provided histological evidence of true periodontal regeneration (Fig. 6.11).

As the evidence for this growth factor continues to appear in the dental literature, we began to combine this potent growth factor with composite bone grafts in the maxillary sinus. Human histology shows favorable formation of new bone surrounding grafted particles during the early healing point of 4 months (Fig. 6.12). This sample was taken from a pneumatized sinus, grafted with rhPDGF + bovine bone + mineralized freeze-dried bone allograft.

Recombinant human bone morphogenic protein (rhBMP) also has significant research supporting its use for large maxillary sinus deficiencies, extraction defects, and peri-implant deficiencies in human and animal studies (Boyne et al. 1997; Cochran et al. 1999; Hanisch et al. 1997; Howell et al. 1997; Jovanovic et al. 2007; Nevins et al. 1996; Sigurdsson et al. 1997; Wikesjö et al. 2001, 2004). This strong recombinant growth factor holds hope for significant

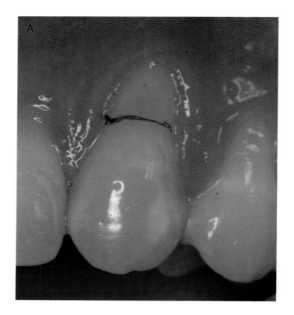

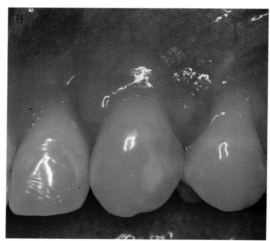

Figure 6.10. a. Before view of test tooth displaying advanced gingival recession. b. Six-month postoperative view of test tooth treated with rhPDGF + β-TCP + collagen membrane (Figs. 6.10a and 6.10b from McGuire and Scheyer 2008c).

regenerative success in clinical practice. Boyne et al. (2005) evaluated recombinant bone morphogenic protein with a collagen carrier in the maxillary sinus, which showed favorable de novo bone formation. Others have published on the power of this growth factor, which is one of the most exciting now available for implant reconstructive therapy (Boyne 2001; Fiorellini et al. 2005).

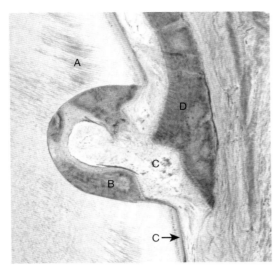

Figure 6.11. Histology from root coverage graft performed with rhPDGF + β-TCP + collagen membrane. a. Tooth root with histological reference notch. b. New cementum. c. Periodontal ligament. d. New bone (from McGuire and Scheyer 2008a).

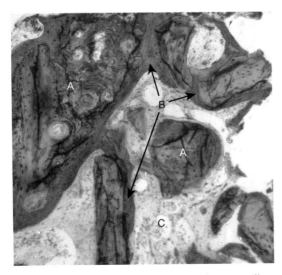

Figure 6.12. Histology of bone core from maxillary sinus grafted with rhPDGF + Bio Oss + FDBA taken at 4.5 months. a. Graft particle. b. Vital new bone. c. Fatty and hematopoietic marrow.

In the future, studies need to validate these growth factors' use in complex extraction defects and alveolar ridge deficiencies. It will

be valuable to evaluate optimal matrices to carry and maintain these growth factors in the wound for the appropriate time period and in efficacious concentrations through additional wound kinetic studies. We realize that during clinical regenerative therapies various factors must be considered to maintain adequate blood supply and provide appropriate scaffolding for new tissue formation (Cochran and Wozney 1999). When utilizing these recombinant growth factors one must understand that it is not only the presence of the growth factor in the initial wound, but that this growth factor remains at the correct concentration and volume—and then must communicate properly with host cells for the appropriate amount of time and work with the host feedback mechanisms to alter activity during the different stages of wound healing. Human recombinant growth factors have a valuable and promising future for reconstructive therapy in both periodontics and implant dentistry by influencing the early stages of wound healing.

Another line of research in soft-tissue engineering has been the implantation of live cell-based skin substitutes or the in vitro construction of a transplantable vital tissue. Historically, one of the first bioengineered skin substitutes consists of autologous expanded fibroblast grown from small biopsies (Isolagen Technologies, Exton, Pennsylvania). One of the first dental studies conducted evaluated autologous fibroblast transplantation in an attempt to expand interdental gingival soft-tissue volumes. In this study, both the investigators' and patients' VAS scores showed statistically significant improvements with the injection of autologous fibroblasts when compared to placebo. Prior to the injection of these expanded fibroblasts, a "priming" procedure was performed in the papillary region to create an inflammatory response. The theory was to develop temporary increased tissue volume, thus enabling the injection of the concentrated cell suspension. The cells were delivered 5–7 days after the priming procedure and then again at two other time points after the first injection. The subjects were assessed at 2, 3, and 4 months after the injections and these preliminary results indicate a novel tissue-engineering technique may hold promise in resolving the open interproximal space (McGuire and Scheyer 2007) (Fig. 6.13).

Further research is under way to evaluate this as a predictable modality of therapy. Historically, there have been other studies conducted at our research center evaluating fibroblasts dermal substitute to treat gingival recession defects where no attached gingiva was present. Although this material is not

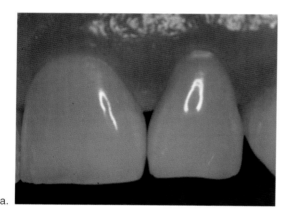

a.

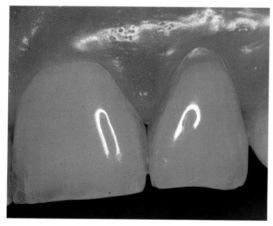

b.

Figure 6.13. a. Preoperative view of open interproximal space. b. Four months after three injections into the papilla with the patient's own expanded and concentrated fibroblast. Note the improved papillary form (Figs. 6.13a and 6.13b from McGuire and Scheyer 2007. Reprinted with permission from the American Academy of Periodontology).

available today, it holds promise in developing new attached gingiva when compared to the free autogenous graft (McGuire and Nunn 2003). Lastly, a current study conducted by McGuire et al. (2008) was to evaluate the safety and efficacy of a bi-layered cell therapy (BCT) (Organogenesis, Inc., Canton, Massachusetts). BCT was compared to a free gingival graft in generating attached gingiva around teeth not requiring root coverage (McGuire et al. 2008). To date preliminary periodontal results appear encouraging and based on these findings a large multicenter trial is under way to determine the clinical efficacy for this live cell technology. These therapies will need to be validated with human histology and other well-controlled clinical trials.

When translating the efficacy of these engineered soft-tissue materials to implant dentistry we must not just consider deficiencies that need to be corrected prior to implant replacement but also existing failures from previous therapy that are sometimes the most challenging defects to correct. It is the author's thought that new technologies will allow us to more predictably restore lost tissues around teeth and integrated dental implants that have suffered tissue losses from pathology and/or treatment failure. Further investigation with recombinant growth factors, extracellular matrices, and live cell therapy needs to be conducted to support these methods for everyday clinical practice. Because of the limited blood supply in the most challenging surgical defects we cannot rely on just the "old" rules for regeneration, but must consider utilizing factors and matrix materials capable of inducing blood flow into and around the defect. Tissue engineering and biosurgery will bring us to new levels of clinical success for periodontics and implant dentistry by providing an active component to our methods.

Implanting live cells is a new dimension of treatment with the idea that live cells will communicate with native cells, optimizing the influx of metabolically active molecules at the appropriate time and in the quantity required by that wound. The field of hard- and soft-tissue engineering is advancing rapidly.

Commercial products are available containing enamel matrix derivatives (Emdogain, Straumann, Basel, Switzerland), rhPDGF + β-TCP (Gem21s-Osteohealth, Shirley, New York), and rhBMP, (Infuse-Medtronic, Memphis, Tennessee). It will not be long before live cell technologies are available to practicing dentists, technologies that not only deliver growth factors but provide a template for cell migration, adhesion, proliferation, and differentiation, thus optimizing the regenerative response. During the next decade we will be able to rewrite some of the rules of regeneration, providing our patients with improved techniques with less morbidity, shorter treatment times, and optimal predictability.

For this clinician, it has been the extensive evidence for regeneration in the small volume periodontal defects that has influenced the use of biologically active molecules for implant-related therapies. As we continue our quest for the ultimate regenerative outcome in both periodontics and implant dentistry, there is no doubt that tissue engineering will play a greater role in our future, providing tomorrow's clinician with bio-active materials that strongly influence the treatment outcome for the patient.

GUIDED BONE REGENERATION WITH OR WITHOUT BONE GRAFTS: FROM EXPERIMENTAL STUDIES TO CLINICAL APPLICATION

Nikolaos Donos

Introduction

Loss of teeth and denture wearing result in a continuous resorption of the residual alveolar ridges that is described as a chronic, gradual, irreversible, and cumulative phenomenon proceeding slowly over a period of time (Atwood 1962; Carlsson and Persson 1967; Tallgren 1967). Nowadays, the use of tita-

nium dental implants is considered a successful and predictable treatment of partial and full edentulism (Adell et al. 1981; Albrektsson et al. 1986). However, a prerequisite for the successful placement of implants in the ideal, prosthodontically driven position is a minimum amount of bone width and height of the recipient site that will provide a functional and cosmetic implant-borne restoration for the patient.

Very often in the everyday clinical practice, it is not possible to place the dental implants in a manner that will avoid the creation of fenestration or dehiscence defects.

Furthermore, the presence of thin alveolar ridges creates the need for further surgical procedures prior to implant placement.

Lateral bone/ridge augmentation procedures are necessary when the width of the recipient alveolar ridge does not present with the adequate dimensions for implant placement that ultimately will provide the masticatory rehabilitation of the patient. A number of surgical procedures have been used for creating adequate bone width and can be performed either in combination with (1) the implant placement (*one-stage/simultaneous approach*)—this would be usually associated with dehiscence or fenestration bone defects; or (2) prior to the surgical placement of the implants and following a period for healing (*two-stage/staged approach*) for thin alveolar ridges. One of the most commonly used procedures for bone regeneration and lateral ridge augmentation is guided bone regeneration (GBR) alone or in combination with grafting procedures.

Development of the GTR/GBR Principle

A series of experimental studies on the regenerative potential of the tissues comprising the periodontium provided the basis for the development of the regenerative treatment modality known as guided tissue regeneration (GTR) (for review, see Karring et al. 1993).

In these experiments it was demonstrated that the exclusion of epithelial and connective tissue cells from the healing process of a periodontal defect may offer the periodontal ligament cells the required space and time to repopulate the root surface and produce a layer of new cementum with inserting collagen fibers (Karring et al. 1993).

The application of the GTR principle in the clinic involves the placement of a membrane adjacent to the root surface, creating a secluded space that can only be repopulated by cells originating from the periodontal ligament or the alveolar bone. At the same time, the membrane acts as a barrier preventing the gingival connective tissue and the oral epithelium from populating the root surface. With this technique, new attachment formation can be achieved predictably, while regeneration of the alveolar bone varies significantly. Nevertheless, this observation indicated that the preservation of a secluded space by a barrier offers the possibility for bone-forming cells emanating from the existent bone surfaces to populate the space and promote bone formation (Karring et al. 1993).

Similarly, the GTR principle with the use of different non-resorbable and resorbable membranes can be used for the regeneration of bone defects or augmentation of deficient sites. For the specific applications, the term GBR is used.

The use of GBR for the healing of critical-size defects (bone defects not healing spontaneously with bone but with fibrous connective tissue) (Schmitz and Hollinger 1986) (Fig. 6.14) has been shown in different experimental animals with bioresorbable and non-bioresorbable membranes to predictably result in the complete regeneration of various defects (Bosch et al. 1995; Dahlin et al. 1988, 1990, 1991, 1993; Donos et al. 2004; Kostopoulos and Karring 1994a, 1994b) (Figs. 6.15–6.17).

Furthermore, the pattern of bone growth and development of the regenerated bone resembles the healthy bone (Schenk et al. 1994). The potential of the GBR principle in experimental animals is similar irrespective of the anatomic location of the defect, and com-

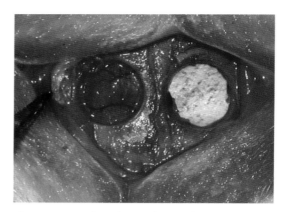

Figure 6.14.   Calvarial critical size defect.

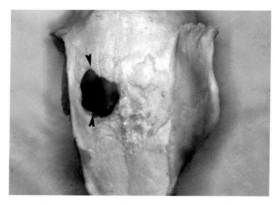

Figure 6.15.   Macerated specimen. One critical size calvarial defect was not treated and remained open during the healing period, whereas the contralateral defect was treated with GBR and presented complete closure with newly formed bone (from Donos et al. 2004).

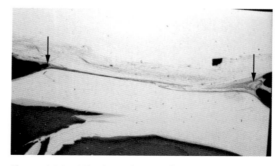

Figure 6.16.   Histological view of an untreated critical size calvarial defect at 120 days following operation (from Donos et al. 2004).

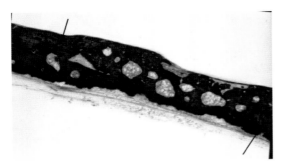

Figure 6.17. Histological view of GBR-treated calvarial defect. At 120 days following operation, complete healing of the defect is observed with newly formed bone (from Donos et al. 2004).

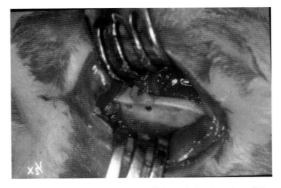

Figure 6.18. Augmentation of the inferior border of the mandible by autogenous mandibular bone graft (from Donos et al. 2002a).

plete bone healing following GBR has been reported in calvarial defects (Bosch et al. 1995; Dahlin et al. 1991; Hämmerle et al. 1992; Lundgren et al. 1992; Mardas et al. 2002), jaw bone defects (Dahlin et al. 1988, 1990, 1994; Kostopoulos and Karring 1994; Schenk et al. 1994), long bone defects (Bluhm and Laskin 1995; Nyman et al. 1995), cleft palate defects (Matzen et al. 1996), and zygomatic arch defects (Mooney et al. 1996).

Provision of space under the membrane is one of the factors that significantly affects the outcome following GBR procedures. It has been reported that collapse of the barrier membranes into the bone defect compromises the amount of newly formed bone by eliminating the space that is necessary for the bone to form (Dahlin et al. 1991; Kostopoulos and Karring 1994a, 1994b). Therefore the use of bone grafts under the occlusive barriers serving as space maintainers reduces the risk for compromised amounts of bone regeneration.

A number of bone grafts combined with GBR have been used in experimental studies in animals for bone regeneration of jaw bone augmentation with varying degrees of success. These include autogenous bone grafts (Alberius et al. 1992; Dahlin et al. 1991; Donos et al. 2002a, 2002b, 2002c, 2002d, 2005; Gordh et al. 1998; Jensen et al. 1995), demineralized bone matrix (Mardas et al. 2003), demineralized freeze-dried bone (DFDBA) (Buser et al. 1998), and xenografts such as deproteinized

bovine bone mineral (Bio-Oss) (Araujo et al. 2002; Donos et al. 2004, 2005; Stavropoulos et al. 2004a), as well as different bone substitutes such as coral-derived hydroxyapatite (HA) granules (Buser et al. 1998), tricalcium phosphate (Buser et al. 1998), bioactive glass (Stavropoulos et al. 2004b), and a biphasic calcium phosphate of HA/TCP (Jensen et al. 2007).

Experimental studies in animals have demonstrated that membranous-origin autogenous bone grafts tend to resorb less and maintain their volume to a greater extent than endochondral bone grafts (Phillips and Rahn 1988; Zins and Whitaker 1983). However, when both types of autogenous bone grafts were combined with GBR for augmentation of the jaws, this resulted in a more significant increase of the jaw dimensions irrespective of the embryonic origin of the graft (Donos et al. 2002d, 2005) (Figs. 6.18–6.24). It is interesting, though, to note that once the membrane was removed a decrease of the bone volume to the initial bone graft dimensions was observed, which was also more pronounced at the endochondral-origin bone grafts (Donos et al. 2005). Nevertheless, the achieved amount of bone formation was still significant and sufficiently adequate to augment a deficient bone site (Donos et al. 2005) (Figs. 6.25, 6.26).

In all these experimental studies it was indicated that the combination of autogenous

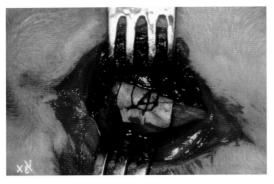

Figure 6.19. Augmentation of the inferior border of the mandible by autogenous mandibular bone graft and a Teflon membrane (from Donos et al. 2002a).

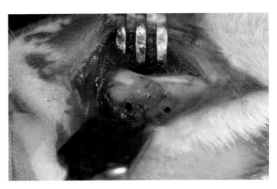

Figure 6.22. Lateral augmentation of the jaw with endochondral origin bone graft (from Donos et al. 2002d).

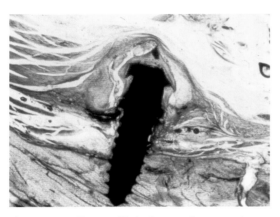

Figure 6.20. The mandibular bone graft presented complete resorption following 180 days of healing (from Donos et al. 2002a).

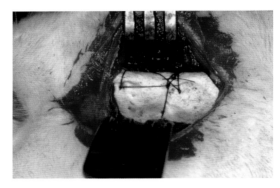

Figure 6.23. Lateral augmentation of the jaw with endochondral origin bone graft and GBR (from Donos et al. 2002d).

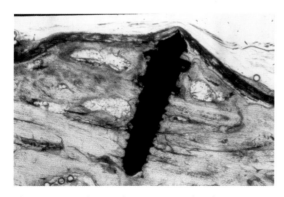

Figure 6.21. The site that was treated with autogenous mandibular bone grafts and GBR presented with integration of the bone graft into newly formed bone and increased jaw dimension at 180 days following operation (from Donos et al. 2002a).

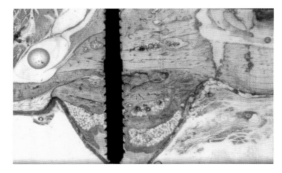

Figure 6.24. The endochondral origin bone graft is encapsulated into newly formed bone under the membrane and the dimensions of the jaw have been significantly increased (from Donos et al. 2002d).

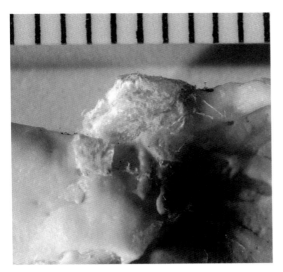

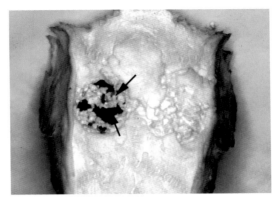

Figure 6.27. The Bio-Oss granules alone did not result in healing of the calvarial defect, whereas when they were combined with GBR the defect presented complete closure (from Donos et al. 2004).

Figure 6.25. Macerated specimen at 5 months following operation. Calvarial bone graft was combined with GBR for augmentation of the inferior border of the rat mandible (from Donos et al. 2005).

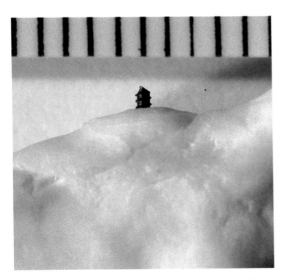

Figure 6.26. Macerated specimen at 11 months following operation and 6 months after membrane removal. The newly formed bone presented resorption to the level of the initial bone graft dimensions (from Donos et al. 2005).

bone grafts with GBR not only decreases the resorption of the bone grafts in comparison to bone grafting alone but also results in complete integration of the bone grafts into newly

formed bone at the recipient site (Alberius et al. 1992; Donos et al. 2002a, 2002b, 2002c, 2002d; Jensen et al. 1995; Lundgren et al. 1997).

In a clinical situation it would be advantageous not to use autogenous bone grafts due to the need for an operation in a second site and the risk for the morbidity of the donor site. The use of xenografts or bone substitutes with optimal bone graft properties (Prolo and Rodrigo 1985) would be an ideal situation when combined with GBR. When deproteinized bovine bone mineral has been used in combination with porcine origin collagen membranes for the treatment of critical-size defects (Donos et al. 2004), for lateral augmentation of the mandible (Araujo et al. 2002), or for augmentation of jaws under Teflon capsules (Donos et al. 2005; Stavropoulos et al. 2001), it was evident that even though clinically the defect/site appeared to be completely healed with newly formed bone (Fig. 6.27), the histological observations (Figs. 6.28, 6.29) indicated only a moderate amount of new bone formed at the base of the graft that was in proximity to the recipient site. As such, it could be suggested that when possible autogenous bone is still the graft of choice.

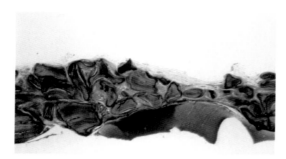

Figure 6.28. The Bio-Oss particles are encapsulated into fibrous connective tissue (from Donos et al. 2004).

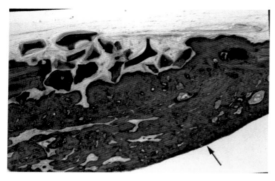

Figure 6.29. Significant intracranial bone formation has been achieved due to the space created by the Bio-Oss particles and the intracranial collagen membrane. At the center of the calvarial defect, though, the Bio-Oss particles are encapsulated into fibrous connective tissue and bone formation is observed only close to the margins of the defect (from Donos et al. 2004).

GBR in Conjunction with Dental Implants

A significant number of studies in experimental animals have demonstrated that the use of GBR alone or in combination with bone grafts results in predictable bone regeneration and coverage of the exposed implant threads when the simultaneous approach is used (Dahlin et al. 1989; Hämmerle et al. 1998; Piatelli et al. 1996; Rasmusson et al. 1997); or that osseointegration successfully takes place in

sites that have been previously regenerated/ augmented with GBR (Buser et al. 1995) as long as primary wound closure and no infection of the membrane is observed during healing.

In recent systematic reviews it has been concluded that the survival rate of implants in regenerated/augmented sites is similar to implants placed conventionally into sites without the need for bone augmentation (Fiorellini and Nevins 2003; Hämmerle et al. 2002). The survival rate of the implants was more than 90% after at least 1 year of function and the success rate of the GBR procedure (simultaneous and staged approach) per se ranged from 60% to 100% (Chiapasco et al. 2006). These procedures are currently used in everyday clinical practice with varying degrees of success (Hämmerle and Hellem 1999).

One of the difficulties in interpreting the data related to the success of the GBR procedure in terms of implant success and long-term preservation of the ridge dimension is that there is a limited number of controlled clinical trials where the success criteria of implants and GBR procedures have been clearly defined, or followed for a long period and compared to other augmentation procedures once the implants have been loaded. Furthermore, in the literature there is a great variety of combined treatments applied (type of membrane and type of bone graft used) as well as evaluation methods that make the long-term clinical outcomes related to GBR difficult to quantify (Chiapasco et al. 2006; Donos et al. 2008).

Taking into account that there is significant evidence in the literature (for review, see Chiapasco et al. 2006) to indicate that simultaneous and staged GBR results in predictable bone regeneration and implant osseointegration, it is important that future controlled clinical trials are performed in order to evaluate the effect of GBR procedure in the long-term success of the implants per se as well as in the long-term maintenance of the dimensions of the augmented site in comparison to other lateral augmentation techniques.

References

Adell R, Lekholm U, Rockler B, Brånemark PI. 1981. A 15-year study of osseointegrated implants in the treatment of the edentulous jaw. *Int J Oral Surg* 10(6): 387–416.

Alberius P, Dahlin C, Linde A. 1992. Role of osteopromotion in experimental bone grafting to the skull: A study in adult rats using a membrane technique. *J Oral Maxillofac Surg* 50(8):829–834.

Albrektsson T, Zarb G, Worthington P, Eriksson AR. 1986. The long-term efficacy of currently used dental implants: A review and proposed criteria of success. *Int J Oral Maxillofac Implants* 1(1):11–25.

Araujo MG, Sonohara M, Hayacibara R, Cardaropoli G, Lindhe J. 2002. Lateral ridge augmentation by the use of grafts comprised of autologous bone or a biomaterial. An experiment in the dog. *J Clin Periodontol* 29(12):1122–1131.

Atwood DA. 1962. Some clinical factors related to rate of resorption of residual ridges. *J Prosthet Dent* 86(2):119–125.

Becker W, Becker BE. 1990. Guided tissue regeneration for implants placed into extraction sockets and for implant dehiscences: Surgical techniques and case reports. *Int J Periodontics Restorative Dent* 10: 377–392.

Bell WH. 1975. Le Fort I osteotomy for correction of maxillary deformities. *J Oral Surg* 33:412–426.

———. 1980. Ridge augmentation as an aid in jaw surgery. In: *Surgical Correction of Dentofacial Deformities*. WH Bell, WR Proffit, and RP White (eds.). Philadelphia: Saunders. 1425–1433.

Blomqvist JE, Alberius P, Isaksson S. 1997. Sinus inlay bone augmentation: Comparison of implant positioning after one- or two-staged procedures. *J Oral Maxillofac Surg* 55:804–810.

Bluhm AE, Laskin DM. 1995. The effect of polytetrafluoroethylene cylinders on osteogenesis in rat fibular defects: A preliminary study. *J Oral Maxillofac Surg* 53(2): 163–166.

Bosch C, Melsen B, Vargervik K. 1995. Guided bone regeneration in calvarial bone defects using polytetrafluoroethylene membranes. *Cleft Palate–Craniofacial J* 32(4): 311–317.

Boyne PJ. 2001. Application of bone morphogenetic proteins in the treatment of clinical oral and maxillofacial osseous defects. *J Bone Joint Surgery America* 82A(Suppl 1 pt2):S146–S150.

Boyne PJ, James RA. 1980. Grafting of the maxillary sinus floor with autogenous marrow and bone. *J Oral Surg* 38: 613–616.

Boyne PJ, Lilly LC, Marx RE, et al. 2005. De Novo bone induction by recombinant human bone morphogenetic protein-2 (rhBMP-2) in maxillary sinus floor augmentation. *J Oral Maxillofac Surg* 63: 1693–1707.

Boyne PJ, Marx RE, Nevins M, et al. 1997. A feasibility study evaluating rhBMP-2/absorbable collagen sponge for maxillary sinus floor augmentation. *Int J Periodontics Restorative Dent* 17:10–25.

Brånemark PI, Zarb GA, Albrektsson T (eds.). 1985. *Tissue-Integrated Prostheses: Osseointegration in Clinical Dentistry.* Chicago: Quintessence.

Buser D, Brägger U, Lang NP, Nyman S. 1990. Regeneration and enlargement of jaw bone using guided tissue regeneration. *Clin Oral Implants Res* 1:22–32.

Buser D, Hoffmann B, Bernard JP, Lussi A, Mettler D, Schenk RK. 1998. Evaluation of filling materials in membrane-protected bone defects. A comparative histomorphometric study in the mandible of miniature pigs. *Clin Oral Implants Res* 9(3): 137–150.

Buser D, Ruskin J, Higginbottom F, Hardwick R, Dahlin C, Schenk RK. 1995. Osseointegration of titanium implants in bone regenerated in membrane-protected defects: A histologic study in the canine mandible. *Int J Oral Maxillofac Implants* 10(6):666–681.

Buser D, Schenk RK, Steinemann S, Fiorellini JP, Fox CH, Stich H. 1991. Influence of surface characteristics on bone integration of titanium implants. A histomorphometric study in miniature pigs. *J Biomed Mater Res* 25:889–902.

Camelo M, Nevins ML, Schenk RK, Lynch S, Nevins M. 2003. Periodontal regeneration in human class II furcations using purified recombinant human platelet-derived growth factor-BB (rhPDGF-BB) with bone allograft. *Int J Periodontics Restorative Dent* 23:213–225.

Carlsson GE, Persson G. 1967. Morphologic changes of the mandible after extraction and wearing of dentures. A longitudinal, clinical, and X-ray cephalometric study covering 5 years. *Odontologisk revy* 18(1): 27–54.

Cawood JI, Stoelinga PJ, Bonus JJ. 1994. Reconstruction of the severely resorbed (class VI) maxilla: A two-step procedure. *Int J Oral Maxillofac Surg* 23:219–225.

Chiapasco M, Zaniboni M, Boisco M. 2006. Augmentation procedures for the rehabilitation of deficient edentulous ridges with oral implants. *Clin Oral Implants Res* 17 Suppl 2:136–159.

Chin M. 1998. The role of distraction osteogenesis in oral and maxillofacial surgery. *J Oral Maxillofac Surg* 56(6):805–806.

Cochran DL, Schenk R, Buser D, Wozney JM, Jones AA. 1999. Recombinant human bone morphogenic protein-2 stimulation of bone formation around endosseous dental implants. *J Periodontol* 70:139–150.

Cochran DL, Wozney JM. 1999. Biological mediators for periodontal regeneration. *Periodontology 2000* 19:40–58.

Dahlin C, Gottlow J, Linde A, Nyman S. 1990. Healing of maxillary and mandibular bone defects using a membrane technique. An experimental study in monkeys. *Scand J Plast Reconstr Surg and Hand Surg* 24(1):13–19.

Dahlin C, Lekholm U, Becker W, Becker B, Higuchi K, Callens A, Van Steenberghe D. 1995. Treatment of fenestration and dehiscence bone defects around oral implants using the guided tissue regeneration technique: A prospective multicenter study. *Int J Oral Maxillofac Implants* 10:312–317.

Dahlin C, Lekholm U, Linde A. 1991. Membrane-induced bone augmentation at titanium implants. A report on ten fixtures followed from 1 to 3 years after loading. *Int J Periodontics Restorative Dent* 11(4):273–281.

Dahlin C, Linde A, Gottlow J, Nyman S. 1988. Healing of bone defects by guided tissue regeneration. *Plastic and Reconstructive Surg* 81(5):672–676.

Dahlin C, Linde A, Rockert H. 1993. Stimulation of early bone formation by the combination of an osteopromotive membrane technique and hyperbaric oxygen. *Scand J Plast Reconstr Surg and Hand Surg* 27(2): 103–108.

Dahlin C, Sandberg E, Alberius P, Linde A. 1994. Restoration of mandibular nonunion bone defects. An experimental study in rats using an osteopromotive membrane method. *Int J Oral Maxillofac Surg* 23(4): 237–242.

Dahlin C, Sennerby L, Lekholm U, Linde A, Nyman S. 1989. Generation of new bone around titanium implants using a membrane technique: An experimental study in rabbits. *Int J Oral Maxillofac Implants* 4(1):19–25.

Davarpanah M, Martinez H, Tecucianu J, Hage G, Lazzara R. 2001. The modified osteotome technique. *Int J Periodontics Restorative Dent* 21:599–607.

Donos N, Kostopoulos L, Karring T. 2002b. Alveolar ridge augmentation by combining autogenous mandibular bone grafts and non-resorbable membranes. *Clin Oral Implants Res* 13(2):185–191.

Donos N, Kostopoulos L, Karring T. 2002c. Alveolar ridge augmentation using a resorbable copolymer membrane and autogenous bone grafts. An experimental study in the rat. *Clin Oral Implants Res* 13(2): 203–213.

Donos N, Kostopoulos L, Karring T. 2002a. Augmentation of the mandible with GTR and onlay cortical bone grafting. An experimental study in the rat. *Clin Oral Implants Res* 13(2):175–184.

Donos N, Kostopoulos L, Karring T. 2002d. Augmentation of the rat jaw with autogeneic cortico-cancellous bone grafts and guided tissue regeneration. *Clin Oral Implants Res* 13(2):192–202.

Donos N, Kostopoulos L, Tonetti M, Karring T. 2005. Long-term stability of autogenous bone grafts following combined application with guided bone regeneration. *Clin Oral Implants Res* 16(2):133–139.

Donos N, Lang NP, Karoussis IK, Bosshardt D, Tonetti M, Kostopoulos L. 2004. Effect of GBR in combination with deproteinized bovine bone mineral and/or enamel matrix proteins on the healing of critical-size defects. *Clin Oral Implants Res* 15(1): 101–111.

Donos N, Mardas N, Chadha V. 2008. Clinical outcomes of implants following lateral bone augmentation: Systematic assessment of available options (barrier membranes, bone grafts, split osteotomy). *J Clin Periodontol*. In press.

Fiorellini JP, Howell TH, Cochran D, et al. 2005. Randomized study evaluating recombinant human bone morphogenetic protein-2 for extraction socket augmentation. *J Periodontol* 76:605–613.

Fiorellini JP, Nevins ML. 2003. Localized ridge augmentation/preservation. A systematic review. *Ann Periodontol* 8(1): 321–327.

Froum SJ, Tarnow DP, Wallace SS, Rohrer MD, Cho S-C. 1998. Sinus floor elevation using anorganic bovine bone matrix (OsteoGraf/N) with and without autogenous bone: A clinical, histologic, radiographic and histomorphometric analysis—part 2 of an ongoing prospective study. *Int J Periodontics Restorative Dent* 18:529–543.

Gelb DA. 1993. Immediate implant surgery: Three-year retrospective evaluation of 50 consecutive cases. *Int J Oral Maxillofac Implants* 8(4):388–399.

Gordh M, Alberius P, Johnell O, Lindberg L, Linde A. 1998. Osteopromotive membranes enhance onlay integration and maintenance in the adult rat skull. *Int J Oral Maxillofac Surg* 27(1):67–73.

Hämmerle CH, Brägger U, Schmid B, Lang NP. 1998. Successful bone formation at immediate transmucosal implants: A clinical report. *Int J Oral Maxillofac Implants* 13(4):522–530.

Hämmerle CH, Hellem S. 1999. Consensus report of Session F. In: *Proceedings of the 3rd European Workshop on Periodontology: Implant Dentistry*. Chicago: Quintessence. 609–614.

Hämmerle CH, Jung RE, Feloutzis A. 2002. A systematic review of the survival of implants in bone sites augmented with barrier membranes (guided bone regeneration) in partially edentulous patients. *J Clin Periodontol* 29(Suppl 3):226–231.

Hämmerle CH, Schmid J, Olah AJ, Lang NP. 1992. Osseous healing of experimentally created defects in the calvaria of rabbits using guided bone regeneration. A pilot study. *Clin Oral Implants Res* 3(3): 144–147.

Hanisch O, Tatakis DN, Boskovic MM, Rohrer MD, Wikesjö UME. 1997. Bone formation and reosseointegration in peri-implantitis defects following surgical implantation of rhBMP-2. *Int J Oral Maxillofac Implants* 12:604–610.

Howell TH, Fiorellini J, Jones A, et al. 1997. A feasibility study evaluating rhBMP-2/absorbable collagen sponge device for local alveolar ridge preservation of augmentation. *Int J Periodontics Restorative Dent* 17:125–139.

Jensen OT, Greer RO, Jr., Johnson L, Kassebaum D. 1995. Vertical guided bone-graft augmentation in a new canine mandibular model. *Int J Oral Maxillofac Implants* 10(3):335–344.

Jensen SS, Yeo A, Dard M, Hunziker E, Schenk R, Buser D. 2007. Evaluation of a novel biphasic calcium phosphate in standardized bone defects: A histologic and histomorphometric study in the mandibles of minipigs. *Clin Oral Implants Res* 18(6): 752–760.

Jovanovic SA, Hunt DR, Bernard GW, Spiekermann H, Wozney JM, Wikesjö UME. 2007. Bone reconstruction following implantation of rhBMP-2 and guided bone regeneration in canine alveolar ridge defects. *Clin Oral Implants Res* 8:224–230.

Karring T, Nyman S, Gottlow J, Laurell L. 1993. Development of the biological concept of guided tissue regeneration—animal and human studies. *Periodontology 2000* 1:26–35.

Kostopoulos L, Karring T. 1994a. Augmentation of the rat mandible using guided tissue regeneration. *Clin Oral Implants Res* 5(2):75–82.

Kostopoulos L, Karring T. 1994b. Guided bone regeneration in mandibular defects in rats using a bioresorbable polymer. *Clin Oral Implants Res* 5(2):66–74.

Kostopoulos L, Karring T, Uraguchi R. 1994. Formation of jawbone tuberosities by guided tissue regeneration. An experimental study in the rat. *Clin Oral Implants Res* 5(4):245–253.

Langer B, Calagna LJ. 1980. The subepithelial connective tissue graft. *J Prosthet Dent* 44(4):363–367.

Langer B, Calagna LJ. 1982. The subepithelial connective tissue graft. A new approach to the enhancement of anterior cosmetics. *Int J Periodontics Restorative Dent* 2(2):22–33.

Langer B, Langer L. 1999. Use of allografts for sinus grafting. In: *The Sinus Bone Graft.* O Jensen (ed.). Chicago: Quintessence. 69–72.

Lazzara RJ. 1989. Immediate implant placement into extraction sites: Surgical and restorative advantages. *Int J Periodontics Restorative Dent* 9:333–343.

Lundgren AK, Lundgren D, Sennerby L, Taylor A, Gottlow J, Nyman S. 1997. Augmentation of skull bone using a bioresorbable barrier supported by autologous bone grafts. An intra-individual study in the rabbit. *Clin Oral Implants Res* 8(2):90–95.

Lundgren D, Nyman S, Mathisen T, Isaksson S, Klinge B. 1992. Guided bone regenera-

tion of cranial defects, using biodegradable barriers: An experimental pilot study in the rabbit. *J Craniomaxillofac Surg* 20(6):257–260.

Mardas N, Kostopoulos L, Karring T. 2002. Bone and suture regeneration in calvarial defects by e-PTFE-membranes and demineralized bone matrix and the impact on calvarial growth: An experimental study in the rat. *J Craniofac Surg* 13(3):453–462.

Mardas N, Kostopoulos L, Stavropoulos A, Karring T. 2003. Osteogenesis by guided tissue regeneration and demineralized bone matrix. *J Clin Periodontol* 30(3):176–183.

Matzen M, Kostopoulos L, Karring T. 1996. Healing of osseous submucous cleft palates with guided bone regeneration. *Scand J Plast Reconstr Surg and Hand Surg* 30(3):161–167.

McGuire MK, Nunn M. 2003. Evaluation of human recession defects treated with coronally advanced flaps and either enamel matrix derivative or connective tissue. I: Comparison of clinical parameters. *J Periodontol* 74:1110–1125.

McGuire MK, Scheyer ET. 2006. Comparison of rhPDGF-BB plus beta tricalcium phosphate and a collagen membrane to subepithelial connective tissue grafting for the treatment of recession defects: A case series. *Int J Periodontics Restorative Dent* 26:127–133.

McGuire MK, Scheyer ET. 2007. A randomized, double-blind, placebo-controlled study to determine the safety and efficacy of cultured and expanded autologous fibroblast injections for the treatment of interdental papillary insufficiency associated with the papilla priming procedure. *J Periodontol* 78:4–17.

McGuire MK, Scheyer ET. 2008c. Evaluation of human recession defects treated with coronally advanced flaps and either BTCP+rhPDGF-BB+collagen membrane or connective tissue. Part I: Comparison of clinical parameters. In press.

McGuire MK, Scheyer ET. 2008a. Evaluation of human recession defects treated with coronally advanced flaps and either BTCP+rhPDGF-BB+collagen membrane or connective tissue. Part II: Human histological analysis. In progress.

McGuire MK, Scheyer ET. 2008b. A prospective, randomized-controlled study of Ossix™ Ossix Plus™ and Bio-Guide™ membranes used in guided bone regeneration of implant dehiscence and fenestration cases. Multi-center clinical trial. In progress.

McGuire MK, Scheyer ET, Nunn ME, Lavin PT. 2008. A pilot study to evaluate a tissue engineered bi-layered cell therapy as an alternative to tissue from the palate. *J Periodontol.* Accepted for publication.

Mellonig JT, Nevins M. 1995. Guided bone regeneration of bone defects associated with implants: An evidence based outcome assessment. *Int J Periodontics Restorative Dent* 15:169–182.

Mooney MP, Mundell RD, Stetzer K, Ochs MW, Milch EA, Buckley MJ, et al. 1996. The effects of guided tissue regeneration and fixation technique on osseous wound healing in rabbit zygomatic arch osteotomies. *J Craniofacial Surg* 7(1):46–53.

Nevins M, Camelo M, Nevins ML, Schenk RK, Lynch SE. 2003. Periodontal regeneration in humans using recombinant human platelet derived growth factor-BB (rhPDGF-BB) and allogeneic bone. *J Periodontol* 74:1282–1292.

Nevins M, Giannobile WV, McGuire MK, et al. 2005. Platelet-derived growth factor stimulates bone fill and rate of attachment level gain: Results of a large multicenter randomized controlled trial. *J Periodontol* 76:2205–2215.

Nevins M, Kirker-Head C, Nevins M, Wozney JA, Palmer R, Graham D. 1996. Bone formation in the goat maxillary sinus induced by absorbable collagen sponge implants impregnated with recombinant human bone morphogenetic protein-2. *Int J Periodontics and Restorative Dent* 16:9–19.

Nyman R, Magnusson M, Sennerby L, Nyman S, Lundgren D. 1995. Membrane-guided bone regeneration. Segmental radius defects studied in the rabbit. *Acta Orthopaedica Scandinavica* 66(2):169–173.

Phillips JH, Rahn BA. 1988. Fixation effects on membranous and endochondral onlay bone-graft resorption. *Plastic Reconstr Surg* 82(5):872–877.

Piattelli M, Scarano A, Piattelli A. 1996. Histological evaluation of freeze-dried dura mater (FDDMA) used in guided bone regeneration (GBR): A time course study in man. *Biomaterials* 17(24):2319–2323.

Prolo DJ, Rodrigo JJ. 1985. Contemporary bone graft physiology and surgery. *Clin Orthopaedics Related Res* 200:322–342.

Rasmusson L, Meredith N, Sennerby L. 1997. Measurements of stability changes of titanium implants with exposed threads subjected to barrier membrane induced bone augmentation. An experimental study in the rabbit tibia. *Clin Oral Implants Res* 8(4):316–322.

Schenk RK, Buser D, Hardwick WR, Dahlin C. 1994. Healing pattern of bone regeneration in membrane-protected defects: A histologic study in the canine mandible. *Int J Oral Maxillofac Implants* 9(1):13–29.

Scheyer ET, Velasquez-Plata D, Brunsvold MA, Lasho DJ, Mellonig JT. 2002. A clinical comparison of a bovine-derived xenograft used alone and in combination with enamel matrix derivative for the treatment of periodontal osseous defects in humans. *J Periodontol* 73(4):423–432.

Schmitz JP, Hollinger JO. 1986. The critical size defect as an experimental model for craniomandibulofacial nonunions. *Clin Orthopaedics Related Res* 205:299–308.

Sigurdsson TJ, Fu E, Tatakis DN, Rohrer MD, Wikesjö UME. 1997. Bone morphogenetic protein-2 for peri-implant bone regeneration and osseointegration. *Clin Oral Implants Res* 8:367–374.

Simion M, Baldoni M, Zaffe D. 1992. Jawbone enlargement using immediate implant placement associated with a split-crest technique and guided tissue regeneration. *Int J Periodontics Restorative Dent* 12:463–473.

Simion M, Jovanovic SA, Trisi P, Scarano A, Piatelli A. 1998. Vertical ridge augmentation around dental implants using a membrane technique and bone auto or allografts in humans. *Int J Periodontics Restorative Dent* 18:9–23.

Stavropoulos A, Kostopoulos L, Mardas N, Nyengaard JR, Karring T. 2001. Deproteinized bovine bone used as an adjunct to guided bone augmentation: An experimental study in the rat. *Clin Implant Dentistry Relat Res* 3(3):156–165.

Stavropoulos A, Kostopoulos L, Nyengaard JR, Karring T. 2004a. Fate of bone formed by guided tissue regeneration with or without grafting of Bio-Oss or Biogran. An experimental study in the rat. *J Clin Periodontol* 31(1):30–39.

Stavropoulos A, Sculean A, Karring T. 2004b. GTR treatment of intrabony defects with PLA/PGA copolymer or collagen bioresorbable membranes in combination with deproteinized bovine bone (Bio-Oss). *Clin Oral Investig* 8(4):226–232.

Summers RB. 1994a. A new concept in maxillary implant surgery: The osteotome technique. *Compend Contin Educ Dent* 15:152–160.

———. 1994b. The osteotome technique. Part 2: The ridge expansion osteotomy (REO) procedure. *Compend Contin Educ Dent* 15:422–436.

Tallgren A. 1967. The effect of denture wearing on facial morphology. A 7-year longitudinal study. *Acta Odontologica Scandinavica* 25(5):563–592.

Tarnow DP, Wallace SS, Froum SJ. 2000. Histologic and clinical comparison of bilateral sinus floor elevations with and without barrier membrane placement in 12 patients: Part 3 of an ongoing prospective study.

Int J Periodontics Restorative Dent 20: 116–125.

Tatum H, Jr. 1986. Maxillary and sinus implant reconstructions. *Dental Clinics of North America* 30:207–229.

Wallace SS, Froum SJ. 2003. Effect of maxillary sinus augmentation on the survival of endosseous dental implants. A systematic review. *Ann Periodontol* 8: 328–343.

Wennerberg A, Albrektsson T, Andersson B, Kroll JJ. 1995. A histomorphometric and removal torque study of screw-shaped titanium implants with three different surface topographies. *Clin Oral Implants Res* 6:24–30.

Wikesjö UME, Qahash M, Thomson RC, et al. 2004. rhBMP-2 significantly enhances guided bone regeneration. *Clin Oral Implants Res* 15:194–204.

Wikesjö UME, Sorensen RG, Kinoshita A, Wozney JM. 2002. RhBMP-2/alphaBSM induces significant vertical alveolar ridge augmentation and dental implant osseointegration. *Clin Implant Dent Relat Res* 4:174–182.

Wikesjö UME, Sorensen RG, Wozney JM. 2001. Augmentation of alveolar bone and dental implant osseointegration: Clinical implications of studies with rhBMP-2. *J Bone Joint Surgery America* 83A(Suppl I): S136–S145.

Yukna RA, Mellonig JT. 2000. Histologic evaluation of periodontal healing in humans following regenerative therapy with enamel matrix derivative. A 10-case series. *J Periodontol* 71:752–759.

Zins JE, Whitaker LA. 1983. Membranous versus endochondral bone: Implications for craniofacial reconstruction. *Plastic Reconstr Surg* 72(6):778–785.

Pre-implant Surgical Augmentation Interventions

HARD-TISSUE AUGMENTATION TO OSSEOINTEGRATE IMPLANTS

Friedrich W. Neukam, Emeka Nkenke, and Rainer Lutz

Introduction

Besides the possibility of augmenting deficient implant sites with autologous bone, which has the drawbacks of limited availability and donor site morbidity, or bone substitute materials that have the risk of infection or immunogenic or foreign body reaction (Nkenke et al. 2002; Raghoebar et al. 2007), local bone can be generated by guided bone formation techniques or distraction osteogenesis. These methods have the disadvantages of being complex and time-consuming, which makes them expensive and only administrable under certain circumstances.

Platelet-Rich Plasma

Growth factors as well as bone morphogenetic proteins can be found in the autologous platelet-rich plasma (PRP). Clinical trials seem to show that the combination of bone substitutes and growth factors such as cytokines contained in PRP may be suitable to enhance bone density (Kassolis et al. 2000; Marx et al. 1998). Fennis et al. (2002) reported an experimental study in goats evaluating a method of mandibular reconstruction with autogenous scaffolds and PRP. In this study, the use of PRP appeared to enhance bone healing considerably. In vitro studies showed that the combination of certain cytokines and growth factors increased osteoblast proliferation and differentiation (Lind 1996). Wiltfang et al. (2003) showed that new bone formation was supported to a small degree when using beta-tricalciumphosphate (TCP) in combination with PRP compared to TCP alone in sinus floor augmentation. New bone formation was 8–10% higher when PRP was applied. Similar results in maxillary sinus lift procedures were found when applying autologous bone in combination with PRP or autologous bone only. At the PRP-treated sites significantly enhanced new bone formation could be detected compared to autologous bone only after 3 months of healing. After 6 months, this effect could no longer be observed (Thor et al. 2007). No significantly positive effects could be found of PRP on the osseointegration of dental implants after maxillary sinus augmentation with autologous bone (Figs. 7.1, 7.2), bioglas (Figs. 7.3, 7.4), or a fluorohydroxyapatite after 1–12 months (Klongnoi et al. 2006a, 2006b).

These results were confirmed by Schlegel et al., who found no significant influence of PRP on the osseointegration of dental implants after maxillary sinus elevation with autologous bone (Figs. 7.5, 7.6) or hydroxyapatite (Fig. 7.7) (Schlegel et al. 2007).

These results corroborate those of other investigators, for example, De Vasconcelos Gurgel et al. (2007), who found no additional effects on bone healing in peri-implant bone defects treated with PRP compared to the control group. The mitogenetic cytokines found in PRP appeared to enhance bone healing considerably in the early phase of bone regeneration. Applying PRP in combina-

tion with autologous bone in critical-size bone defects in an established pig model, a significantly accelerating effect on early bone regeneration after 2 weeks was found (Schlegel et al. 2004). This effect was not evident when PRP was added to bovine collagen. After 4 weeks, mineralization values of autogenous bone grafting were significantly lower if PRP was added to the graft. After 12 weeks post-surgery, no difference could be seen between autologous bone graft with or without PRP (Schlegel et al. 2004). In this experimental setting PRP modulated the expression of the bone matrix proteins collagen I, osteocalcin, osteonectin, and osteopontin, but showed no long-term effects on bone formation (Thorwarth et al. 2006). In the same model, combination of xenogenic bone substitutes with PRP hardly influenced bony regeneration, degradation of the substitute materials, or cytokine expression (Wiltfang et al. 2004). Finally, PRP promotes new bone

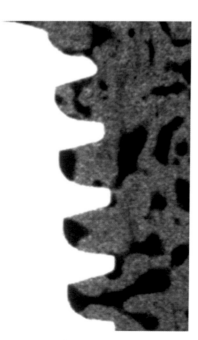

Figure 7.1. Microradiographic image of augmentation using autogenous bone at 12 months. From Klongnoi et al. 2006a.

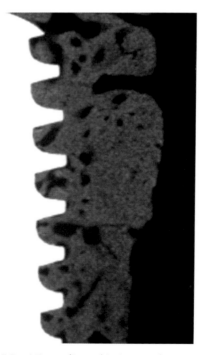

Figure 7.2. Microradiographic image of augmentation using autogenous bone with platelet-rich plasma at 12 months (×1.25). From Klongnoi et al. 2006a.

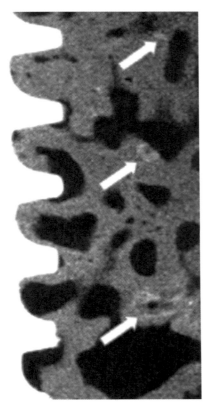

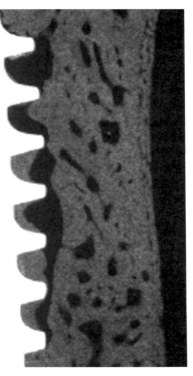

Figure 7.3. Microradiographic image of augmentation using Biogran® at 8 months (×1.25). Some particles of the Biogran® (arrows) could be partly identified. From Klongnoi et al. 2006a.

Figure 7.4. Microradiographic image of augmentation using Biogran® with platelet-rich plasma at 12 months (×1.25). Biogran® particles at this period were hardly identified. The newly formed bone did not exhibit a density comparable to that in the autogenous bone group. From Klongnoi et al. 2006a.

Figure 7.5. a. Microradiographic image of a sinus augmented with autogenous bone plus PRP at the final observation period of 52 weeks (×1.25). b. Same specimen in light microscopic image (toluidine blue O, original magnification × 1.25). From Schlegel et al. 2007.

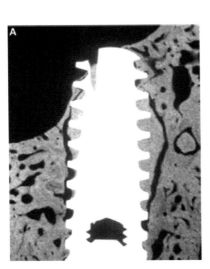

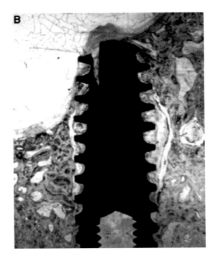

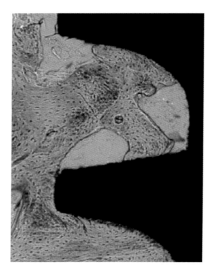

Figure 7.6. Autogenous bone plus PRP, light microscopy at 4 weeks. Graft material is already not clearly detectable (toluidine blue O, original magnification × 10). From Schlegel et al. 2007.

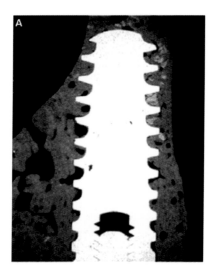

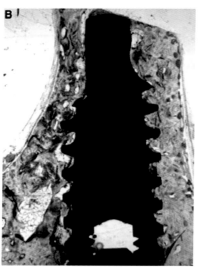

Figure 7.7. a. Microradiographic image of a sinus augmented with Bio-Oss plus PRP at the final observation period of 52 weeks (×1.25). b. Same specimen in light microscopic image (toluidine blue O, original magnification × 1.25). From Schlegel et al. 2007.

formation at an early stage of bone regeneration but shows no effects on long-term results. So one must question whether the use of PRP in combination with autologous bone grafting or bone substitute materials in hard-tissue augmentation is really worth the effort.

Bone Morphogenetic Proteins

An alternative of growing interest is the use of appropriate growth factors to induce new bone formation. Within the growth factors, bone morphogenetic proteins (BMPs) as a member of the TGF-β superfamily represent a group of proteins with mitogenetic and morphogenetic properties and therefore play an important role in bone regeneration (Urist et al. 1983). Since its discovery by Urist (1965), many attempts have been made to use BMP to heal or reconstruct bone. The establishment of techniques to clone recombinant human (rh) BMP simplified the production of BMP and made it available for clinical use

(Urist and Mikulski 1979; Urist et al. 1983). Currently, rhBMP is used clinically and results have shown that several BMP devices are promising for clinical use (Wang et al. 1990). An osteogenic capacity has been shown for the members of the BMP subfamily BMP-2, BMP-4 through 7, and BMP-9 (Wang et al.

1990; Wozney et al. 1988). BMP-2 is a potent osseoinductive factor (Wang et al. 1990) shown to induce osteogenic differentiation of mesenchymal cells, and further administration of recombinant BMP-2 protein in vivo is known to induce orthotopic and ectopic de novo bone formation (Cook et al. 1995; Govender et al. 2002). After demonstration of efficacy and safety in spinal-fusion cases the FDA approved the use of rhBMP-2 in human spine fusion procedures (Sucato et al. 2004). Regarding the use of BMPs in combination with dental implants, one has to distinguish between pre-implant augmentations, bone regeneration around compromised implants, and (due to lack of bone quantity) only partially inserted implants. Pre-implant augmentation of the alveolar ridge intends to create a quantitatively and qualitatively sufficient amount of bone for primary stable implant placement. Recently Dickinson et al. (2008) compared the healing process of BMP-2/resorbable collagen matrix constructs versus conventional iliac bone grafting in skeletally mature cleft patients. They found increased bone regeneration (95% vs. 63% defect filling) and fewer complications (11% vs. 50%) in the BMP-2 group. The patients in the BMP-2 group, of course, had no donor site morbidity, the mean length of stay was shorter, and the mean overall costs of the treatment were lower (Dickinson et al. 2008). Boyne (2001) could show complete regeneration of large continuity critical-sized defects (simulated hemimandibulectomy) after application of rhBMP in a collagen carrier with titanium orthopedic mesh fixation in Macaca monkeys after 5–6 months. In the same model, implants were applied in the regenerated bone and functionally loaded for 8 months. Increased bone density, bone volume, and thickness of the trabecular pattern were found, both in young and in older (>20 years) animals (Boyne 2001). Similar results were shown by Jovanovic et al. (2007), who found complete bone regeneration after application of rhBMP-2 combined with a collagen carrier in alveolar ridge defects. Partially inserted implants require primary stable inserted

implants and a stable carrier in order to induce peri-implant bone formation (Stenport et al. 2003). Another possibility is to release the BMP directly from the implant surface (Liu et al. 2007; Schliephake et al. 2005). Sailer and Kolb (1994) showed that purified, concentrated BMP preparations are able to achieve implant osseointegration in patients with compromised bone or soft-tissue conditions. However, long-term results on the performance of bone generated by BMPs are not presently available. Although encouraging results have been achieved with BMP-2 and other recombinant human BMPs (rhBMPs) in animal experiments and clinical applications, several problems, such as relatively high protein doses as well as a short protein half-life, are obstacles that still have to be overcome (Sellers et al. 2000). One possibility for overcoming these obstacles is to apply BMP-DNA via gene therapy and have the required BMP produced in the required defect site.

BMP Gene Therapy

Gene therapy can be applied with viral or nonviral vectors (Mehrara et al. 1999; Park et al. 2003). Although methods using adenoviruses and retroviruses are very efficient, they carry some risks, including possible immunological reactions and compromised safety. Retroviruses, in particular, promote long-term expression that is hard to control and has the risk of insertial mutagenesis. Although non-viral gene transfer provides only limited, transient gene expression (Bebök et al. 1996), the relatively short-term expression of a target protein using liposomal gene delivery, ranging from a few days to a few weeks, was shown to be sufficient for inducing bone regeneration in a critical-sized bone defect (Ono et al. 2004, Park et al. 2003). BMP gene therapy provides the possibility of applying BMP-2 cDNA to local cells, which then begin to produce and secrete BMP-2 protein. This has the advantage of continuous levels of BMP-2 protein secretion over a defined time period rather than a single administration of a large amount of protein (Baltzer and Lieberman 2004). Park et al. (2007) showed that direct application of the BMP-2 gene using a liposomal vector enhances bone regeneration in peri-implant defects, and gene delivery in combination with bone grafts leads to an efficient transfection (Fig. 7.8); this induces rapid bone regeneration (Fig. 7.9) and osseointegration of the bone-implant interface with enhanced bone-to-implant contact rates (Fig. 7.10) (Lutz et al. 2008).

These findings are comparable to the results of another examination using non-viral vectors in combination with a porous hydroxyapatite carrier. Efficient gene delivery was mainly achieved in mobilized cells surrounding the hydroxyapatite carrier (Ono et al. 2004). At present gene therapy is not used

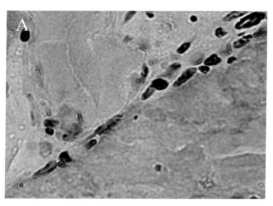
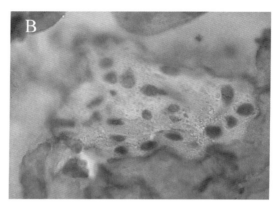

Figure 7.8. Most of the cells in the trabecular lining seemed to be osteoblasts and were still tightly bound to the bone chip surface. These cells stained positively for BMP-2 after immunohistochemical staining of the autologous/liposomal group at week 1; a: autologous bone graft/liposomal group, and b: autologous bone graft group. From Park et al. 2007.

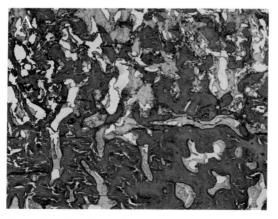
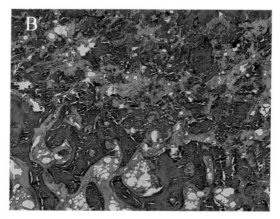

Figure 7.9. Rapid new bone matrix organization in a combined treatment of autologous bone graft/liposomal gene delivery. In the early stages of wound healing after bone graft, there was a clear difference in the bone matrix reorganization of particulated bone chips between the autologous bone graft/liposomal group (a) and the autologous bone graft group (b). One week after bone graft, new bone trabeculae were emerging directly from the particulated bone chips, and new bone matrix had already begun to be organized. From Park et al. 2007.

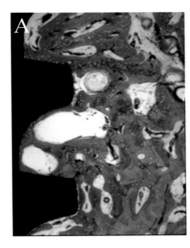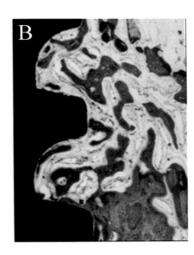

Figure 7.10. An enhanced bone-to-implant contact could be detected the collagen/BMP-2 liposmal vector group (a) compared to the collagen-only group (b). From Lutz et al. 2008.

in implant dentistry, but as there is a growing requirement for superior solutions to treat bone loss and improve implant osseointegration in compromised bone, it is conceivable that gene therapy approaches will reach the clinical settings within the next few years to decades. Till then much work remains to be done. If we intend to use these methods for clinical treatment we have to ensure that there are no risks to the patient's health. For that purpose liposomal vectors seem to be a promising approach.

Carrier Materials

Whether applying BMP as protein or BMP-DNA combined with a vector system the carrier plays an important role (Sigurdsson et al. 1996; Wikesjö et al. 1998). As the optimal carrier does not yet exist, some research also has to be done in this area. For spacing defects, for example, in sinus lifts, alveolar cleft defects, or peri-implant defects, collagen carriers have proven to be sufficient (Boyne et al. 1997; Dickinson et al. 2008; Li and Sun 2007; Park et al. 2007). Nevertheless, Stenport et al. (2003) could not induce supracrestal bone growth around partially inserted titanium implants with BMP combined with a collagen carrier, covered by a titanium mesh for stability, in a dog model after 16 weeks. It could be concluded that non-spacing defects require carrier materials with mechanical stability, such as hydroxyapatite (HA) or TCP, which bring the disadvantages of conventional bone substitute materials, even though it has been reported that addition of BMP speeds the degradation of the substitute materials and increases the amount of newly formed bone (Jung et al. 2003; Maus et al. 2008; Zhou et al. 2007). Here mechanically stable, resorbable materials with non-toxic degradation products and with defined releasing kinetics could decrease the amount of BMP required, making the therapy more effective and reducing the costs and possible side effects for the patients (Hosseinkhani et al. 2007; Schliephake et al. 2008).

Perspectives

The beneficial effects of BMPs in bone regeneration have been shown in several animal and preclinical studies. In the future one important aspect of research will be to determine the exact molecular mechanism of the influence of BMPs on bone regeneration. Understanding the pharmacodynamics of

BMPs in higher mammals will help to determine the optimal concentrations and releasing kinetics of BMPs, and also support development of superior carriers for BMP and gene therapy. Until now BMPs have been used in a pharmacological dosage, which is much higher than the physiological one. Possibly gene therapy could make the BMP therapy more similar to the physiological processes. As in nature, information in the form of DNA is delivered and the responsive cells produce the desired protein in a more biological concentration, enabling smart bone regeneration. Nowadays BMPs often are applied after conventional methods have failed. In the future BMP therapy could reduce the number of autologous bone grafts and the use of bone substitute materials in bone regeneration.

ONLAY AND INLAY GRAFTING IN IMPLANT REHABILITATION: CLINICAL ASPECTS

Karl-Erik Kahnberg

With clinical experience traversing over 40 years, implant rehabilitation has proven to be a safe and reliable procedure. Both edentulous jaws and partially dentated situations can be rehabilitated with success rates between 90 and 100% (Adell et al. 1990a; Albrektsson et al. 1986; Lindquist et al. 1996). Although the mandible provides the better quality bone, the maxilla also has enough bone volume to give a predictable outcome with conventional implant surgery. However, in cases with resorption of the alveolar process owing to loss of teeth from trauma, periodontitis, or caries, the situation becomes less predictable. But in the mandible, even in cases with severely resorbed jaw bones, it is usually possible to perform conventional implant therapy between the mental foramen. In the posterior mandible, the mandibular canal with the inferior alveolar nerve sets the limit for conventional implant surgery in resorption cases. In the maxilla, the bone is much more spongious and fragile than in

the mandible, owing to the fact that the mandible has the muscle insertion and is the mobile part in the chewing system. Furthermore, the nasal cavity and the maxillary sinus cavity occupy a large space in the maxilla and limit the volume of bone in the alveolar process.

Consequently, the indications for bone grafting are focused mostly on maxillary situations.

Onlay Grafting

The first attempt to increase the bone volume in severely resorbed maxillas was onlay grafting by use of bone blocks from the iliac bone (Adell et al. 1990b; Kahnberg et al. 1989; Nyström et al. 2002). The grafted bone was modeled to fit onto the crest, and the cortical bone in the crest was also perforated to facilitate bone healing. Large blocks of bone were attached to the residual crest with implant screws. Initially, these were one-stage surgical procedures with a healing time of 6 months or more. The clinical results in long-term follow-up varied between 70% and 85% implant survival and success rates. Problems that always arise in onlay procedures are soft-tissue closure and tension in the flap. If the flap is stretched too much the vascularization is compromised and there will be dehiscence, with eventual loss of bone graft. It can be technically difficult with large onlay grafts to cover the bone block satisfactorily without getting any entrances into the grafted area from the mouth, with subsequent inflammation. The one-stage surgical technique is also somewhat risky because the osseointegration of the implant does not occur until the grafted bone has become vascularized, so the integration period is prolonged. Yet there are many situations that call for onlay grafting, such as thin alveolar crests or defects due to trauma or infection, where buccal onlays are perfectly suitable. The two-stage technique is preferable, with bone graft healing as a first step and the implant surgery some months later.

Covering of the bone graft with resorbable membranes is, of course, possible but not always necessary.

Inlay Grafting

The bone grafting techniques have in many respects used orthognathic surgical techniques for bone augmentation in atrophied maxillas. The maxillary osteotomy according to Le Fort I (Sailer 1989) has been successful in both restoring the sagittal relation between the upper and lower jaws while at the same time providing the possibility of filling the sinus recesses and the nasal floor with bone graft material (Kahnberg et al. 1999, 2005). In addition to the conventional Le Fort I osteotomy technique, other techniques for attaching the bone graft and doing one- or two-stage surgery have varied among surgeons. Two-stage surgery with bone grafting and repositioning of the maxilla in one stage and 4 months later doing the implant installation is a safe and predictable technique with success and implant survival rates between 90% and 100%. Furthermore, the implants can be easily positioned in the direction optimal for the prosthetic rehabilitation.

The two-stage procedure is also more predictable with regard to the osseointegration process (Kahnberg et al. 2005).

The long-term outcome of bone grafts and implants concerning resorption of bone graft with the inlay method has been shown to be only minor resorption of the bone graft (1–1.5 mm) over 5 years in a prospective study (Kahnberg et al. 2005). Thus, functional loading of the inlay grafts is highly predictable. In cases of partial dentition of the upper jaw, where teeth are missing in the posterior maxilla and the volume of bone in the alveolar crest below the sinus cavity is minimal, the sinus lifting technique is advisable (Figs. 7.11, 7.12).

The sinus lifting technique is another inlay grafting technique. Sinus lift can be performed with many variations. The most common

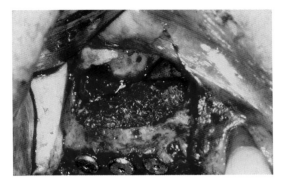

Figure 7.11. One-stage sinus lifting procedure with implants connected to the bone graft.

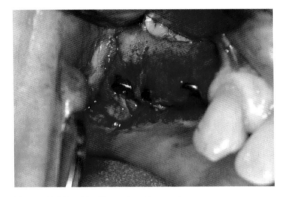

Figure 7.12. Healing after 6 months.

method is the buccal window technique, in which a circumferential window is made with a round or diamond burr or piezoelectric surgery on the buccal aspect of the sinus cavity. The idea is to approach the sinus membrane without perforating it. If it is perforated it has to be repaired with collagen membrane or, if possible, by suturing it.

After careful lifting of the sinus membrane, thereby exposing the sinus cavity bottom, bone graft material is placed in the sinus recess.

The methods of attaching the bone graft material vary from clinic to clinic; some surgeons do not immobilize their graft material while others use screws, plates, or wires (Fig. 7.13).

The method may also vary depending on the clinical situation. The sinus lifting

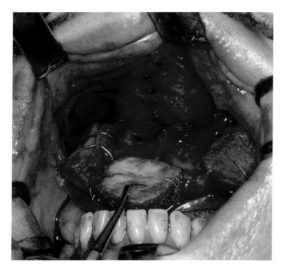

Figure 7.13. Maxillary osteotomy with bone graft attached to the sinus recesses and nasal cavity by use of wires.

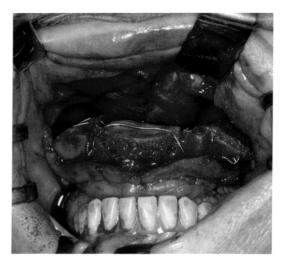

Figure 7.14. The alveolar crest reconstructed with bone graft.

procedure can be done either as a one-stage or two-stage procedure. In a one-stage procedure implants are placed simultaneously with the bone graft material (Kahnberg et al. 2001; Keller et al. 1999; Wannfors et al. 2000).

With one-stage protocol the bone tissue below the sinus cavity has to have a certain volume—at least 6–7 mm if not more—to stabilize the implants, otherwise there may be mobility in the graft material with the implants, initiating an inflammatory process with subsequent loss of both bone graft and implants.

The two-stage procedure with grafting first, then allowing for healing for about 4 months, and then implant placement is the most common (Kahnberg and Vannas-Löfqvist 2008; Krekmanov and Heimdahl 2000). This procedure is successful according to most publications, with implant survival and success rates between 85% and 100%. The complication that may arise is, of course, when there is a perforation of the sinus membrane. If the perforation is limited in size (3–4 mm) it is normally possible to cover it with a collagen membrane and still succeed with the operation. The sinus cavity is a closed space with drainage only through the osteum,

which is why infections can easily be established in sinus lifting procedures. Local sinus lifting can be done when a single tooth is missing in the posterior maxilla and the sinus cavity has extended down in to the alveolar process. For a local sinus lift we recommend using the implant as a tent pin to hold the sinus membrane, reserving the space around the implant for bone filling (Figs. 7.14–7.18).

The use of biomaterial instead of autologous bone is becoming increasingly popular. Bio-Oss and similar products function very well. The only criticism is that healing time is extended to almost 2–3 times that of natural bone. With the use of zygoma fixtures in resorbed maxillary cases, there are indications for use of this kind of implant. Zygoma implants should preferably be used in edentulous cases with available bone in the anterior region, for placement of three to four conventional implants. A combination of two zygoma implants and two to three conventional implants has a good success and implant survival rate (97%) (Kahnberg et al. 2007). However, the weak points of zygoma implants are the positioning of the implant from a prosthetic point of view and the passage through the alveolar process into the sinus

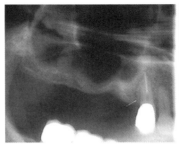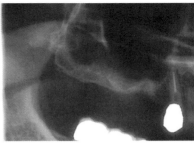

Figure 7.15. Maxillary sinus occupying the posterior part of a partially edentulous maxilla.

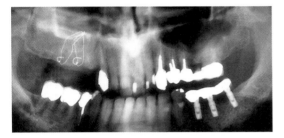

Figure 7.16. Bone graft reconstruction of the right posterior maxilla by sinus lifting procedure.

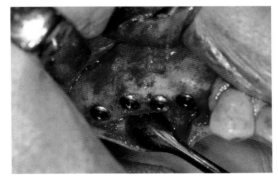

Figure 7.17. Complete healing of the bone graft after 4 months with implants inserted.

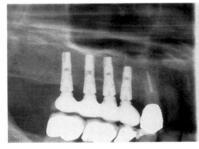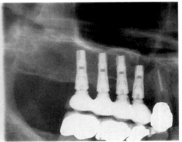

Figure 7.18. Radiograph with implants and bridge in place.

cavity, which, with sinus fistulas, can occasionally be problematic.

Summary

The use of bone grafts in implant rehabilitation will continue to play an important role for patients with bone deficiency. Although new and better implant surfaces are being developed, a certain amount of vital bone is still necessary in demanding cases. For extremely demanding cases necessitating major reconstructions, bone grafts will always be a key factor in the rehabilitation process.

IS AUTOGENOUS BONE STILL THE "GOLD STANDARD" FOR GRAFTING? CURRENT OPINION ON THE USE OF AUTOGRAFT IN IMPLANT DENTISTRY

Craig M. Misch

Introduction

Autogenous bone grafting is a well-documented procedure for reconstruction of the atrophic maxilla and mandible for restoration with implant prostheses. In many cases autogenous bone grafts continue to remain the gold standard for repair of jaw atrophy and bone defects, especially when there are larger bone defects and/or severe atrophy. However, clinical studies have found autogenous bone may not be necessary in the management of smaller intraosseous defects, localized bone augmentation procedures, and sinus bone grafting (Aghaloo and Moy 2007; Wallace and Froum 2003). A systematic review of the literature on hard-tissue augmentation techniques concluded that many alveolar ridge augmentation procedures lack detailed documentation or long-term follow-up studies (Aghaloo and Moy 2007). Comparing clinical studies on the use of autogenous bone versus bone substitutes and various graft techniques (i.e., guided bone regeneration vs. block bone grafting) is difficult. Many alveolar augmentation procedures are technique-sensitive and dependent on operator experience (Aghaloo and Moy 2007).

Advancements in biological engineering will produce alternatives to autogenous bone grafts that may well exceed existing clinical outcomes and replace traditional indications for their use (Boyne et al. 2005; Fiorellini et al. 2005). However, fewer clinical studies are available to evaluate the efficacy of tissue engineering for osseous reconstruction. In addition, the increased costs of technology can be an obstacle to routine use of new products. Autogenous bone grafting offers a well-proven, predictable method for ridge augmentation and defect repair for dental implant placement.

The use of autogenous bone with dental implants was originally discussed by Brånemark et al. (1975). Early studies focused on the use of iliac bone grafts in the treatment of the atrophic edentulous maxilla and mandible (Breine and Brånemark 1980). Although the iliac crest is most often used for major jaw reconstruction, it has the disadvantages of the need for hospitalization, general anesthesia, and alteration of ambulation. Additional donor sites have been evaluated including the calvarium, proximal tibia, and maxillofacial regions such as the mandibular symphysis and ramus. Autogenous bone can be used in several forms including cancellous marrow, particulate bone chips, or cortical and cortico-cancellous blocks. The timing of graft placement and implant insertion has been well researched. The preferred approach in most cases of onlay bone grafting is delayed implant placement into the healed bone graft. Earlier studies of machined screw-type implants often found lower survival rates in grafted bone (Breine and Brånemark 1980). The use of implants with enhanced microtextured surface features has improved outcomes in regenerated bone with success rates comparable to those in native bone (Wallace and Froum 2003).

Bone Graft Incorporation

Some clinicians are critical of block autograft techniques with concerns about graft resorption. Graft resorption to some degree is a necessary sequela of graft incorporation to the host site. The graft must be revascularized and remodeled through osteoclastic and osteoblastic activity (Burchardt 1983). The subject of embryologic origin of autologous bone grafts has received much attention regarding graft incorporation and resorption. Membranous bone grafts, from the mandible or calvarium, have been found to reveal less resorption than grafts from endochondral sites, such as the iliac crest (Hardesty and Marsh 1990; Smith and Abramson 1974; Zins and Whitaker 1983). Most studies examining the influence of graft origin on resorption refer to onlay augmentation with block bone grafts. It is important to make a distinction between the graft morphology (particulate, block) and whether the graft is used for onlay or interpositional placement. Interpositional bone grafts typically resorb less than bone used for onlay augmentation. Sinus floor augmentations are more comparable to interpositional rather than onlay bone grafts and therefore less resorption would be expected. More recent studies examining graft loss have challenged the hypothesis of embryologic origin and emphasize the microarchitecture of the bone used for grafting (Ozaki and Buchman 1998). Ozaki and Buchman (1998) found that regardless of their embryologic origin, cortical bone grafts reveal less volume loss than cancellous bone grafts. Cortical bone grafts from the mandible exhibit minimal resorption. Clinical studies have found cortical onlay grafts show a volume loss of less than 20% (Proussaefs et al. 2002). Upon incorporation they maintain their dense quality, making them ideal for onlay augmentation prior to implant placement (Misch et al. 1992).

The routine need for barrier membranes over block bone grafts has been debated. Cortical bone grafts exhibit minimal resorption and do not typically require membrane protection (Dongieux et al. 1998; Misch et al. 1992; Ozaki and Buchman 1998; Proussaefs et al. 2002). Grafts with a larger cancellous component and particulate grafts are more susceptible to volume loss. The use of a barrier membrane may improve the incorporation of the peripheral particulate graft around the block (Figs. 7.19–7.24).

Membranes should always be used with particulate grafts for ridge augmentation. Collagen membranes are preferred, as they are associated with fewer complications such as exposure and infection than PTFE membranes (Von Arx and Buser 2006). Another approach for particulate cancellous bone is to

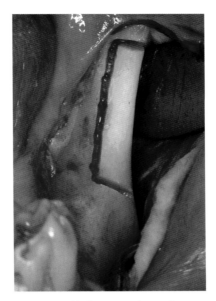

Figure 7.19. Mandibular ramus donor site.

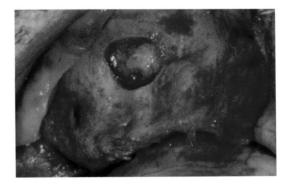

Figure 7.20. Maxillary sinus graft window.

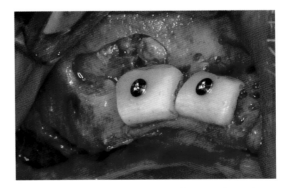

Figure 7.21. Cortical block onlay bone grafts and particulate sinus graft.

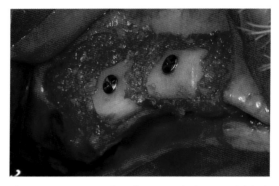

Figure 7.22. Particulate bone packed around block bone grafts.

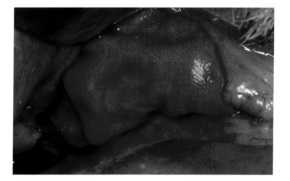

Figure 7.23. Collagen barrier membrane over bone graft site.

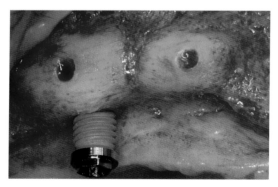

Figure 7.24. Four months graft healing for implant placement.

use titanium mesh to support and protect the graft during healing (Boyne and Peetz 1997).

The addition of supplemental autologous growth factors, such as platelet-rich plasma,

has been reported to enhance and accelerate the incorporation of autologous cancellous bone grafts (Marx et al. 1998). In addition, platelet-rich plasma may be useful as a matrix for soft-tissue repair, adhesion of bone graft particles, and for improving surgical hemostasis. Adding a prepared concentrate of the patient's platelets to the bone grafted site can also enhance and accelerate soft-tissue wound healing. The various cytokines and mediators found in the alpha granules of the platelets promote angiogenesis and collagen synthesis (Cromack et al. 1990). This may diminish the risk of wound dehiscence and bone graft exposure to the oral cavity.

Smoking has been associated with a high rate of wound dehiscence and graft failure (Levin and Schwartz-Arad 2005). A smoking cessation protocol is followed, including the use of prescription medications such as bupropion and the nicotine patch. Patients are instructed to quit 1 week prior to surgery and told not to smoke at least until the incision is completely closed approximately 2 weeks later.

Autogenous Bone Graft Donor Sites

Mandibular Symphysis

The symphysis of the mandible has been used extensively for sinus and onlay bone grafting (Jensen et al. 1994; Khoury 1999; Lundgren et al. 1996; Misch 1997; Misch et al. 1992). The symphysis donor site offers the greatest volume of intraoral bone. The average interforaminal distance is approximately 5.0 cm and the depth of the anterior mandible usually exceeds 1.0 cm (Buhr and Coulon 1996). The ease of surgical access is another advantage of the symphysis region.

The mandibular symphysis is associated with a higher incidence of postoperative complications than other intraoral donor sites (Hallman et al. 2002; Nkenke et al. 2001; Raghoebar et al. 2001). Altered sensation of the lower anterior teeth is a relatively common postoperative symptom when bone blocks are removed (Hallman et al. 2002; Misch et al. 1992; Nkenke et al. 2001; Raghoebar et al. 2001). Patients describe dullness in sensation of the incisors, which usually resolves within 6 months. The need for endodontic treatment of anterior teeth is very rare. Neurosensory disturbances in the chin region also may be encountered, even when a sulcular incision is used (Hallman et al. 2002; Nkenke et al. 2001; Raghoebar et al. 2001). The incidence of temporary mental nerve paraesthesia for symphysis graft patients is usually low but has been found to be as high as 43% (Raghoebar et al. 2001). Although the vast majority of these nerve injuries recover, they are disconcerting to patients. It is prudent to discuss the possibility of temporary altered sensation of the teeth and chin prior to surgery. Although no postoperative alteration in soft-tissue chin contour has been reported, patients are often concerned with the possible aesthetic consequences of bone removal from this area. Filling the donor site with a resorbable bone substitute can help alleviate the patient's concerns (Misch et al. 1992).

Mandibular Ramus

The posterior mandible is an excellent donor site for bone harvest. Although the ramus donor site provides a thinner cortical graft than the symphysis the peripheral dimensions of a graft can approach 4.0 × 1.5 cm. The buccal cortex of the posterior mandible measures 3.0–4.0 mm, making this donor site ideal for veneer onlay grafting (Smith et al. 1991). The ramus is the preferred donor site for single tooth and small segment defects requiring width augmentation (Misch 1996, 2000). It is also the preferred harvest area for the narrow posterior mandible, as the donor and recipient sites are in the same surgical field (Misch 1996, 2000).

Compared with the symphysis region, the ramus donor site is associated with a much lower incidence of complications (Misch 1996, 1997, 2000). Patients have shown less

concern with bone removal from the ramus area. The masseter muscle provides soft-tissue bulk and augmentation of this donor site has been unnecessary. Neurosensory disturbances from bone harvest are uncommon if osteotomies are properly planned around the position of the mandibular canal (Misch 1996, 2000). Ramus graft patients appear to have fewer difficulties with managing postoperative edema and pain compared with chin graft surgery (Misch 1997). Patients may experience trismus following surgery and should be placed on postoperative glucocorticoids and non-steroidal anti-inflammatory medications to help reduce dysfunction. The mandibular ramus has significantly less morbidity than the symphysis and has become the preferred donor site of many clinicians (Peleg et al. 2004).

Tibia

The proximal tibial metaphysis provides an excellent source of cancellous bone for grafting (Catone et al. 1992; Mazock et al. 2004; O'Keefe et al. 1991). This donor site offers up to 40 ml of cancellous bone with low reported morbidity (Catone et al. 1992; Mazock et al. 2004). The surgery may be performed in an office environment. The most common approach to the donor site is laterally at Gerdy's tubercle, a bony protuberance located 1.5 cm below the articulating surface of the tibia (Catone et al. 1992; Mazock et al. 2004). There has been a low reported incidence of significant complications with this procedure (Catone et al. 1992; Chen et al. 2006; Mazock et al. 2004; O'Keefe et al. 1991). Complications may include hematoma formation, wound dehiscence, infection, and, rarely, fracture.

Ilium

The grafting of larger areas of bone deficiency often requires bone harvest from the ilium. As the tibia offers a convenient site for harvesting cancellous bone, the ilium is most often reserved for cases requiring corticocancellous block grafting. In most cases adequate bone may be harvested using an anterior approach to the hip. A posterior approach to the ilium is less often required and is usually reserved for major reconstructive surgeries requiring large amounts of cancellous bone. In addition, the need to rotate the patient after posterior bone harvest is an inherent disadvantage. Although posterior bone harvest is reported to result in lower postoperative pain (Nkenke et al. 2004), the use of an anesthetic pain pump can minimize the problem with anterior harvest (Hahn et al. 1996). The iliac crest is usually cut along its length for unicortical bone harvest, leaving the opposing cortex intact. When thicker pieces of bone are needed for vertical bone augmentation a bicortical bone graft may be harvested from the entire width of the crest. This graft geometry is typically used for reconstructing the severely atrophic premaxilla.

Sinus Bone Grafting

Over the years numerous bone graft materials including autografts, allografts, alloplasts, xenografts, and combinations have been successfully used for sinus grafting. The 1996 Sinus Graft Consensus evaluated retrospective data on various graft materials and concluded that they all seemed to perform well (Jensen et al. 1998). However, the data analysis did not factor the amount of residual bone below the sinus. Three systematic reviews of the literature on sinus bone grafting have determined that implants placed into sinuses grafted with autogenous bone and/or bone substitutes produce high implant survival rates (Aghaloo and Moy 2007; Del Fabbro et al. 2004; Wallace and Froum 2003). At this time, comparative studies using different graft materials (i.e., autograft vs. xenograft) may be of less value (Aghaloo and Moy 2007). Although de novo bone growth has been reported with the use of recombinant human

bone morphogenetic protein, the dental implant survival rate was much lower than numerous studies using bone substitutes (84%) (Boyne et al. 2005). It may be concluded that the choice of bone substitutes for sinus grafting may be considered in most cases.

There are many advantages in using some autologous bone in sinus grafts, especially when minimal bone remains below the sinus floor (Block and Kent 1997; Misch 2002). Several studies have found an increase in bone formation when autologous bone is used alone or added to other grafting materials in sinus grafts (Block and Kent 1997; Froum et al. 1998; Jensen and Sennerby 1998; Lorenzetti et al. 1998). Froum et al. (1998) found a statistically significant increase in vital bone formation when as little as 20% autologous bone was added to bovine-derived grafts. The use of a barrier membrane over the sinus window has also been advocated to increase bone formation when bone substitutes are used (Tarnow et al. 2000). A membrane may not be necessary when a significant portion of the graft is autologous bone.

The healing time requirements of autologous bone grafts are shorter, compared to bone substitutes, especially in larger pneumatized sinuses. The healing period for sinuses grafted with autologous bone can be as short as 3–4 months compared to the 8–10 months often recommended for bone substitutes (Froum et al. 1998) (Figs. 7.25–7.27).

The addition of autologous bone to composite bone grafts can also shorten healing times (Froum et al. 1998; Hallman et al. 2002). This offers a significant advantage, as patients often object to extended treatment lengths. Froum et al. (1998) found a mean vital bone formation of 27.1% at 6–9 months after sinus grafting with mostly bovine hydroxylapatite and a small amount of autogenous bone (20%).

It is also beneficial to use autologous bone for sinus grafting when additional simultaneous onlay augmentation is desired. However, implants placed in sinuses augmented with particulate grafts show higher survival rates

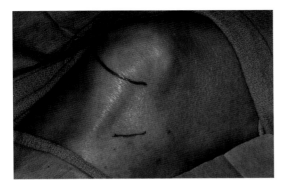

Figure 7.25. Proximal tibia cancellous bone graft donor site.

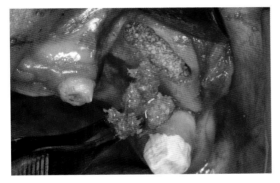

Figure 7.26. Composite graft of cancellous autograft and bovine hydroxylapatite used for sinus augmentation in a pneumatized sinus.

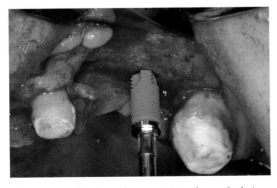

Figure 7.27. Implant placement into the grafted sinus after 4 months healing.

than those placed into sinuses augmented with block grafts (Wallace and Froum 2003). The posterior maxilla resorbs medially following tooth loss and this pattern of bone loss often results in an unfavorable ridge relationship with the opposing lower dentition. It is not unusual to require sinus bone grafting to increase the vertical bone dimension as well as onlay bone grafting to augment the ridge width and/or correct bone deficiencies in the posterior maxilla. Autologous bone may be harvested for sinus bone grafting and simultaneous residual ridge reconstruction using autologous block grafts. The healing period of the onlay block and sinus bone grafts will be similar, allowing for earlier implant placement. This approach may be preferred to a staged reconstruction where sinus grafting is performed first using bone substitutes and autologous block bone grafts are placed at a later date. Not only do autologous bone grafts heal faster than bone substitutes, the quality of the regenerated bone is often better. Histological studies have shown greater bone formation and higher bone-implant contact when autologous bone grafts are used compared with allografts (Jensen and Sennerby 1998). This improved bone formation at an earlier time can allow for shorter implant healing periods compared to the use of bone substitutes.

Ridge Augmentation

In the reconstruction of larger bone defects and severe atrophy autogenous bone has been the preferred graft material. Bone substitutes, such as allografts, alloplasts, and xenografts, lack the regenerative capacity required for large volumes of bone regeneration. Although guided bone augmentation techniques utilizing barrier membranes have proven to be useful in managing localized defects, they have limited application in large areas of bone loss (Aghaloo and Moy 2007). The use of tissue engineering with growth factors, such as rhBMP-2, holds great promise for

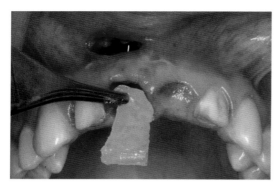

Figure 7.28. rhBMP-2 used with a collagen sponge for socket defect repair.

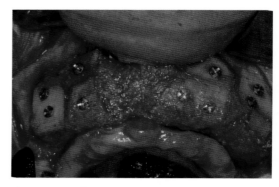

Figure 7.29. Iliac corticocancellous block bone grafts used to reconstruct the maxilla following facial fractures and tooth avulsion.

replacing the need for autogenous bone harvest. However, onlay augmentation requires structural integrity of the graft matrix especially when soft-tissue compression is present.

The development of suitable carriers for the growth factors with proper scaffold properties will be necessary for reconstructing larger defects (Wozney and Wikesjö 2008). The collagen sponge appears to be a suitable matrix for interpositional bone grating such as socket defects (Fig. 7.28).

Implant Placement in Onlay Bone Grafts

Reconstruction of the atrophic jaws for implant placement is usually staged, with implant placement after graft healing. Previous studies on simultaneous bone graft and implant placement reveal lower success rates, unpredictable bone remodeling, and diminished bone-to-implant contact (Adell et al. 1990b; Breine and Brånemark 1980; Jensen et al. 1994). Onlay bone grafts should be allowed to incorporate prior to dental implant placement. Enough time should elapse for graft incorporation, but implants should be inserted early enough to stimulate and maintain the regenerated bone (Nyström et al. 1996) (Figs. 7.29–7.31).

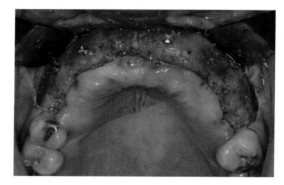

Figure 7.30. Incorporation of the bone graft after 4 months healing.

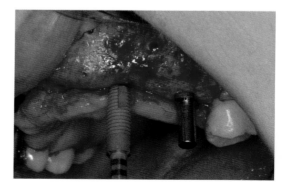

Figure 7.31. Placement of implants into the onlay grafted maxilla after graft remodeling.

Autogenous block grafts should heal for approximately 4 months before implant placement (Matsumoto et al. 2002; Misch et al. 1992). Particulate cancellous bone grafts with barrier membranes or titanium mesh used for ridge augmentation often require longer healing periods of at least 6 months.

The placement of implants into healed bone grafts is similar to their use in sites that have not been grafted. However, the implant site is often at the junction between the block and host bone. The surgeon should be careful not to displace the block from the ridge during the implant osteotomy and placement. Fixation screws are usually removed prior to implant insertion. Elevation of large flaps simply for screw removal is discouraged as this disrupts the vascular supply to the healed graft. Small mucosal incisions over the screw heads allows for easy retrieval. If a fixation screw is not in the path of implant insertion it may be left intact, especially if it will provide added stability to the graft.

The healing period of implants placed into incorporated bone grafts is similar to native bone. Microtextured implant surfaces have diminished healing implant periods to as little as 6 weeks (Attard and Zarb 2005). Immediate implant loading in grafted bone may even be considered if primary implant stability is adequate. Additional graft resorption following implant placement and delayed loading has not been noted radiographically (Buser et al. 2002).

References

Adell R, Eriksson B, Lekholm U, Brånemark PI, Jemt T. 1990a. A long-term follow-up study of osseointegrated implants in the treatment of totally edentulous jaws. *Int J Oral Maxillofac Implants* 5:347–359.

Adell R, Lekholm U, Gröndahl K, Brånemark PI, Lindström J, Jacobsson M. 1990b. Reconstruction of severely resorbed edentulous maxillae using osseointegrated fixtures in immediate autogenous bone grafts. *Int J Oral Maxillofac Implants* 5: 233–246.

Aghaloo TL, Moy PK. 2007. Which hard tissue augmentation techniques are the most successful in furnishing bony support for implant placement? *Int J Oral Maxillofac Implants* 22(Suppl):49–70.

Albrektsson T, Zarb G, Worthington P, Eriksson A. 1986. The long-term efficacy of currently used dental implants: A review and proposed criteria of success. *Int J Oral Maxillofac Implants* 1:11–25.

Attard NJ, Zarb GA. 2005. Immediate and early implant loading protocols: A literature review of clinical studies. *J Prosthet Dent* 94:242–258.

Baltzer AW, Lieberman JR. 2004. Regional gene therapy to enhance bone repair. *Gene Ther* 11(4):344–350.

Bebök Z, Abai AM, Dong JY, King SA, Kirk KL, Berta G, Hughes BW, Kraft AS, Burgess SW, Shaw W, Felgner PL, Sorscher EJ. 1996. Efficiency of plasmid delivery and expression after lipid-mediated gene transfer to human cells in vitro. *J Pharmacol Exp Ther* 279(3):1462–1469.

Block MS, Kent JN. 1997. Sinus augmentation for dental implants: The use of autogenous bone. *J Oral Maxillofac Surg* 55: 1281–1286.

Boyne PJ. 2001. Application of bone morphogenetic proteins in the treatment of clinical oral and maxillofacial osseous defects. *J Bone Joint Surg Am* 83-A Suppl 1 (Pt 2):S146–150.

Boyne PJ, Lilly LC, Marx RE, Moy P, Nevins M, Spagnoli DB, Triplett RG. 2005. De novo bone induction by recombinant human bone morphogenic protein-2 (rhBMP-2) in maxillary sinus floor augmentation. *J Oral Maxillofac Surg* 63: 1693–1707.

Boyne PJ, Marx RE, Nevins M, Triplett G, Lazaro E, Lilly LC, Alder M, Nummikoski P. 1997. A feasibility study evaluating rhBMP-2/absorbable collagen sponge for maxillary sinus floor augmentation. *Int J Periodontics Restorative Dent* 17(1): 11–25.

Boyne PJ, Peetz M. 1997. *Osseous Reconstruction of the Maxilla and Mandible: Surgical Techniques Using Titanium Mesh and Bone Mineral.* Carol Stream, IL: Quintessence. 1–100.

Brånemark PI, Lindstrom J, Hallen O. 1975. Reconstruction of the defective mandible. *Scand J Plast Reconstr Surg* 9:116–128.

Breine U, Brånemark PI. 1980. Reconstruction of alveolar jaw bone. An experimental and clinical study of immediate and preformed autologous bone grafts in combination with osseointegrated implants. *Scand J Plast Reconstr Surg* 14(1):23–48.

Buhr W, Coulon JP. 1996. Limits of the mandibular symphysis as a donor site for bone grafts in early secondary cleft palate osteoplasty. *Int J Oral Maxillofac Surg* 25: 389–393.

Burchardt H. 1983. The biology of bone graft repair. *Clin Orthop Relat Res* 174:28–42.

Buser D, Ingimarsson S, Dula K. 2002. Long-term stability of osseointegrated implants in augmented bone: A 5-year prospective study in partially edentulous patients. *Int J Periodontics Restorative Dent* 22: 108–117.

Catone GA, Reimer LB, McNeir D. 1992. Tibial autogenous cancellous bone as an alternative donor site in maxillofacial surgery: A preliminary report. *J Oral Maxillofac Surg* 50:1258–1263.

Chen YC, Chen CH, Chen PL, Huang IY, Shen YS, Chen CM. 2006. Donor site morbidity after harvesting of proximal tibia bone. *Head Neck* 28(6):496–500.

Cook SD, Wolfe MW, Salkeld SL, Rueger DC. 1995. Effect of recombinant human osteogenic protein-1 on healing of segmental defects in non-human primates. *J Bone Joint Surg Am* 77(5):734–750.

Cromack DT, Porras-Reyes B, Mustoe TA. 1990. Current concepts in wound-healing: Growth-factor and macrophage interaction. *J Trauma* 30(12):S129–133.

De Vasconcelos Gurgel BC, Goncalves PF, Pimentel SP, Ambrosano GM, Nociti FH, Jr., Sallum EA, Casati MZ. 2007. Platelet-rich plasma may not provide any additional effect when associated with guided bone regeneration around dental implants in dogs. *Clin Oral Implants Res* 18(5): 649–654.

Del Fabbro M, Testori T, Francetti L, Weinstein R. 2004. Systematic review of survival rates for implants placed in the grafted maxillary sinus. *Int J Periodontics Restorative Dent* 24:565–577.

Dickinson BP, Ashley RK, Wasson KL, O'Hara C, Gabbay J, Heller JB, Bradley JP. 2008. Reduced morbidity and improved healing with bone morphogenic protein-2 in older patients with alveolar cleft defects. *Plast Reconstr Surg* 121(1):209–217.

Dongieux JW, Block MS, Morris G, Gardiner D. 1998. The effect of different membranes on onlay bone graft success in the dog mandible. *Oral Surg Oral Med Oral Pathol Oral Radiol Endod* 86:145–151.

Fennis JP, Stoelinga PJ, Jansen JA. 2002. Mandibular reconstruction: A clinical and radiographic animal study on the use of autogenous scaffolds and platelet-rich plasma. *Int J Oral Maxillofac Surg* 31(3): 281–286.

Fiorellini JP, Howell TH, Cochran D, et al. 2005. Randomized study evaluating recombinant human bone morphogenetic protein-2 for extraction socket augmentation. *J Periodontol* 76:605–613.

Froum SJ, Tarnow DP, Wallace SS, Rohrer MD, Cho SC. 1998. Sinus floor elevation using anorganic bovine bone matrix (OsteoGraf/N) with and without autogenous bone: A clinical, histologic, radiographic and histomorphometric analysis—Part 2 of an ongoing study. *Int J Periodont Rest Dent* 18:529–543.

Govender S, Csimma C, Genant HK, Valentin-Opran A, Amit Y, Arbel R, Aro H, Atar D, et al. 2002. Recombinant human bone morphogenetic protein-2 for treatment of open tibial fractures: A prospective, controlled, randomized study of four hundred and fifty patients. *J Bone Joint Surgery America* 84-A(12):2123–2134.

Hahn M, Dover MS, Whear NM, Moule I. 1996. Local bupivacaine infusion following bone graft harvest from the iliac crest. *Int J Oral Maxillofac Surg* 25(5): 400–401.

Hallman M, Hedin M, Sennerby L. 2002. A prospective 1-year clinical and radiographic study of implants placed after maxillary sinus floor augmentation with bovine hydroxylapatite and autogenous bone. *J Oral Maxillofac Surg* 60:277–284.

Hardesty RA, Marsh JL. 1990. Craniofacial onlay bone-grafting: A prospective evaluation of graft morphology, orientation, and embryonic origin. *Plast Reconstruct Surg* 85:5–14.

Hosseinkhani H, Hosseinkhani M, Khademhosseini A, Kobayashi H. 2007. Bone regeneration through controlled release of bone morphogenetic protein-2 from 3-D tissue engineered nano-scaffold. *J Control Release* 117(3):380–386.

Jensen J, Sindet-Petersen S, Oliver AJ. 1994. Varying treatment strategies for reconstruction of maxillary atrophy with implants: Results in 98 patients. *J Oral Maxillofac Surg* 52:210–216.

Jensen OT, Sennerby L. 1998. Histological analysis of clinically retrieved titanium microimplants placed in conjunction with maxillary sinus floor augmentation. *Int J Oral Maxillofac Implants* 13:513–521.

Jensen OT, Shulman LB, Block MS, Iacono VJ. 1998. Report of the Sinus Consensus Conference of 1996. *Int J Oral Maxillofac Implants* 13(Suppl):11–45.

Jovanovic SA, Hunt DR, Bernard GW, Spiekermann H, Wozney JM, Wikesjo UM. 2007. Bone reconstruction following implantation of rhBMP-2 and guided bone regeneration in canine alveolar ridge defects. *Clin Oral Implants Res* 18(2): 224–230.

Jung RE, Glauser R, Scharer P, Hammerle CH, Sailer HF, Weber FE. 2003. Effect of rhBMP-2 on guided bone regeneration in humans. *Clin Oral Implants Res* 14(5): 556–568.

Kahnberg KE, Ekestubbe A, Gröndahl K, Nilsson P, Hirsch J-M. 2001. Sinus lifting procedure. I: One-stage surgery with bone transplant and implants. *Clin Oral Implants Res* 12:478–487.

Kahnberg KE, Henry PJ, Hirsch J-M, Öhrnell LO, Andreasson L, Brånemark PI, Chiapasco M, Gynther G, Finne K, Higuchi KW, Isaksson S, Malevez C, Neukam FW, Sevetz E, Jr., Urgell JP, Widmark G, Bolind P. 2007. Clinical evaluation of the zygoma implant: 3-year follow-up at 16 clinics. *J Oral Maxillofac Surg* 65:2033–2038.

Kahnberg KE, Nilsson P, Rasmusson L. 1999. Le Fort I osteotomy with interpositional bone grafts and implants for rehabilitation of the severely resorbed maxilla: A 2-stage procedure. *Int J Oral Maxillofac Implants* 14:571–578.

Kahnberg KE, Nyström E, Bartholdsson L. 1989. Combined use of bone grafts and Brånemark fixtures in the treatment of severely resorbed maxillae. *Int J Maxillofac Implants* 4:297–304.

Kahnberg KE, Vannas-Löfqvist L. 2005. Maxillary osteotomy with interpositional bone graft and implants for reconstruction of the severely resorbed maxilla. A clinical report. *Int J Oral Maxillofac Implants* 20: 938–945.

Kahnberg KE, Vannas-Löfqvist L. 2008. Sinus lifting procedure using a two-stage surgical technique. I: Clinical and radiographic study up to 5 years. In manuscript.

Kassolis JD, Rosen PS, Reynolds MA. 2000. Alveolar ridge and sinus augmentation utilizing platelet-rich plasma in combination with freeze-dried bone allograft: Case series. *J Periodontol* 71(10):1654–1661.

Keller EE, Tolman DE, Eckert SE. 1999. Maxillary antral-nasal inlay autogenous bone graft reconstruction of compromised maxilla: A 12-year retrospective study. *Int J Oral Maxillofac Implants* 14: 707–721.

Khoury F. 1999. Augmentation of the sinus floor with mandibular bone block and simultaneous implantation: A 6-year clinical investigation. *Int J Oral Maxillofac Implants* 14:557–601.

Klongnoi B, Rupprecht S, Kessler P, Thorwarth M, Wiltfang J, Schlegel KA.

2006a. Influence of platelet-rich plasma on a bioglass and autogenous bone in sinus augmentation. An explorative study. *Clin Oral Implants Res* 17(3):312–320.

Klongnoi B, Rupprecht S, Kessler P, Zimmermann R, Thorwarth M, Pongsiri S, Neukam FW, Wiltfang J, Schlegel KA. 2006b. Lack of beneficial effects of platelet-rich plasma on sinus augmentation using a fluorohydroxyapatite or autogenous bone: An explorative study. *J Clin Periodontol* 33(7):500–509.

Krekmanov L, Heimdahl A. 2000. Bone grafting to the maxillary sinus from the lateral side of the mandible. *Brit J Oral Maxillofac Surg* 38:617–619.

Levin L, Schwartz-Arad D. 2005. The effect of cigarette smoking on dental implants and related surgery. *Implant Dent* 14: 357–361.

Li XS, Sun JJ. 2007. [Reconstruction of maxillary sinus lateral bone wall and mucosa defect with collagen sponge and acellular cancellous bone combined with bone morphogenetic protein-2]. *Zhonghua Yi Xue Za Zhi* 87(18):1276–1278.

Lind M. 1996. Growth factors: Possible new clinical tools. A review. *Acta Orthop Scand* 67(4):407–417.

Lindquist L, Carlsson GE, Jemt T. 1996. A prospective 15-year follow-up study of mandibular fixed prostheses supported by osseointegrated implants. Clinical results and marginal bone loss. *Clin Oral Implants Res* 7:329–336.

Liu Y, Huse RO, De Groot K, Buser D, Hunziker EB. 2007. Delivery mode and efficacy of BMP-2 in association with implants. *J Dent Res* 86(1):84–89.

Lorenzetti M, Mozzati M, Campanino PP, Valente G. 1998. Bone augmentation of the inferior floor of the maxillary sinus with autogenous bone or composite bone grafts: A histologic-histomorphometric preliminary report. *Int J Oral Maxillofac Implants* 13:69–76.

Lundgren S, Moy P, Johansson C, Nilsson H. 1996. Augmentation of the maxillary sinus floor with particulated mandible: A histo-

logic and histomorphometric study. *Int J Oral Maxillofac Implants* 11:760–766.

Lutz R, Park J, Felszeghy E, Wiltfang J, Nkenke E, Schlegel A. 2008. Bone regeneration after topical BMP-2-gene delivery therapy in circumferential peri-implant bone defects. *Clin Oral Implants Res* 19(6):590-599.

Marx RE, Carlson ER, Eichstaedt RM, Schimmele SR, Strauss JE, Georgeff KR. 1998. Platelet-rich plasma: Growth factor enhancement for bone grafts. *Oral Surg Oral Med Oral Pathol Oral Radiol Endod* 85(6):638–646.

Matsumoto MA, Filho HN, Francishone CE. 2002. Microscopic analysis of reconstructed maxillary alveolar ridges using autogenous bone grafts from the chin and iliac crest. *Int J Oral Maxillofac Implants* 17: 507–516.

Maus U, Andereya S, Gravius S, Ohnsorge JA, Siebert CH, Niedhart C. 2008. BMP-2 incorporated in a tricalcium phosphate bone substitute enhances bone remodeling in sheep. *J Biomater Appl* 22(6):559–576.

Mazock JB, Schow SR, Triplett RG. 2004. Proximal tibia bone harvest: Review of technique, complications, and use in maxillofacial surgery. *Int J Oral Maxillofac Implants* 19(4):586–593.

Mehrara BJ, Saadeh PB, Steinbrech DS, Dudziak M, Spector JA, Greenwald JA, Gittes GK, Longaker MT. 1999. Adenovirus-mediated gene therapy of osteoblasts in vitro and in vivo. *J Bone Miner Res* 14(8): 1290–1301.

Misch CM. 1996. Ridge augmentation using mandibular ramus bone grafts for the placement of dental implants: Presentation of a technique. *Pract Periodont Aesthet Dent* 8:127–135.

———. 1997. Comparison of intraoral donor sites for onlay grafting prior to implant placement. *Int J Oral Maxillofac Implants* 12:767–776.

———. 2002. Discussion. A prospective 1-year clinical and radiographic study of implants placed after maxillary sinus floor augmentation with bovine hydroxylapatite

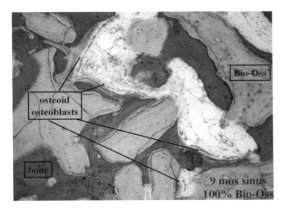

Figure 8.1. Sinus core 100% Bio-Oss at 9 months. Stevenel's blue, picric fuchsin. Orig mag × 20.

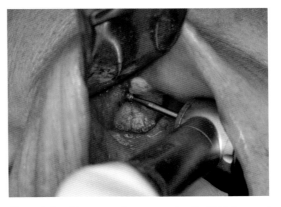

Figure 8.2. Osteotomy (antrostomy) with #8 high-speed diamond bur.

Concerns that long-term results may not be favorable due to the prolonged presence of the non-vital xenograft in the sinus are not founded. Histological studies by Iezzi et al. (2008) at 5 years and Traini et al. (2007) at 9 years both show residual xenograft, ongoing active bone remodeling, and a lack of contact between the xenograft with the implant surfaces.

Today's Surgical Protocols

With less reliance on autogenous bone grafts, lateral window techniques today are usually performed as an in-office procedure rather than a hospital-based procedure. The choice between simultaneous and delayed implant placement today is made by the clinician based upon the ability to achieve primary stability of the implant in the residual crestal bone. If this stability is achieved, the Wallace and Froum review showed no difference in implant survival between simultaneous and delayed placement.

The traditional rotary technique involves lateral window preparation with a high-speed or surgical hand piece, elevation of the membrane across the sinus floor and up the medial wall, grafting with a particulate bone replacement graft, and the placement of a barrier

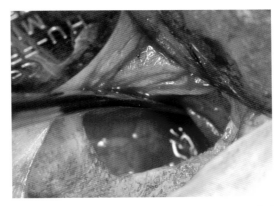

Figure 8.3. Elevation of the membrane up the medial wall.

membrane over the lateral window (Figs. 8.2–8.5)

The lateral window procedure is usually favored when residual crestal bone height is 4–5 mm or less. Today we have alternative techniques that allow us to utilize less invasive procedures when greater amounts of crestal bone are available. Summers (1994) introduced the osteotome sinus elevation technique, which is a transcrestal approach. Since that time a large number of transcrestal techniques have been introduced that utilize a modified Summers technique (Davarpanah et al. 2001), crestal bone core elevation (Toffler 2001), hydraulic sinus floor elevation

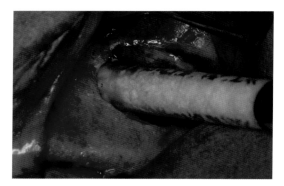

Figure 8.4. Placement of particulate bone replacement graft.

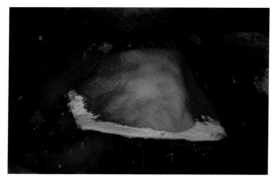

Figure 8.5. Bioabsorbable barrier membrane over the window.

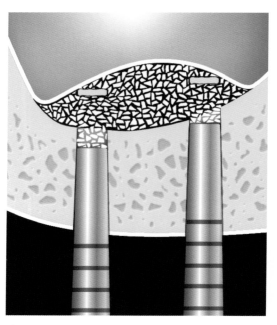

Figure 8.6. Summers osteotome technique.

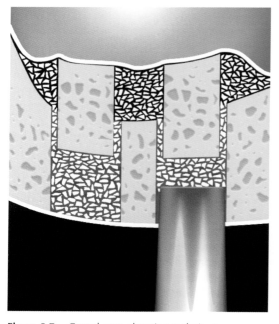

Figure 8.7. Crestal core elevation technique.

(Chen and Cha 2005), and balloon sinus floor elevation (Kfir 2007). It is difficult to assess the universal outcome for many of these newer procedures, as each is only documented by minimal or only a single clinical study. There are, however, two evidence-based reviews for the osteotome procedure. The Wallace and Froum review (five studies; 445 implants) reported an implant survival rate of 93.5%. The review by Emmerich et al. (eight studies; 1,137 implants) reported implant survival rates of 98.2%, 97.5%, 95.7%, and 90.9% at 6, 12, 24, and 36 months, respectively (Emmerich et al. 2005) (Figs. 8.6–8.9).

The most exciting innovation in recent years for sinus augmentation surgery is the utilization of piezoelectric surgery for lateral

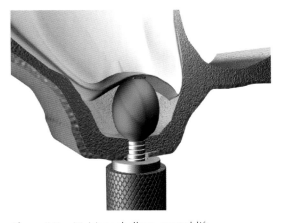

Figure 8.8.   Meisinger balloon control lift.

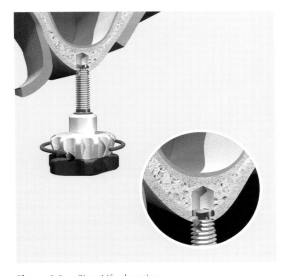

Figure 8.9.   Sinu-Lift elevation.

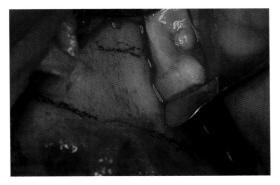

Figure 8.10.   Osteoplasty insert to thin the lateral wall.

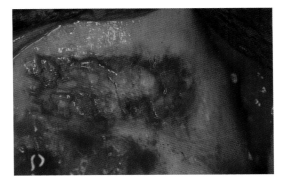

Figure 8.11.   Osteoplasty completed.

window osteotomy preparation and sinus membrane elevation (Vercellotti et al. 2001). The technique was introduced by Vercellotti in Europe 9 years ago, but it has only been utilized in North America for 3 years. Its popularity can be attested to by the fact that, as of this writing, four piezoelectric surgical devices are available in North America and others will be introduced in the near future.

Piezoelectric surgery, due to its low ultrasonic frequency of vibration (less than 30 kHz), can only cut hard tissue. This promises a reduction of intraoperative complications due to bleeding and sinus membrane perforations. A study by Wallace has shown a reduction in the membrane perforation rate from the average of 25% to 5% in a hundred consecutive cases (Wallace et al. 2007). Animal studies by Preti et al. have shown superior wound healing in bone when piezoelectric surgery is compared to rotary instrumentation (Preti et al. 2007). Figures 8.10–8.12 show the piezoelectric technique utilized in sinus surgery. Figure 8.13 demonstrates the dissection of the posterior superior alveolar artery from the lateral wall, and Figure 8.14 shows the initial elevation of the sinus membrane with a non-cutting elevator.

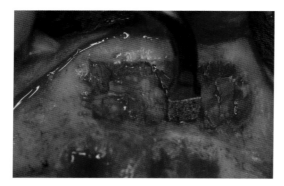

Figure 8.12.   Osteotomy to refine window.

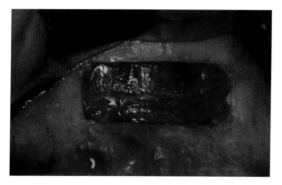

Figure 8.13.   Dissection of artery from the lateral wall.

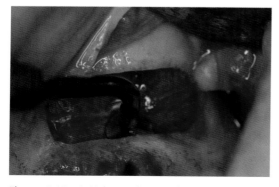

Figure 8.14.   Initial membrane elevation with non-cutting elevator.

Future Directions

Regardless of the successful outcomes that are being achieved today, clinicians and researchers are always seeking new techniques and technologies that may result in improved bone quality and/or a reduction in graft maturation times. Research has been ongoing to provide answers to these clinical issues. Patient-derived (autologous) growth factors (PRP, PRGF) have been in use for many years in the hope of improving patient outcomes. Over the past decade we have also seen the growth of genetic therapies that have led to the development of recombinant growth factors (rh-PDGF) and bone morphogenetic proteins (rh-BMP-2) for use in dental surgery today. Also currently being investigated is the use of tissue-engineered bone and stem cell cultures.

PRP and PDGF

Both platelet-rich plasma (PRP) and plasma rich in growth factors (PRGF) clinically produce platelet concentrations on the order of four to six times that found in whole blood. The concentrates contain all of the growth factors found in plasma including PDGF, TGF-β, FGF, VEGF, EGF, IGF-1, and HGF, as well as fibronectin, osteonectin, and fibrin. Extensive evidence exists showing enhanced soft-tissue healing in treating diabetic ulcers, burns, and other skin lesions (Aldecoda 2001). While positive results have been seen in soft tissue healing for both PRP and PRGF, statistically significant increases in vital bone formation have only infrequently been reported (Kassolis and Reynolds 2005; Marx et al. 1998). Other researchers have reported less successful results (Froum et al. 2002; Thor et al. 2005), and it is the conclusion of a recent evidence-based review by Boyapati and Wang that there is insufficient evidence to support the utilization of platelet-rich plasma as an adjunctive therapy for increasing bone formation in maxillary sinus grafting (Boyapati and Wang 2006).

rh-PDGF

After being introduced by Lynch et al., recombinant human platelet-derived growth factor has become the most extensively studied protein-signaling molecule in dentistry (Lynch et al. 1989). It is currently available for dental use as GEM 21S® (OsteoHealth, Shirley, New York) in combination with the carrier β-TCP. PDGF is naturally present in the alpha granules of platelets, where it is released following injury. Once released, PDGF enhances chemotaxis and mitogenesis of osteoprogenitor cells and osteoblasts and also plays an active role in promoting angiogenesis. In comparison to PRP, which increases the concentration of PDGF four to six times that found in whole blood, the recombinant PDGF in GEM 21S® achieves a concentration of 1,000 times that of the PRP or PRGF concentrate. Clinical efficacy in treating periodontal defects has been reported in studies by Camelo and Nevins, and GEM 21S® has been FDA approved for this purpose (Camelo et al. 2003; Nevins et al. 2003). Its use in sinus grafting is currently an off-label use. Studies are ongoing to demonstrate clinical efficacy in sinus grafting and ridge augmentation (Simion et al. 2007).

BMP-2

Bone morphogenetic proteins comprise a family of osteoinductive proteins that are capable of stimulating the existing host mesenchymal cells to form bone. A multicenter randomized controlled trial by Boyne et al. compared the bone morphogenetic protein BMP-2 in two concentrations (.75 and 1.5 mg/ml) with a sinus bone graft control. Implant success rates after 36 months of loading for the control group, the .75 mg/ml group, and the 1.5 mg/ml group were 81%, 88%, and 79%, respectively. This was a study done at a very high level of investigative rigor. What seem like lower-than-expected success rates were influenced by the high drop-out rate that accompanies a study of 5 years' duration. Of further interest, however, was the fact that 15% of the test cases did not produce sufficient bone volume for the placement of dental implants and, when the lower dose was utilized, the maturation time prior to implant placement had to be increased (Boyne et al. 2005).

One of the major shortcomings experienced with the use of 100% autogenous bone in sinus grafts is the observed tendency of this graft to resorb (Johansson et al. 2001). This may result in partial re-pneumatization of the sinus with resultant loss in graft volume accompanied by a decrease in density. Using the above rationale, one might speculate that the results with BMP-2/ACS might be improved by the addition of a slowly resorbable or non-resorbable bone replacement graft.

The authors (Wallace and Froum) are presently investigating two clinical applications of the addition of bone replacement grafts to the BMP-2/ACS system to address the aforementioned concerns regarding low density and loss of volume. The first application presented here utilizes Bio-Oss particles rolled in the absorbable collagen sponges (ACS) and placed into the sinus (Fig. 8.15). The second application cuts the hydrated ACS into small strips

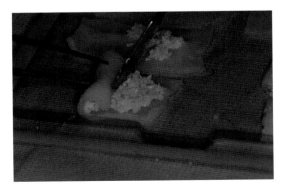

Figure 8.15.   Rollatini technique.

before adding the Bio-Oss to form a composite prior to insertion into the sinus (Fig. 8.16). The preoperative condition is seen in Figure 8.17. The immediate postoperative DentaScan panoramic view (Fig. 8.18) shows the distribution of the graft for both the rollatini technique on the right and the composite technique on the left.

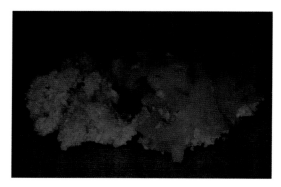

Figure 8.16. "Composite" graft technique.

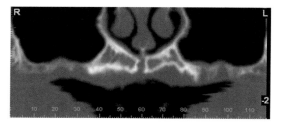

Figure 8.17. Preoperative DentaScan.

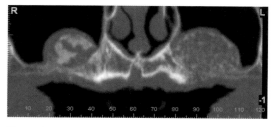

Figure 8.18. Postoperative DentaScan.

Conclusion

The evidence-based literature reviews tell us that implants placed in the maxillary sinus after lateral window sinus augmentation surgery experience an average survival rate of approximately 92%. By using an evidence-based decision-making process we can increase that survival rate to over 98%. Further, we have seen new sinus augmentation techniques such as the osteotome sinus elevation that, under certain conditions of available crestal bone height, is equally effective. The large ranges of implant survival, 61.2–100% with the lateral window technique and 88.6–100% with the osteotome technique, remind us that we are still seeking direction.

Our direction for the future, therefore, is multi-factorial and should encompass the following goals:

1. We must re-investigate in a more rigorous manner much of the work of the past with regard to surgical protocols and graft materials. The resulting decision-making processes would then lead to a higher survival rate with a smaller range.
2. We must conduct research in new directions and adopt new techniques and technologies only *after* they have been proven to be effective in improving outcomes.
3. Likewise, we must be willing to change our mindset and utilize these new techniques and technologies, even when they seem to go against our past training.
4. Finally, we must realize, as both researchers and clinicians, that our ultimate goal is the provision of the highest level of patient care. Our responsibility, therefore, is to develop, refine, and utilize therapies that provide our patients with the highest predictability. But, as health care providers, we must do this in a caring manner, and we can do this by adopting the least complicated and least demanding solutions to our patients' dental problems.

Our future is as close as tomorrow and we must endeavor, through both scientific rigor and concern for our patients, to make it as bright as possible.

BONE AUGMENTATION IN THE SEVERELY RESORBED MAXILLA

Lars Rasmusson

Bone augmentation procedures before or in conjunction with implant placement are today routine procedures utilized to create the required bone volume necessary to adequately house the implants. Implant placement in the posterior maxilla is a special problem due to a relatively fast resorption of alveolar bone after tooth loss. But before any augmentation procedures are planned, one important question must be asked. How much bone do we need for a successful result? It has been claimed that there is an almost linear relationship between implant length and survival rate. According to Ferrigno et al. (2006), 8 mm implants placed in the posterior maxilla had a survival rate of 88.9%, and 12 mm implants had a survival rate of 93.4% (12-year cumulative survival rate). It appears that a usable residual alveolar bone height of around 10 mm should remain for an improved long-term implant survival rate.

Not only poor quantity but also deficient bone quality is frequently seen in aging patients, in whom osteoporosis is common and due to annual loss of bone mass. Loss of bone occurs in men as well as women, but osteoporotic fractures are more common in women, since men have greater original bone mass than do women. Additionally, wear from dentures is frequently observed, and for patients who have had dentures for many years maxillary resorption could be extreme. There is no definite consensus on the definition of bone quality, but factors such as bone mineral density and thickness of the cortical lamina have been suggested as important by several investigators. It is agreed that the combination of severe resorption and demineralization (*poor bone quality*) increases the risk of implant failure.

The anterior part of the maxilla usually loses width, while the posterior part loses height, both from the superior (sinus) and inferior (crestal) directions. The buccal resorption of the anterior maxilla will subsequently result in a sagittal discrepancy between the jaws and, in severe cases, a Le Fort I osteotomy may be the best option to correct the prognathism and at the same time augment the maxilla with interpositional bone blocks. In less severe cases, a combination of sinus inlay and lateral onlay could be the method of choice. The use of Le Fort I osteotomy in conjunction with autogenous bone graft placement was originally described by Keller et al. (1987) and has yielded promising results. However, a considerable amount of bone usually has to be harvested and particulated grafts cannot be used since the sinus membrane is lacerated during the osteotomy (Fig. 8.19).

Onlay grafting was originally proposed by Breine and Brånemark in 1980. They recommended at that time the simultaneous placement of a horseshoe-shaped graft with implants to stabilize the transplant and at the same time reduce the overall treatment time. A two-stage protocol was later suggested by Rasmusson and co-workers (1999). However, except for donor site morbidity, the healing of these grafts takes several months and there is a considerable degree of resorption during the maturation process of the augmented area. Bone resorption in the buccal/palatal

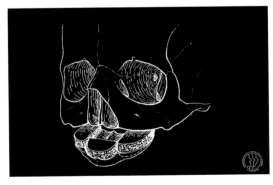

Figure 8.19. Le Fort I osteotomy with interpositional block bone graft (schematic).

direction for lateral onlay grafts could be as much as 60% during the first year according to some authors (Johansson et al. 2001; Widmark et al. 1997). Autogenous bone is grafted in cortical, cancellous, or cortico-cancellous form and can be placed onto the recipient bed either as a piece, en bloc, or particulated (Fig. 8.20).

The transplanted bone can then become a piece of partially necrotic tissue that over time goes through various stages of resorption and later acts as a scaffold for new bone formation. On the other hand, a swift and gentle handling of the graft with resultant cell survival may lead to revitalization of the graft in situ. Since osteocytes are dependent on a vascular supply at a distance not further than 0.1 mm, a cortical bone graft may only have small potential to exhibit surviving cells. The cells of a cancellous graft, however, may be

more prone to survival due to the structure and possible diffusion of nutrients and revascularization from the recipient bed.

The use of allografts and xenografts such as frozen or freeze-dried mineralized or demineralized bone are alternatives to the autogenous bone graft in reconstructive maxillary surgery. Many new products in this field have been introduced to the market in recent years. These are usually far more resistant to resorption when compared to autogenous bone, but they are, on the other hand, only osteoconductive.

Local Growth Factors

In order to stimulate new bone formation and a faster healing of autogenous bone grafts,

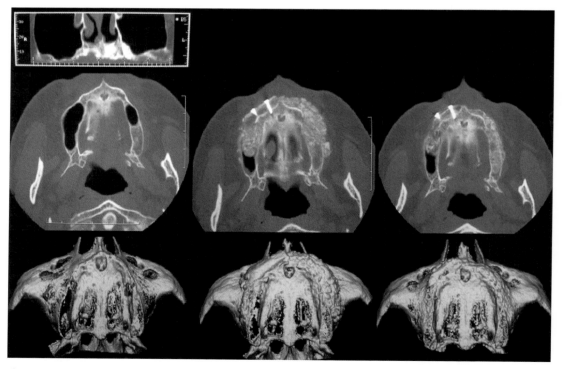

Figure 8.20. Radiograph showing a resorbed maxilla before treatment, immediately after grafting (lateral onlay block bone on patient's right side and particulate bone anterior left side + sinuses bilaterally), and after 6 months of healing.

growth factors have been studied extensively. In 1938 Levander observed ectopic bone formation around periosteal and surface layer–free bone grafts in non-skeletal sites, and much later Urist identified protein extracts from demineralized bone matrix that were able to induce bone formation. In 1971 Urist named this bone morphogenetic protein (BMP). The BMPs form a subgroup of the TGF-β super family, which is a large group of proteins that affect cell growth, migration, and differentiation including regulatory roles in tissue homeostasis and repair in adult organisms.

Platelets are the second most abundant unit in blood and they are 1.5–3.0 μm in diameter. Their role in hemostasis is central and they are vital to wound healing and inflammation. In a resting state they circulate in blood for 9–10 days. At least three types are released upon activation; α-granules, dense core granules, and lysosomes. The lysosomes contain glycosidases, proteases, and cationic proteins. The dense granules contain nucleotides such as adenine and guanine but also amines such as serotonin and histamine.

The α-granules are well known in regenerative surgery. They contain *adhesion molecules, protease inhibitors, coagulation factors* (e.g., fibrinogen, plasminogen, and factors V, VII, XI, and XIII), and finally *mitogenic factors* such as PDGF, VEGF, IGF and TGF-β.

The use of autologous local growth factors derived from the patient's own platelets (platelet-rich plasma or PRP) to enhance the healing of autogenous bone grafts in maxillofacial reconstruction was first described by Marx et al. in 1998 and later others (Grageda 2004; Thor et al. 2005). The idea is to concentrate platelets at the wound-healing site to facilitate healing and counteract resorption. The gel formed by the platelets can be added to particulated bone, producing a moldable graft that is easily placed at the recipient site.

PRP is usually prepared by perioperative withdrawal of 50–450 ml whole blood from a peripheral vein. The blood is then transferred to a gradient cell separator (centrifuge)

and the separation is done in two steps. The second preparation is to finally extract the platelets in a concentrated form in plasma. To achieve anticoagulation during the process, citrate phosphate dextrose is usually added. When the PRP is ready to use with the particulated bone, coagulation is initiated with 10% calcium chloride. The PRP-bone mix, now a moldable graft, is then immediately applied in the sinus floor or applied laterally to augment height and the width of the alveolar crest (Figs. 8.21, 8.22).

The implants can be placed after a healing period of between 4 and 6 months. If the graft maturation time is too short, a soft and immature graft may result. If the maturation time is too long, the graft volume may decrease due to resorption. In order to analyze the possible effect of the PRP, a platelet count must be performed before and after separation. Generally, the increase in number of platelets/unit will be four-fold after a correct separation. In many studies this has been the only attempt to correlate platelet count with effect, the assumption being that the number

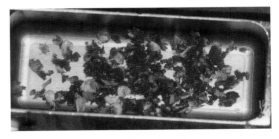

Figure 8.21. Particulate bone from the iliac crest.

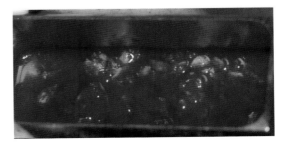

Figure 8.22. The same bone mixed with PRP.

of platelets also correlates with levels of released growth factors. However, activation of platelets and the subsequent release of growth factors is a complex situation that does not always coincide with platelet numbers.

In a series of studies, Thor and co-workers have tried to investigate the healing process of autogenous particulated bone grafts harvested from the hip and mixed with either PRP or whole blood. In a clinical study where sinus inlay grafts were compared, biopsies showed significantly more new bone formation on the PRP side compared to the control side. The biopsies were harvested after 3 months of healing and it was concluded that PRP had a positive influence on the healing process during the initial phase of the remodelling of the grafts (Figs. 8.23, 8.24).

After an additional healing period of 3 months (total 6 months), new biopsies were harvested at the time of implant installation. At this time point no difference between test and control could be observed in the histologic slides. Resonance frequency analysis (Fig. 8.25) was used to measure implant stability at implant placement, after 6 months (abutment connection), and after 1 year in function. There was a tendency of higher stability for implants installed in the PRP-treated

sinuses but the difference was not statistically significant.

No statistical differences were seen in marginal bone level alterations and only 2 out of 152 implants failed during the observation period (1 year post-loading).

It can be concluded that local growth factors administrated via a concentrate of the patients own platelets (PRP) resulted in a significant improvement in the early phase of graft healing. However, a routine use of PRP must be questioned since there is little or no

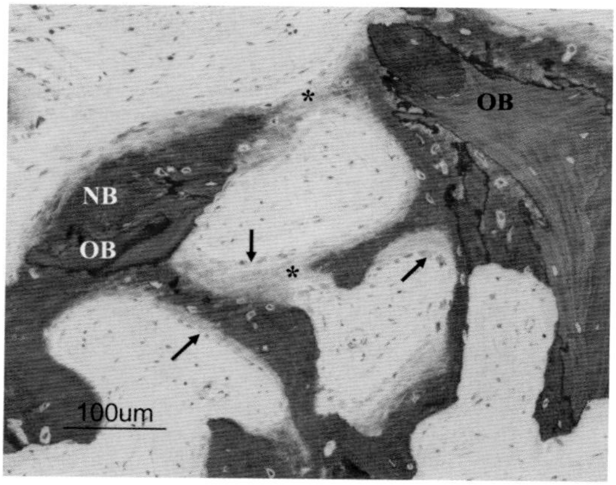

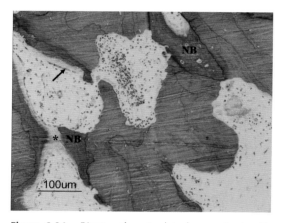

Figure 8.24. Biopsy of particulate bone mixed with whole blood used for sinus floor augmentation, harvested after 3 months of healing. NB = new bone formation, OB = old (not yet remodelled) bone.

Figure 8.23. Biopsy of particulate bone mixed with PRP used for sinus floor augmentation taken after 3 months of healing. NB = new bone formation, OB = old (not yet remodelled) bone.

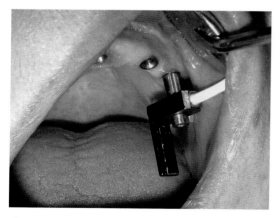

Figure 8.25. Resonance frequency analysis for stability measurements.

clinical benefit in the long-term treatment outcome, except for an improved handling of the particulated bone graft.

Activation of Platelets with Titanium

One hypothesis about the superior osseointegration properties of titanium over other materials is that its superiority is due to its thrombogenicity. Activation of the coagulation cascade is predictable when titanium (but also other materials) comes in contact with hard and soft tissues during installation. Whole blood, PRP, and PPP (platelet poor plasma) have been tested in a slide chamber model. Activation of the coagulation system, as reflected in the generation of TAT (thrombin-antithrombin complex) showed that the activation was most pronounced with whole blood (Fig. 8.26).

When compared to baseline values, the TAT increased 3,000-fold with whole blood, 2-fold with PRP, and not at all with PPP. In addition, the platelet activation showed a similar pattern with a 15-fold higher release of β-TG (β-thrombo-globulin) in whole blood compared to baseline values. With PRP and PPP the β-TG values remained at initial levels. These somewhat surprising results were not able to be repeated when a portion of the erythrocytes was left in the PRP. The erythrocytes consequently have not only a role in oxygen transportation but are also deeply involved in the activation of the platelets.

In conclusion, PRP in conjunction with grafting of particulated bone to the severely resorbed edentulous maxilla does not improve the integration and clinical function of dental implants installed after 6 months of healing. However, significantly more new bone has been observed in biopsies of maxillary sinuses grafted with autogenous bone and PRP compared to controls without PRP after 3 months of healing. Whole blood, not PRP, displays significantly stronger activation of the coagulation system with respect to generation of thrombin and platelet activation due to the lack of erythrocytes in PRP. The relationship between the potential effects of PRP in a dose-dependent way on cell proliferation in experimental cell cultures should be further evaluated.

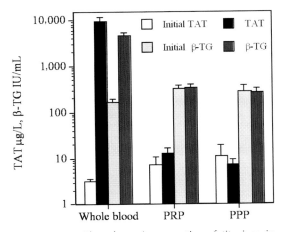

Figure 8.26. Thrombogenic properties of titanium in contact with whole blood, PRP, and PPP. Results reflect the generation of TAT and the release of β-TG in plasma.

References

Aghaloo TL, Moy PK. 2007. Which hard tissue augmentation techniques are the most successful in furnishing bony support for implant placement? *Int J Oral Maxillofac Implants* 22(Suppl):49–70.

Aldecoda EA. 2001. A new approach to bone regeneration: Plasma rich in growth factors (PRGF). *Vitoria-Spain: Puesta Al Dia Publicaciones, S.L.*

Becktor J, Isaksson S, Sennerby L. 2007. Endosseous implants and bone augmentation in the partially edentulous maxilla. *J Oral Maxillofac Implants* 22:603–608.

Blomqvist JE, Alberius P, Isaksson S. 1996. Retrospective analysis of one-stage maxillary sinus augmentation with endosseous implants. *Int J Oral Maxillofac Implants* 11:512–521.

Blomqvist JE, Alberius P, Isaksson S. 1998. Two-stage maxillary sinus reconstruction with endosseous implants: A prospective study. *Int J Oral Maxillofac Implants* 13: 758–766.

Boyapati L, Wang HL. 2006. The role of platelet-rich plasma in sinus augmentation: A critical review. *Implant Dent* 15: 160–170.

Boyne PJ, James RA. 1980. Grafting of the maxillary sinus floor with autogenous marrow and bone. *J Oral Surg* 38: 613–616.

Boyne PJ, Lilley LE, Marx RE, Moy PK, Nevins M, Spagnoli DB, Triplett RG. 2005. De novo bone induction by recombinant human bone morphogenetic protein-2 in maxillary sinus floor augmentation. *J Oral Maxillofac Surg* 63:1693–1707.

Breine U, Brånemark PI. 1980. Reconstruction of alveolar jaw bone. An experimental and clinical study of immediate and preformed autologous bone grafts in combination with osseointegrated implants. *Scand J Plast Reconstr Surg* 14:23–48.

Camelo M, Nevins ML, Schenk RK, Lynch SE, Nevins M. 2003. Periodontal regeneration in human class II furcations using purified recombinant platelet-derived growth factor-BB (rhPDGF-BB) with bone allograft. *Int J Periodontics Restorative Dent* 23(3):213–225.

Chen L, Cha J. 2005. An 8-year retrospective study: 1,100 patients receiving 1,557 implants using the minimally invasive hydraulic sinus condensing technique. *J Periodontol* 76(3):482–491.

Davarpanah M, Martinez H, Lazzara R, et al. 2001. The modified osteotome technique. *Int J Periodontics Restorative Dent* 21: 599–607.

Del Fabbro M, Testori T, Francetti L, Weinstein R. 2004. Systematic review of survival for implants placed in the grafted maxillary sinus. *Int J Periodontics Restorative Dent* 24(6):565–577.

Emmerich D, Att W, Stappert C. 2005. Sinus floor elevation using osteotomes: A systematic review and meta-analysis. *J Periodontol* 76:1237–1251.

Ferrigno N, Laureti M, Fanali S. 2006. Dental implants placed in conjunction with osteotome sinus floor elevation: A life table analysis from a study on 588 ITI implants. *Clin Oral Implants Res* 17:194–205.

Froum SJ, Wallace SS, Tarnow DP, Cho SC. 2002. Effect of platelet-rich plasma on bone growth and osseointegration in human maxillary sinus grafts: Three bilateral case reports. *Int J Periodontics Restorative Dent* 22:45–53.

Grageda E. 2004. Platelet-rich plasma and bone graft materials: A review and a standardized research protocol. *Implant Dent* 13:301–309.

Iezzi G, Scarano A, Piattelli A. 2008. Histologic results from a human implant retrieved due to fracture 5 years after insertion in a sinus augmented with anorganic bovine bone. *J Periodontol* 79:192–198.

Jensen J, Sindet-Petersen S. 1991. Autogenous mandibular bone grafts and osseointegrated implants for reconstruction of the severely atrophied maxilla. *J Oral Maxillofac Surg* 49:1277–1287.

Johansson B, Grepe A, Wannfors K, Hirsch JM. 2001. A clinical study of changes in the volume of bone grafts in the atrophic maxilla. *Dentomaxillofac Radiol* 30: 157–161.

Johansson B, Wannfors K, Ekenbäck J, Smedberg J-I, Hirsch J. 1999. Implants and sinus inlay bone grafts in a 1-stage procedure on severely atrophied maxillae: Surgical aspects of a 3-year follow-up study. *Int J Oral Maxillofac Implants* 14:811–818.

Kahnberg K-E, Ekestubbe A, Gröndahl K, Nilsson P, Hirsch J-M. 2001. Sinus lifting procedure: One-stage surgery with bone transplant and implants. *Clin Oral Implants Res* 12:479–487.

Kassolis JD, Reynolds MA. 2005. Evaluation of the adjunctive benefits of platelet-rich plasma in subantral sinus augmentation. *J Craniofac Surg* 16(2):280–287.

Keller EE, Eckert SE, Tolman DE. 1994. Maxillary antral and nasal one-stage inlay composite bone graft: Preliminary report on 30 recipient sites. *J Oral Maxillofac Surg* 52:438–447.

Keller EE, Eckert SE, Tolman DE. 1999. Maxillary antral-nasal autogenous bone graft reconstruction of the compromised maxilla: A 12-year retrospective study. *Int J Oral Maxillofac Implants* 14:707–721.

Keller EE, Van Roekel NB, Desjardins RP, Tolman DE. 1987. Prosthetic-surgical reconstruction of the severely resorbed maxilla with iliac bone grafting and tissue-integrated prostheses. *Int J Oral Maxillofac Implants* 2:155–165.

Kent JN, Block MS. 1989. Simultaneous maxillary sinus floor bone grafting and placement of hydroxyapatite coated implants. *J Oral Maxillofac Surg* 47:238–242.

Kfir E. 2007. Minimally invasive antral membrane balloon elevation: Report of 36 procedures. *J Periodontol* 78:2032–2035.

Levander G. 1938. A study of bone regeneration. *Surg Gynecol Obstet* 67:705–714.

Lynch SE, Williams RC, Polson AM. 1989. A combination of platelet-derived growth factor and insulin-like growth factor enhances periodontal regeneration. *J Clin Periodontol* 16:545–548.

Marx RE, Carlson ER, Eichstraedt RM, Schimmele SR, Strauss JE, Georgeff KR. 1998. Platelet-rich plasma: Growth factor enhancement for bone grafts. *Oral Surg Oral Med Oral Pathol Oral Radiol Endod* 85:638–646.

Nevins M, Camelo M, Nevins ML, Schenk RK, Lynch SE. 2003. Periodontal regeneration in humans using recombinant human platelet-derived growth factor-BB (rhPDGF-BB) and allogenic bone. *J Periodontol* 74(9):1282–1292.

Preti G, Martinasso G, Peirone B, Scheirano G, et al. 2007. Cytokines and growth factors involved in the osseointegration of oral titanium implants positioned using piezoelectric bone surgery versus a drill technique: A pilot study in minipigs. *J Periodontol* 78:716–722.

Raghoebar GM, Brouwer TJ, Reintsema H, Van Oort RP. 1993. Augmentation of the maxillary sinus floor with autogenous bone for the placement of dental implants. *J Oral Maxillofac Surg* 51:1198–1203.

Rasmusson L, Meredith N, Cho I, Sennerby L. 1999. The influence of simultaneous vs. delayed placement on the stability of titanium implants in onlay bone grafts. *Int J Oral Maxillofac Surg* 28:224–231.

Simion M, Rocchietta I, Dellavia C. 2007. Three-dimensional ridge augmentation with xenograft and recombinant human platelet-derived growth factor-BB in humans: Report of two cases. *Int J Periodontics Restorative Dent* 27:109–115.

Smiler DG, Holmes RE. 1987. Sinus lift procedure using porous hydroxyapatite: A preliminary clinical report. *J Oral Implantol* 13:239–253.

Smiler DG, Johnson PW, Lozada JL, Misch C, Rosenlicht JL, Tatum OH, Wagner JR. 1992. Sinus lift grafts and endosseous implants. *Dent Clin North Am* 36:151–186.

Summers R. 1994. A new concept in maxillary implant surgery: The osteotome technique. *Compend Contin Educ Dent* 15:152–162.

Tarnow DP, Wallace SS, Froum SJ. 2000. Histologic and clinical comparison of bilateral sinus floor elevations with and without barrier membrane placement in 12 patients: Part 3 of an ongoing prospective study. *Int J Periodontics Restorative Dent* 20:116–125.

Tatum H. Maxillary and sinus implant reconstruction. 1986. Dent *Clin North Am* 30:207–229.

Thor A, Franke Stenport V, Johansson C, Rasmusson L. 2007. Early bone formation in human bone grafts treated with platelet-rich plasma. *Int J Oral Maxillofac Surg* 36:1164–1171.

Thor A, Rasmusson L, Wennerberg A, Thomsen P, Hirsch JM, Nilsson B, Hong J. 2007. The role of whole blood in thrombin generation in contact with various titanium surfaces. *Biomaterials* 28:966–974.

Thor A, Wannfors K, Sennerby L, Rasmusson L. 2005. Reconstruction of the severely resorbed maxilla with autogenous bone, platelet-rich plasma, and implants: 1-year results of a controlled prospective 5-year study. *Clin Implant Dent Relat Res* 7(4):209–220.

Toffler M. 2001. Site development in the posterior maxilla using osteocompression and apical alveolar displacement. *Compend Contin Educ Dent* 22:782–790.

Traini T, Valentini P, Iezzi G, Piattelli A. 2007. A histologic and histomorphometric evaluation of anorganic bovine bone retrieved 9 years after a sinus augmentation procedure. *J Periodontol* 78:955–961.

Urist MR, Strates BS. 1971. Bone morphogenetic protein. *J Dent Res* 50:1392–1406.

Vercellotti T, De Paoli S, Nevins M. 2001. The piezoelectric bony window osteotomy and sinus membrane elevation: Introduction of a new technique for simplification of the sinus augmentation procedure. *Int J Periodontics Restorative Dent* 21: 561–567.

Wallace SS, Froum SJ, Cho S-C, Elian N, Kim BS, Tarnow DP. 2005. Sinus augmentation utilizing anorganic bovine bone (Bio-Oss) with absorbable and non-absorbable membranes over the lateral window: A histomorphometric and clinical analysis. *Int J Periodontics Restorative Dent* 25: 551–559.

Wallace SS, Froum SJ. 2003. Effect of maxillary sinus augmentation on the survival of endosseous dental implants. A systematic review. *Ann Periodontol* 8:328–343.

Wallace SS, Mazor Z, Froum SJ, Cho SC, Tarnow DP. 2007. Schneiderian membrane perforation rate during sinus elevation using piezosurgery: Clinical results of 100 consecutive cases. *Int J Periodontics Restorative Dent* 27:413–419.

Widmark G, Andersson B, Ivanoff CJ. 1997. Mandibular bone graft in the anterior maxilla for single-tooth implants. *Int J Oral Maxillofac Surg* 26:106–109.

Biomaterials and Substances for Site Optimizing

ALVEOLAR AUGMENTATION: PAST, PRESENT, AND FUTURE

Ulf M.E. Wikesjö, Massimo Simion, and Michael S. Reddy

Twenty-five years ago dental implant reconstruction was largely prosthetically managed with implants placed into the available residual ridge. Although the clinicians of the time realized that soft tissue and bone loss were consequences of tooth loss, it was given very little consideration other than its replacement with acrylic and ceramic dental materials. The predominant literature of the era addressed implant surface and load distribution and studies on various blade-form implants. At that time, the concept of osseointegration was introduced to North American dentists, along with the merits of osseointegration to improve implant prosthetic treatment as well as traditional restorative approaches.

In 1982 it was well known that following extraction of teeth the empty alveolar extraction sockets filled with blood, which sequentially clotted and organized into bone (Carlsson and Persson 1967). However, if the process were that simple and stopped there, dentures that were initially fitted to the ridge in a meticulous fashion would remain stable. We now know extraction of teeth disrupts the homeostasis of the alveolar bone and that the physiologic response is a complex process leading to further remodeling, resulting in a net loss of bone. Radiographic studies based on longitudinal cephalometric images provided excellent visualization of the gross patterns of destruction of alveolar bone that are induced following the loss of teeth (Atwood and Coy 1971; Hedegård 1962; Tallgren 1972). From these studies the mean rate of alveolar ridge resorption was found to be four times greater in the mandible than in the maxilla (Atwood and Coy 1971; Tallgren 1972). Further, in the most severe cases of residual ridge resorption, over 4 mm of vertical bone was lost during the first year after the extraction of mandibular teeth (Carlsson and Persson 1967).

At the time, it was postulated that residual ridge resorption was a multi-factorial biomechanical disease that resulted from a combination of anatomic, metabolic, and mechanical determinants. While it was ill-defined, it was and remains a significant clinical problem brought on by the loss of the natural dentition. Twenty-five years ago approximately 30% of the North American population over the age of 65 was completely edentulous. Retention of natural teeth has increased but remains a significant problem, with 25% of older adults being completely edentulous. Osseointegration concepts and implant-retained restorations became the answer to the clinical suffering. The report of a 15-year study of a clinically rigid restoration corresponding microscopically to a direct bone-implant interface without intervening fibrotic tissue represented a major announcement of significant clinical impact (Adell et al. 1981). The placement of endosseous implants provided for a stable restoration that would function much like natural teeth. The minimal bone loss found around the osseointegrated implant translated into maintenance of the residual alveolar bone. In cases of severely atrophic mandibular arches, the restoration from an edentulous state to a fixed hybrid prosthesis resulted in a reversal of the resorption process and the potential for functional regeneration of the atrophic mandible (Reddy et al. 2002).

After the Toronto Conference implant dentistry focused on using biocompatible materials to obtain a fixed restoration. This bone-preserving approach exercised specific surgical principles based on preserving alveolar bone. This preservation, rather than a regenerative approach, is still the basis for much of the current implant surgery techniques. Most surgery techniques are founded in creating minimal trauma to the bone. The use of copious irrigation and slow speed drills limits the zone of bone devitalization and aids in the subsequent phase of osseointegration. Precise fit and primary stability of the implant was and still is a key step to a successful progression to osseointegration. Aseptic techniques and anti-infective procedures kept the implant free from infection that might interfere with the implant stability and viability of the bone at the implant interface.

The concept of ridge augmentation or site development was largely not considered,

and site preparation was limited to resective surgery aimed at modifying the edentulous ridge area. The common concept was to flatten the ridge to a dimension of at least 1 mm wider than the implant diameter. Osteoplasty was used to remove bone and reduce the edentulous ridge to fit the implant dimensions or prosthesis. The common diameter of the implant was approximately 3.75 mm, with a variety of lengths. The surgical approach was resective with very little attention given to alveolar regeneration. Even with a resective treatment approach the results were profound and had promising long-term outcomes. In a 20-year follow-up study evaluating 273 standard implants (3.75 × 10 mm) in 47 patients placed in 1982, 30 subjects were available for follow-up. The cumulative survival rate for these implants was 98.9% with a mean crestal bone loss of 1.6 mm (Ekelund et al. 2003). Thirty-seven implants available for follow-up demonstrated exposure of two threads over 20 years. The incidence of unresolved peri-implantitis was as low as 3%. Importantly, all 30 subjects had continuous prosthesis function, two subjects having had their prosthesis remade during the 20-year observation period.

Lateral Alveolar Augmentation: GBR and a Composite Bone Biomaterial

The most common form of tooth loss is a partially edentulous state. Therefore, this also represents the most common indication for implant-based prosthetic reconstruction. This is particularly challenging when ridge resorption has taken place in only one segment of the mouth. Without intervention alveolar ridge resorption, even at a single tooth site, appears rapid, often occurring within 6 months (Bartee 2001; Lekovic et al. 1998). This leads to a variety of acquired ridge deformities that may preclude or limit the ability to restore the patient with implants. One of the most common current approaches to ridge augmentation is the application of a bone graft in combination with a barrier membrane (Fiorellini and Nevins 2003; Hämmerle and Karring 1998). This guided bone regeneration (GBR) method is based on the ability of the membrane to provide space for bone formation (Hämmerle and Karring 1998). In order to regenerate bone there is a need for cells to migrate into the space, the expression of growth factors, an adequate blood supply, and a scaffold to support the bone growth. Most current clinical GBR therapeutic approaches rely on the bone graft itself to provide growth factors and serve as a scaffold, while the membrane selectively allows repopulation with cells advantageous for bone growth.

In a recent study evaluating GBR, a bioresorbable synthetic membrane based on 67% polyglycolic acid and 33% trimethylene carbonate (PGA/TMC) was used to cover a bone biomaterial containing assayed demineralized bone matrix and cortical cancellous allogenic bone chips in a thermoplastic carrier (Geurs et al. 2008). The two-center study enrolled 38 subjects with inadequate ridge width for placement of dental implants. The ridge width was measured with ridge-mapping calipers at the crest and 4 mm below the crest during ridge augmentation surgery, and at 6 months post-augmentation at implant placement using a surgical guide to identify the position of the augmented sites. At the time of implant placement a 2 mm trephine biopsy was harvested from each implant site to be processed for histometric analysis. Trephines containing the block were embedded in methylmethacrylate resin and sectioned through the center of the trephine, stained with Paragon stain, and analyzed for the proportions of new bone and residual biomaterial. Figures 9.1 and 9.2 show representative examples of change in alveolar ridge width.

Clinical recordings showed a statistically significant 2.8 ± 1.7 mm mean increase in ridge width at the crest and a 3.1 ± 1.9 mm mean increase in ridge width 4 mm below the crest ($p < 0.001$). The change in ridge width for the individual sites is represented in Figures 9.3 and 9.4.

Figure 9.5 shows representative photomicrographs from the biopsies obtained at 6 months post-augmentation at implant placement showing new bone formation surrounding implanted biomaterials. The histometric evaluation estimated new bone formation comprising $20.6 \pm 8.8\%$ of the biopsies, bone biomaterials $36.2 \pm 15\%$, and marrow and other tissues $49.9 \pm 17.3\%$.

In this study a long-term synthetic bioresorbable PGA/TMC membrane was used

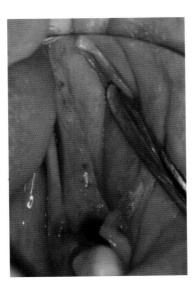
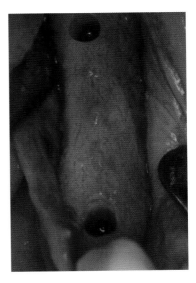

Figure 9.1. Mandibular lateral ridge augmentation using a PGA/TMC membrane combined with assayed demineralized bone matrix (DBM) and cortical cancellous allogenic bone chips uniformly dispersed in a thermoplastic carrier. Left panel shows the ridge prior to surgery. Right panel shows the site at 6 months post-surgery following harvesting of biopsies with a 2 mm trephine. Figures from Geurs et al. 2008, copyrighted by and reproduced with permission from the American Academy of Periodontology.

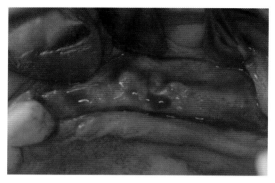
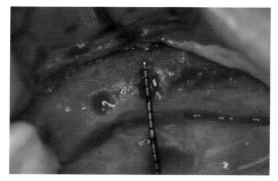

Figure 9.2. Maxillary lateral ridge augmentation using a PGA/TMC membrane combined with assayed DBM and cortical cancellous allogenic bone chips uniformly dispersed in a thermoplastic carrier (left). The right panel shows the augmented site at 6 months post-surgery following harvesting of biopsies with a 2 mm trephine. Figures from Geurs et al. 2008, copyrighted by and reproduced with permission from the American Academy of Periodontology.

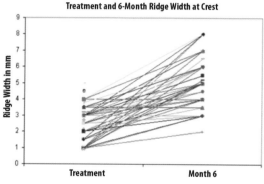

Figure 9.3. Individual measurements (by site) of alveolar ridge width at the crest prior to and at 6 months post-augmentation (n = 72 sites).

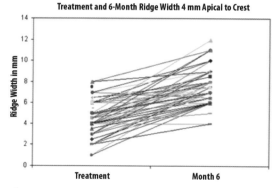

Figure 9.4. Individual measurements (by site) of the alveolar ridge 4 mm apical to the crest prior to and at 6 months post-augmentation (N = 72).

combined with an osteoinduction-assayed bone biomaterial. The bone biomaterial was suspended in a gelatin matrix that was thermoplastic and set to a rubbery consistency when cooled to body temperature. After setting, the biomaterial was more rigid than commonly used particulate bone biomaterials. These features facilitated subsequent placement of the membrane because the biomaterial was dimensionally stable and tacks were not required to stabilize the membrane and prevent displacement during healing. The membrane itself had excellent surgical handling and bioresorptive characteristics. Moreover, the PGA/TMC membrane may lend itself to incorporation of biologic or antimicrobial agents. Collectively, these properties suggest that use of the PGA/TMC membrane combined with the composite bone biomaterial may represent a predictable treatment for lateral ridge augmentation procedures.

Vertical Alveolar Augmentation: Techniques and Trends

The prime prerequisite to predict long-term success for osseointegrated implants is a sufficient bone volume at the recipient site.

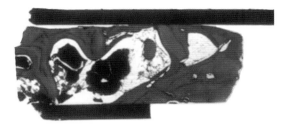

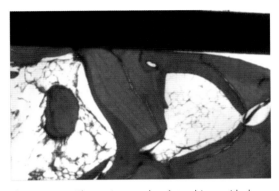

Figure 9.5. Photomicrograph of trephine with bone core from an augmented ridge at 6 months post-surgery; the high power (10×) view showing new bone and marrow surrounding the DBM particles. Figures from Geurs et al. 2008, copyrighted by and reproduced with permission from the American Academy of Periodontology.

Nevertheless, a sufficient amount of bone is frequently lacking as a consequence of trauma or advanced periodontitis. A number of different techniques have been deployed to reconstruct alveolar ridges to allow implant placement using immediate or staged approaches. In perspective, vertical bone loss in partially edentulous patients appears to be a major challenge due to anatomical limitations and technical difficulties. GBR concepts applied to partially edentulous atrophic mandibles to achieve vertical bone regeneration using titanium reinforced non-resorbable expanded polytetrafluoroethylene (ePTFE) membranes were first reported by Simion et al. (1994a). By the late 1990s, small variations in surgical techniques were applied, such as adding autogenous or a bone biomaterial including demineralized freeze-dried bone under the membrane with the intent to enhance vertical bone growth. Vertical alveolar augmentation ranging up to 7 mm was reported in a study following these concepts (Tinti et al. 1996; Fig. 9.6). The long-term implant stability and resorption pattern of bone regenerated with this technique has been reported in a retrospective multicenter study following 1–5 years of prosthetic loading evaluating 123 implants (Simion et al. 2001).

However, extra- or intraoral harvesting of autogenous bone constitutes a high degree of patient discomfort and morbidity. Hence, efforts have been applied to decrease the volume of autogenous bone harvested by applying a 1:1 ratio of deproteinized bovine bone and autogenous bone under the GBR ePTFE membranes for vertical bone regeneration (Simion et al. 2007a). Although the results reported have been shown to be successful, this technique still requires autogenous bone harvesting and the use of a non-resorbable membrane, which in turn demands expert operator skills or the surgical site may be prone to wound dehiscences and subsequent infection (Simion et al. 1994b).

Advances in tissue engineering may offer solutions that resolve bone volume deficits and periodontal defects while at the same time eliminating concerns imposed by current techniques. Among a number of matrix, growth, and differentiation factors, recombinant platelet derived growth factor (rhPDGF-BB) has been extensively evaluated for orthopedic and periodontal indications. The principal aim in using a growth factor such as rhPDGF-BB is to eliminate the need for autogenous bone harvesting and possibly the use of membranes. A proof-of-principle study recently evaluated rhPDGF-BB for alveolar augmentation (Simion et al. 2006). A deproteinized bovine bone block infused with rhPDGF-BB was used for vertical augmentation in a canine model to support bone regeneration in the three dimensions (Fig. 9.7).

The observations from this study translate to the possibility to regenerate bone vertically by using a xenograft as a scaffold infused with a potent growth factor without the need

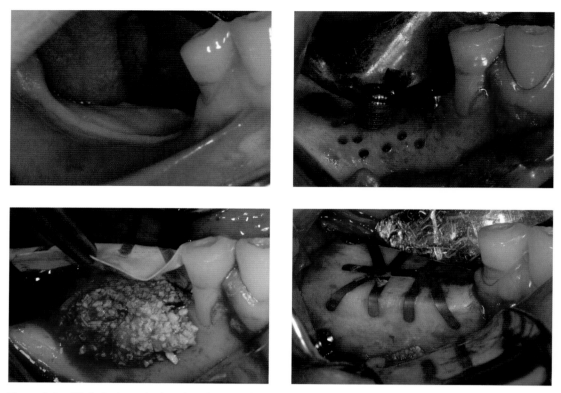

Figure 9.6. Clinical view of edentulous lower right mandible exhibiting severe atrophy and minimal keratinized mucosa (top left). Cortical perforations performed with a diamond round bur to enhance bleeding. Two titanium implants are inserted to support a membrane and composite graft (top right). Autogenous bone chips mixed in a 1:1 ratio with deproteinized bovine bone particles (lower left). Re-entry at 6 months. The titanium-reinforced membrane appears stable with the fixation screws in place (lower right).

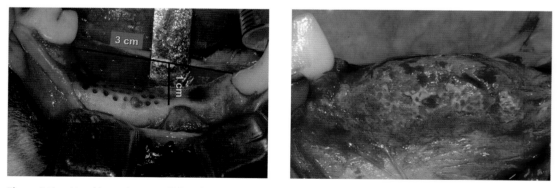

Figure 9.7. Atrophic canine mandible prior to augmentation surgery (left). Clinical re-entry of a deproteinized bovine block + rhPDGF-BB site following 4 months of submerged healing (right). Implants are covered by a large tissue mass resembling bone.

to harvest autogenous bone or use a membrane. Two atrophic human alveolar defects were successfully treated using the same protocol (Simion et al. 2007b). These recent studies point to trends of less invasive treatments minimizing complications and side effects of the surgery, decreasing patient morbidity, and increasing success rates while decreasing technical difficulties. The application of tissue-engineering concepts to clinical surgical procedures will indeed create a new paradigm.

Alveolar Augmentation and rhBMP-2

Recombinant human bone morphogenetic protein 2 (rhBMP-2) in an absorbable collagen sponge (ACS) carrier (INFUSE® Bone Graft, Medtronic Sofamor Danek, Memphis, Tennessee) was approved for orthopedic indications including spine fusion and long bone fracture repair in 2002 and has since reached rapid market acceptance. INFUSE® Bone Graft was approved for oral/maxillofacial indications in 2007 (http://www.fda.gov/cdrh/mda/docs/p050053.html) following extensive evaluation (Huang et al. 2008). Studies have shown that rhBMP-2/ACS may induce clinically relevant bone formation for inlay indications including augmentation of the subantral space, advanced vertical/horizontal peri-implantitis defects, and extraction socket sites. Advanced saddle-type alveolar ridge defects have been reconstructed using rhBMP-2/ACS to allow placement and long-term functional loading of endosseous dental implants. rhBMP-2/ACS and rhBMP-2 combined with other carrier technologies have been evaluated for vertical/horizontal alveolar ridge augmentation. Several studies have evaluated BMP technologies for alveolar augmentation and endosseous implant osseointegration. The following represents selected critical preclinical studies demonstrating the biologic basis, the clinical potential, and the versatility of BMP technologies for alveolar augmentation and osseointegration as exemplified by rhBMP-2.

Using a discriminating canine model for vertical alveolar ridge augmentation (Wikesjö et al. 2006), our laboratory first showed that a BMP construct used as an onlay has the potential to induce clinically relevant alveolar bone augmentation and osseointegration (Sigurdsson et al. 1997). rhBMP-2/ACS or ACS control was applied to critical-sized, 5 mm, supraalveolar, peri-implant defects in contralateral jaw quadrants. The defect sites were subject to histometric evaluation following a 16-week healing interval. Sites receiving rhBMP-2 showed significant bone formation and osseointegration, with newly formed bone approaching or exceeding the implant platform. Controls showed limited, if any, bone formation (Fig. 9.8).

These observations appear even more pertinent when compared to those evaluating decalcified, freeze-dried, allogeneic bone (DFDBA) combined with GBR or GBR alone in the same model (Caplanis et al. 1997). The DFDBA biomaterial remained unaltered in all sites receiving this treatment, solidified within a dense connective tissue matrix and in close contact to the titanium implant surface without evidence of bone formation and osseointegration (Fig. 9.9).

Bone formation was limited and clinically irrelevant for both GBR/DFDBA and GBR alone. In contrast to that observed for rhBMP-2, the results from this study suggest that DFDBA has no relevant osteoinductive, osteoconductive, or other adjunctive effect to GBR and that GBR has limited potential to support osteogenesis at least for onlay indications (vertical alveolar augmentation). It should be noted that the canine model should have greater healing potential than clinical patients; thus if healing is not observed in this model, it should not be expected in clinical settings. Conversely, clinically relevant bone formation and osseointegration in this model is expected to have clinical significance.

Subsequent studies evaluated a space-providing, porous ePTFE device to support rhBMP-2/ACS induced bone formation using

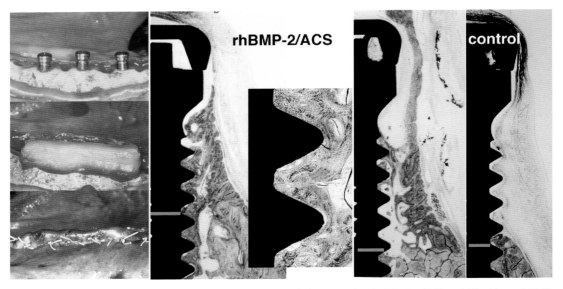

Figure 9.8. Critical-sized, 5-mm, supraalveolar, peri-implant defect treated with rhBMP-2/ACS or ACS without rhBMP-2 (control). Clinical photographs show the supraalveolar defect implanted with rhBMP-2/ACS before and after wound closure for primary intention healing. The left photomicrographs show defect sites having received rhBMP-2/ACS exhibiting bone formation reaching or exceeding the implant platform, the newly formed bone showing osseointegration to the machined titanium implant surface (high magnification insert). Control sites show limited, if any, bone formation. Green lines delineate the level of the surgically reduced alveolar crest. Healing interval 16 weeks. Figures copyrighted by and modified with permission from Blackwell Munksgaard Ltd. Source: Sigurdsson et al. 1997.

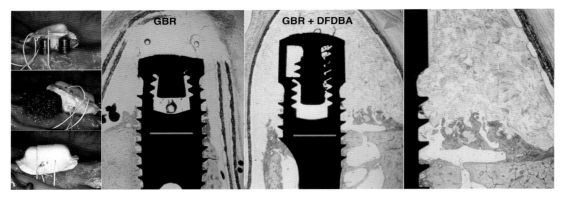

Figure 9.9. Critical-sized, 5 mm, supraalveolar, peri-implant defect treated with GBR (occlusive space-providing ePTFE membrane; green arrowheads) with or without a DFDBA. The clinical panels show the supraalveolar defect with the GBR membrane, with DFDBA rehydrated in autologous blood, and with the membrane in place prior to wound closure for primary intention healing. Note limited regeneration of alveolar bone in absence and presence of DFDBA suggesting (1) that the innate regenerative potential of alveolar bone is limited, and (2) that the DFDBA biomaterial has limited, if any, osteoinductive and/or osteoconductive properties to support bone regeneration. Green lines delineate the level of the surgically reduced alveolar crest. Healing interval 16 weeks. Figures copyrighted by and modified with permission from Quintessence Publishing. Source: Caplanis et al. 1997.

the canine supraalveolar, peri-implant defect model (Wikesjö et al. 2003, 2004). The concept behind the design was to provide an unobstructed space allowing vascular and cellular elements from the gingival connective tissue to support rhBMP-2 induced bone formation, the geometry of which was outlined by a porous ePTFE device. Four animals received the space-providing, dome-shaped device alone or combined with rhBMP-2/ACS in contralateral jaw quadrants. Four animals similarly received rhBMP-2/ACS solo versus rhBMP-2/ACS combined with the porous ePTFE device. The implant sites were subject to histometric analysis following an 8-week healing interval. GBR alone limitedly enhanced bone formation (Fig. 9.10).

rhBMP-2/ACS alone induced significant augmentation of the alveolar ridge; however, the geometry of induced bone was highly irregular. In contrast, the dome-shaped, space-providing, porous ePTFE device–rhBMP-2/ACS combination predictably produced bone formation filling the large space provided by the device. This study points to important tissue engineering principles; BMP bone formation follows the outline or design of the matrix.

Recent studies have evaluated alternative BMP carrier technologies to ACS exhibiting structural integrity for onlay indications. rhBMP-2 in a DFDBA/fibrin carrier as a stand-alone therapy induced clinically relevant vertical alveolar augmentation for

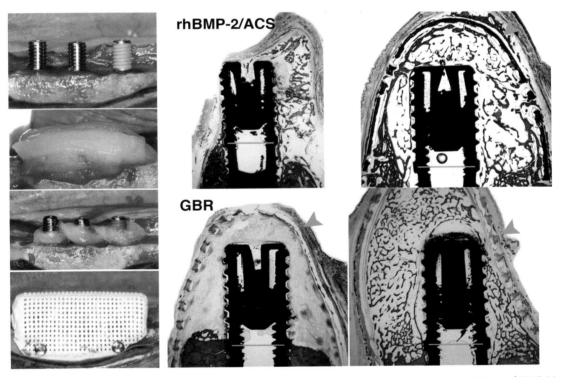

Figure 9.10. Critical-sized, 5 mm, supraalveolar, peri-implant defects treated with rhBMP-2/ACS, GBR, or rhBMP-2/ACS combined with GBR using a porous, space-providing ePTFE membrane. The clinical panels show the supraalveolar defect with rhBMP-2/ACS and with the porous GBR membrane. Note how rhBMP-2 induced bone fills the space provided by the membrane (green arrowheads), whereas rhBMP-2/ACS alone provides very irregular bone formation (top left). GBR alone (bottom left) provides for limited, if any, regeneration of alveolar bone. Green lines delineate the level of the surgically reduced alveolar crest. Healing interval 8 weeks. Figures copyrighted by and modified with permission from Blackwell Munksgaard Ltd. Sources: Wikesjö et al. 2003 and Wikesjö et al. 2004.

placement and osseointegration of dental implants (Sigurdsson et al. 2001). Using the canine model, bilateral, critical-sized, horizontal alveolar ridge defects received an rhBMP-2/DFDBA/fibrin onlay. Ten-mm implants were placed into the rhBMP-2 induced alveolar ridge at 8 and 16 weeks. The implant sites were subject to a histometric evaluation at 24 weeks. Ninety percent of the bone-anchoring surface was invested in rhBMP-2 induced bone (Fig. 9.11).

Osseointegration approximated 55% in rhBMP-2 induced and in resident bone of similar density, emphasizing the clinical relevance of this candidate treatment. Nevertheless, the use of cadaver-sourced biomaterials such as DFDBA may have difficulty in receiving public acceptance and thus synthetic carrier technologies for alveolar indications are to be preferred.

A second study evaluating a synthetic calcium phosphate cement matrix (α-BSM) as a candidate carrier for rhBMP-2 found this to be an effective stand-alone protocol for vertical alveolar ridge augmentation (Wikesjö et al. 2002). Using the supraalveolar peri-implant defect model, three animals received rhBMP-2/α-BSM in contralateral jaw quadrants (rhBMP-2 at 0.40 and 0.75 mg/mL), and three animals received α-BSM alone (control). In defect sites subject to histometric evaluation following a 16-week healing interval, rhBMP-2/α-BSM induced clinically relevant alveolar ridge augmentation (Fig. 9.12).

Vertical bone augmentation comprised the entire 5 mm exposed implant, the newly formed bone exhibiting bone density approximating 60% (type II bone) with established cortex and osseointegration approximating 27%. Control sites exhibited limited, if any, bone formation. This synthetic technology shows considerable promise since α-BSM may be shaped to the desired contour and set to provide space for rhBMP-2 induced bone formation. In addition, α-BSM is injectable for inlay and has minimally invasive indications and may prove to be an amazing technology for maxillary sinus augmentation in conjunction with placement of oral implants, pinpointing bone formation at the implant body.

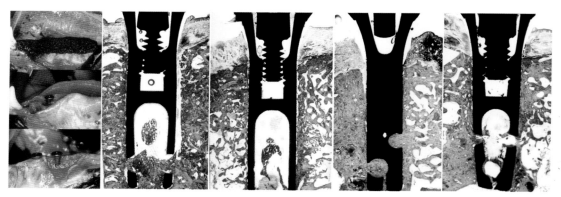

Figure 9.11. Surgically created horizontal alveolar ridge defect implanted with rhBMP-2 combined with DFDBA rehydrated in autologous blood. The clinical panels show the rhBMP-2/DFDBA/fibrin construct placed onto the surgically reduced flat alveolar ridge prior to wound closure for primary intention healing. Transmucosal oral titanium implants were placed into the rhBMP-2 induced alveolar ridge at weeks 8 and 16 post-surgery. The animals were euthanized 24 weeks following the ridge augmentation procedure. The left photomicrographs show implants placed at week 8 and the right photomicrographs show implants placed at week 16. Approximately 90% of the bone-anchoring surface of the implants was housed in rhBMP-2 induced bone exhibiting limited evidence of crestal resorption. There was no significant difference in bone density between rhBMP-2 induced and the contiguous resident bone. Also, osseointegration (approximately 55%) was similar in induced and resident bone irrespective of whether the implants were placed at week 8 or 16. Figures copyrighted by and modified with permission from Quintessence Publishing. Source: Sigurdsson et al. 2001.

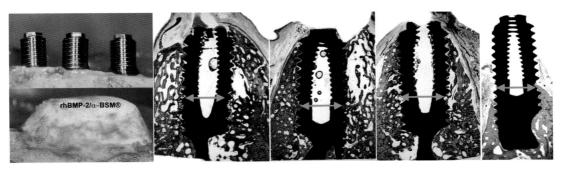

Figure 9.12. Critical-sized, 5 mm, supraalveolar peri-implant defect treated with rhBMP-2 in a calcium phosphate cement (α-BSM) or α-BSM without rhBMP-2 (control). The clinical panels show the supraalveolar peri-implant defect before and after application of α-BSM. The photomicrographs show representative observations for jaw quadrants receiving rhBMP-2/α-BSM, in this particular jaw quadrant rhBMP-2 at 0.4 mg/mL. Note substantial new bone formation at sites treated with rhBMP-2/α-BSM compared to the control (far right) exhibiting limited, if any, evidence of new bone formation. The rhBMP-2 induced bone exhibits similar trabeculation, osseointegration, and cortex formation as the contiguous resident bone. Also note no evidence of residual biomaterial. Green arrows delineate the apical extension of the supraalveolar peri-implant defects. Healing interval 16 weeks. Figures copyrighted by and modified with permission from Blackwell Munksgaard Ltd. Source: Wikesjö et al. 2002.

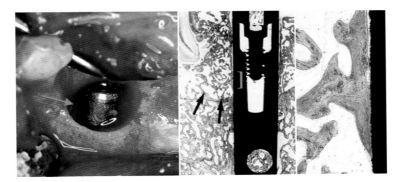

Figure 9.13. Re-osseointegration following treatment of chronic peri-implantitis defect with rhBMP-2/ACS. The clinical panel shows the debrided peri-implantitis defect prior to treatment with rhBMP-2/ACS; the green arrow points to the aspect of the implant shown in the photomicrographs. Black arrows delineate the apical aspect of the peri-implantitis defect; the green bracket depicts a high magnification area (right) showing re-osseointegration. Note that the rhBMP-2 induced bone exhibits qualities of the contiguous resident bone. Healing interval 16 weeks. Figures copyrighted by and modified with permission from Quintessence Publishing. Source: Hanisch et al. 1997.

rhBMP-2/ACS has also been shown to support re-osseointegration of endosseous implants exposed to peri-implantitis (Hanisch et al. 1997). Ligature-induced peri-implantitis lesions created around hydroxyapatite-coated titanium implants in the posterior mandible and maxilla over 11 months in non-human primates exhibiting a microbiota similar to that of advanced human peri-implantitis and complex defect morphology were treated with rhBMP-2/ACS following flap elevation and defect debridement. Control defects received buffer/ACS. Histometric analysis performed following a 16-week healing interval showed clinically relevant three-fold greater vertical bone gain in sites receiving rhBMP-2/ACS including convincing evidence of re-osseointegration (Fig. 9.13).

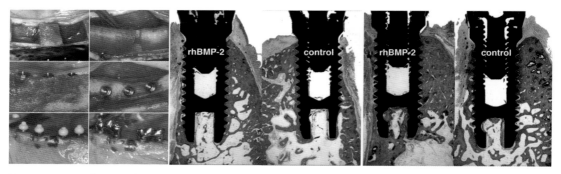

Figure 9.14. Evaluation of titanium implants placed into rhBMP-2 induced bone subject to 12 months of functional loading. The clinical panels show surgically induced mandibular, saddle-type (~15 × 10 mm), full-thickness alveolar ridge defects (two per jaw quadrant). The defects were immediately implanted with rhBMP-2/ACS with or without a barrier membrane. Healing progressed for 3 months when endosseous oral implants were installed into the rhBMP-2/ACS induced bone and into the contiguous resident bone (control). Following 4 months of osseointegration, the implants received abutments and prosthetic reconstruction. Prosthetically reconstructed implants were then subject to functional loading for 12 months. The photomicrographs show implants placed into rhBMP-2 induced and resident bone following 12 months of functional loading. There is no discernable difference in bone formation and osseointegration between rhBMP-2 induced and resident bone. Figures copyrighted by and modified with permission from Blackwell Munksgaard Ltd. Source: Jovanovic et al. 2003.

The results suggest that surgical implantation of rhBMP-2 may have considerable clinical utility in the reconstruction of peri-implantitis defects and alveolar defects of lesser complexity.

A decisive test for any technology aimed at alveolar augmentation and osseointegration of endosseous implants is functional loading. Jovanovic et al. (2003) showed that rhBMP-2/ACS induces normal physiologic bone allowing installation, osseointegration, and long-term functional loading of endosseous implants. Mandibular, alveolar ridge, full-thickness, saddle-type defects were surgically created in a canine model. The defect sites were immediately implanted with rhBMP-2/ACS. Endosseous implants were placed into the rhBMP-2 induced and adjoining resident bone (control) following a 12-week healing interval. The implants were subject to prosthetic reconstruction following 16 weeks of osseointegration and were then exposed to functional loading for 12 months, at which point the implant sites were subject to histometric analysis. rhBMP-2 induced bone exhibited features of the resident bone including a re-established cortex (Fig. 9.14). There were no significant differences between implants placed into rhBMP-2 induced and resident bone for any parameter evaluated. The implant sites exhibited some crestal resorption and, importantly, clinically relevant osseointegration (50% in rhBMP-2 induced and 75% in resident bone) supporting functional loading over 12 months. While previous reported studies demonstrated clinically relevant alveolar bone augmentation and osseointegration following surgical implantation of rhBMP-2/ACS, this study was the first to show the functional utility of rhBMP-2 induced bone for implant dentistry.

The observations reflected in this chapter on alveolar augmentation point to a significant paradigm shift in implant dentistry. Surgical placement of implants can today be facilitated through a number of protocols and technologies. It is clear that never before have clinicians had such an immediate access to technologies that predictably support bone formation and osseointegration for strategic relevant positioning of dental implants for prosthetic reconstruction. Only long-term studies, clinical experience, and patient acceptance will determine the most successful approaches.

References

Adell R, Lekholm U, Rockler B, Brånemark PI. 1981. A 15-year study of osseointegrated implants in the treatment of the edentulous jaw. *Int J Oral Surg* 10: 387–416.

Atwood DA, Coy WA. 1971. Clinical cephalometric and densitometric study of reduction of residual ridges. *J Prosthet Dent* 26:280–295.

Bartee BK. 2001. Extraction site reconstruction for alveolar ridge preservation. Part 1: Rationale and materials selection. *J Oral Implantol* 27:187–193.

Caplanis N, Sigurdsson TJ, Rohrer MD, Wikesjö UME. 1997. Effect of allogeneic, freeze-dried, demineralized bone matrix on guided bone regeneration in supraalveolar peri-implant defects in dogs. *Int J Oral Maxillofac Implants* 12:634–642.

Carlsson GE, Persson G. 1967. Morphologic changes of the mandible after extraction and wearing of dentures. *Odontologisk Revy* 18:27–54.

Carlsson GE, Thilander H, Hedegård B. 1967. Histologic changes in the upper alveolar process after extractions with or without insertion of an immediate full denture. *Acta Odontol Scand* 25:1–23.

Ekelund JA, Lindquist LW, Carlsson GE, Jemt T. 2003. Implant treatment in the edentulous mandible: A prospective study on Brånemark system implants over more than 20 years. *Int J Prosthodont* 16:602–608.

Fiorellini JP, Nevins ML. 2003. Localized ridge augmentation/preservation. A systematic review. *Ann Periodontol* 8:321–327.

Geurs NC, Korostoff J, Vassilopoulos PJ, et al. 2008. Clinical and histological assessment of lateral alveolar ridge augmentation using a synthetic long-term bioabsorbable membrane and an allograft. *J Periodontol*. In press.

Hämmerle CH, Karring T. 1998. Guided bone regeneration at oral implant sites. *Periodontology 2000* 17:151–175.

Hanisch O, Tatakis DN, Boskovic MM, Rohrer MD, Wikesjö UME. 1997. Bone formation and reosseointegration in peri-implantitis defects following surgical implantation of rhBMP-2. *Int J Oral and Maxillofac Implants* 12:604–610.

Hedegård B. 1962. Some observations on tissue changes with immediate maxillary dentures. *Dental Practitioner and Dental Record* 13:70–79.

Huang Y-H, Polimeni G, Qahash M, Wikesjö UME. 2008. Bone morphogenetic proteins and osseointegration. Current knowledge—future possibilities. *Periodontology 2000*. In press.

Jovanovic SA, Hunt DR, Bernard GW, Spiekermann H, Nishimura R, Wozney JM, Wikesjö UME. 2003. Long-term functional loading of dental implants in rhBMP-2 induced bone. A histologic study in the canine ridge augmentation model. *Clin Oral Implants Res* 14:793–803.

Lekovic V, Camargo PM, Klokkevold PR, Weinlaender M, Kenney EB, Dimitrijevic B, Nedic M. 1998. Preservation of alveolar bone in extraction sockets using bioabsorbable membranes. *J Periodontol* 69:1044–1049.

Reddy MS, Geurs NC, Wang I-C, Liu P-R, Hsu Y-T, Jeffcoat RL, Jeffcoat MK. 2002. Mandibular growth following implant restoration: Does Wolff's Law apply to residual ridge resorption? *Int J Periodontics Restorative Dent* 22:315–321.

Sigurdsson TJ, Fu E, Tatakis DN, Rohrer MD, Wikesjö UME. 1997. Bone morphogenetic protein-2 for peri-implant bone regeneration and osseointegration. *Clin Oral Implants Res* 8:367–374.

Sigurdsson TJ, Nguyen S, Wikesjö UME. 2001. Alveolar ridge augmentation with rhBMP-2 and bone-to-implant contact in induced bone. *Int J Periodontics Restorative Dent* 21:461–473.

Simion M, Fontana F, Rasperini G, Maiorana C. 2007a. Vertical ridge augmentation by expanded-polytetrafluoroethylene membrane and a combination of intraoral autogenous bone graft and deproteinized anorganic bovine bone (Bio-Oss). *Clin Oral Implants Res* 18:620–629.

Simion M, Jovanovic SA, Tinti C, Parma-Benfenati S. 2001. Long-term evaluation of osseointegrated implants inserted at the time or after vertical ridge augmentation. A retrospective study on 123 implants with 1–5 year follow-up. *Clin Oral Implants Res* 12:35–45.

Simion M, Rocchietta I, Dellavia C. 2007b. Three-dimensional ridge augmentation with xenograft and rhPDGF-BB in humans: Report of three cases. *Int J Periodontics and Restorative Dent* 27: 109–115.

Simion M, Rocchietta I, Kim D, Nevins M, Fiorellini J. 2006. Vertical ridge augmentation by means of deproteinized bovine bone block and rhPDGF-BB. A histological study in a dog model. *Int J Periodontics and Restorative Dent* 26:415–423.

Simion M, Trisi P, Maglione M, Piattelli A. 1994b. A preliminary report on a method for studying the permeability of expanded polytetrafluoroethylene membrane to bacteria in vitro: A scanning electron microscopic and histological study. *J Periodontol* 65:755–761.

Simion M, Trisi P, Piattelli A. 1994a. Vertical ridge augmentation using a membrane technique associated with osseointegrated implants. *Int J Periodontics and Restorative Dent* 14:496–511.

Tallgren A. 1972. The continuing reduction of the residual alveolar ridges in complete denture wearers: A mixed longitudinal study covering 25 years. *J Prosthet Dent* 27:120–132.

Tinti C, Parma-Benfenati S, Polizzi G. 1996. Vertical ridge augmentation: What is the limit? *Int J Periodontics and Restorative Dent* 16:220–229.

Wikesjö UME, Qahash M, Thomson RC, Cook AD, Rohrer MD, Wozney JM, Hardwick WR. 2003. Space-providing expanded polytetrafluoroethylene devices define alveolar augmentation at dental implants induced by recombinant human bone morphogenetic protein-2. *Clin Implant Dent and Relat Res* 5:112–123.

Wikesjö UME, Qahash M, Thomson RC, Cook AD, Rohrer MD, Wozney JM, Hardwick WR. 2004. rhBMP-2 significantly enhances guided bone regeneration. *Clin Oral Implants Res* 15:194–204.

Wikesjö UME, Sorensen RG, Kinoshita A, Wozney JM. 2002. rhBMP-2/α-BSM® induces significant vertical alveolar ridge augmentation and dental implant osseointegration. *Clin Oral Implants Res* 4:173–181.

Wikesjö UME, Susin C, Qahash M, Polimen G, Leknes KN, Shanaman RH, Prasad HS, Rohrer MD, Hall J. 2006. The critical-size supraalveolar peri-implant defect model: Characteristics and use. *J Clin Periodontol* 33:846–854.

Implant Surgery Interventions

10

THREE-DIMENSIONAL REVERSE TISSUE ENGINEERING FOR OPTIMAL DENTAL IMPLANT RECONSTRUCTION

Michael A. Pikos and Albert H. Mattia

The three-dimensional loss of soft- and hard-tissue contour in the oral cavity compromises implant restoration of aesthetics and function, and creates a myriad of prosthetic, surgical, and cosmetic challenges for the implant team (Elian et al. 2007). Compromised implant angulation and off-axis loading negatively impact case success and longevity (Misch and Bidez 1994). Three-dimensional reverse tissue engineering is a state-of-the-art protocol for the objective design and surgical implementation of digitally engineered soft- and hard-tissue augmentation for optimal dental implant reconstruction.

This chapter will outline a contemporary team approach to dental implant rehabilitation, integrating classic clinical diagnostic protocols with interactive cone-beam CT technology and the most current soft- and hard-tissue reconstruction techniques.

Digitally Guided Bone Augmentation (DGBA®) will be presented as a proprietary approach for three-dimensional reconstruction and restoration of complex aesthetic zone defects. Pre- and post-grafting digital prosthetic workup, reverse tissue engineering with interactive CT graft assessment, and prosthetic-driven implant planning with stent-driven implant placement is featured.

The creation of an implant prosthesis-fixture-tissue complex that restores form, function, and aesthetics is the goal of modern implant dentistry. Case planning must engineer a biomechanical advantage to the complex that will dissipate masticatory forces at a physiologically acceptable level to achieve predictability and longevity (Isidor 1996). Failure in design of the system can result in prosthetic and implant failure and further breakdown of hard and soft tissue.

Advances in CT imaging and interactive diagnostic software allow for three-dimensional implant planning of unprecedented accuracy, and the objective quantification of necessary bone grafting for a predictable outcome (Sarment et al. 2003). The practical clinical application from this development has been to precisely communicate engineered parameters of virtual tissue grafting to the real-time surgical reality of the patient. With integration of rapid prototype technology and state-of-the-art surgical regenerative concepts, a digitally guided surgical conduit can be established to direct virtually planned 3-D bone augmentation.

Phase I: Diagnostic Planning

The optimally engineered implant reconstruction begins with establishing the 3-D aesthetic and functional requirements of the proposed dental implant restoration. From a conventional laboratory diagnostic workup, restoration parameters are communicated through a custom-fabricated CT scanning appliance to a 3-D digital DICOM data volume (Rosenfeld et al. 2006) (Fig. 10.1).

After CT imaging with the appliance in place, interactive CT software is utilized to initiate a sequential diagnostic protocol, where patient hard- and soft-tissue anatomy are interpreted from the perspective of the proposed restoration (Fig. 10.2).

Implants can then be planned with optimal 3-D axial orientation, including fixture length and diameter for optimal biomechanical prosthetic loading (Fig 10.3).

Virtual Tissue Regeneration

Once implant size and trajectory are established, virtual anatomic regenerative graft planning can be performed. Next, the objective hard-tissue augmentation volumes are designed to support the implant plan (Figs. 10.4, 10.5).

This represents a significant paradigm shift from conventional planning for maximum utilization of available bone, which often limits implants to unfavorable fixture size and

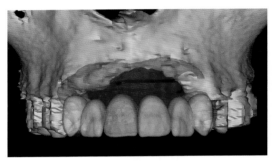

Figure 10.2. DICOM data volume segmentation allows visualization of the proposed restoration and interpretation of bony anatomy with interactive 3-D surface renderings.

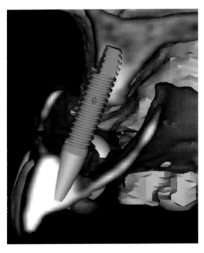

Figure 10.3. Scanning template interpretation is essential for 3-D implant planning to optimize biomechanical support for the proposed restoration.

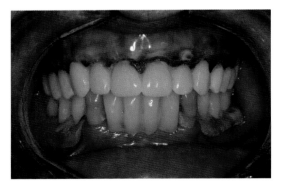

Figure 10.1. Customized scanning template appliances communicate 3-D restoration parameters to the CT DICOM data volume.

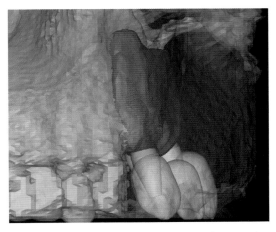

Figure 10.4. Interactive interpretation of restoration tissue volume parameters is necessary for virtually engineered augmentations and 3-D quantification of planned surgical bone grafts.

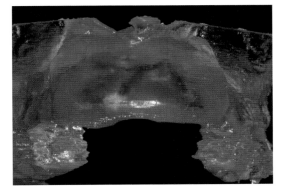

Figure 10.6. Rapid prototyping is utilized to create three-dimensional stereolythographic resin models that accurately reflect the virtually planned augmentation (DGBA model).

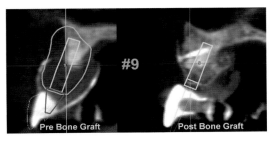

Figure 10.5. Interactive cross-sectional imagery contrasts the planned virtual bone augmentation with the completed DGBA.

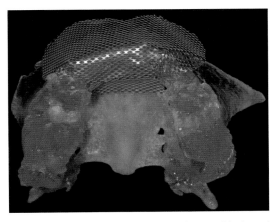

Figure 10.7. Titanium mesh can be modified and shaped on the DGBA model to predictably communicate the three-dimensional graft plan to the surgical graft site.

trajectories, as well as to negative biomechanical force factors (Yokoyama et al. 2004).

DGBA/Rapid Prototyping/3-D Modeling

DGBA® describes the process whereby virtual bone grafting is communicated to clinical surgical augmentation. Once the bone graft has been fabricated in the virtual phase, rapid prototype manufacturing technology can create 3-D hard models that reflect the virtual grafting volumes created in the software planning phase (Fig. 10.6).

Using an intaglio concept, the surgeon can mold titanium mesh to matrix the 3-D volumetric aspects of the graft area, and offer a direct transfer of the virtual plan to the surgical graft recipient site (Fig. 10.7).

Pre-Graft Soft-Tissue Augmentation

Complex three-dimensional bony defects command large volumes of bony augmenta-

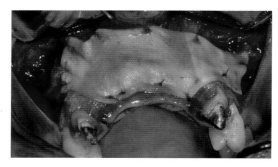

Figure 10.8. Human dermal tissue augmentation provides increased soft-tissue volume to allow adequate flap release and avoid graft dehiscence.

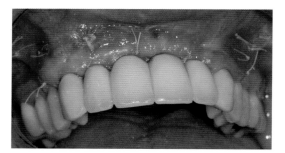

Figure 10.9. Two-week healing of the soft tissue augmentation prior to DGBA grafting.

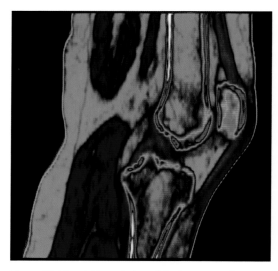

Figure 10.10. 3-D rendering of the knee joint depicting the medullary bone volume of the tibial head.

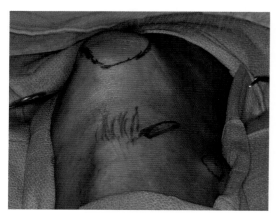

Figure 10.11. Gerdy's tubercle is utilized as the lateral bony anatomic landmark in tibial harvest with access incision lateral to the patellar tendon.

tion that require tension-free soft-tissue closure to maintain blood supply to the grafted area (Jensen et al. 2004). This also prevents incision line opening, the number one complication of large alveolar bone grafts (Pikos 2005).

Preliminary soft-tissue augmentation utilizes both allogeneic tissue (freeze-dried human dermis), as well as autogenous tissue (palatal connective tissue), to prevent vestibular dehiscence, another common complication following alveolar bone grafts. Three months of healing is required prior to bone grafting (Figs. 10.8, 10.9).

Autogenous Bone Grafting

The efficacy of autogenous bone grafting is well documented (Esposito et al. 2006).

Compared to the hip, the tibial bone harvest offers a greater volume of autogenous marrow with comparatively lower morbidity (O'Keeffe et al. 1991), and the convenience of an in-office protocol (Figs. 10.10, 10.11).

A slow resorbing bovine-derived xenograft is added to the autogenous marrow to minimize graft resorption and provide for long-term graft volume maintenance (Fig. 10.12).

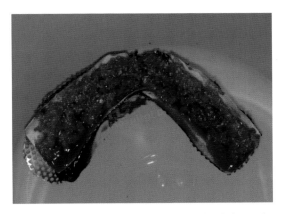

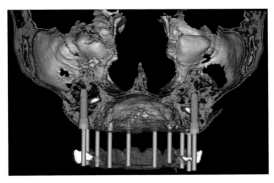

Figure 10.12.   Graft marrow complex is loaded into the mesh framework with a collagen membrane barrier between graft and mesh.

Figure 10.14.   Phase II scanning demonstrates the accurate transfer of the virtual graft plan to the patient and the presence of regenerated bone volume necessary for optimal implant biomechanics.

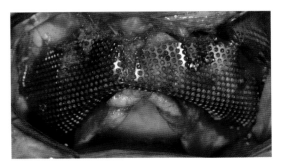

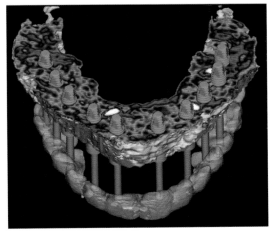

Figure 10.13.   The intaglio surface of the titanium mesh matrixes the bone graft against the recipient bony defect and communicates the virtual graft plan to the patient.

Figure 10.15.   Axial clipping of surface rendered 3-D model illustrates the predictable 3-D reconstruction of bone for implants to support a full arch fixed prosthesis.

Platelet-rich plasma is also used to accelerate wound healing and stimulate graft incorporation (Marx et al. 1998). The graft complex is then added to the preformed titanium matrix along the intaglio surface against a slow resorbing collagen membrane (Fig. 10.13).

Phase II: Implant Planning

A second interactive diagnosis is performed after graft healing to assess progress of the phase I tissue grafting, and to finalize a guided surgical implant plan. New models and records and a modified or new CT scanning appliance are utilized with a second CT image to allow for a restoration-driven interpretation of the new grafted bone anatomy. Optimized implant planning is now performed a second time with attention to a guided surgical protocol (Fig. 10.14).

Interactive software planning is then performed to allow for selective segmentation of 3-D models and removal of the graft matrix scaffold in virtual planning. This allows implant planning to be performed on the actual bony architecture (Fig. 10.15).

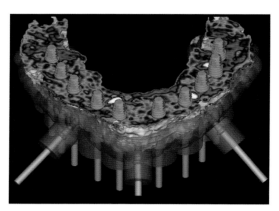

Figure 10.16. Software engineering allows virtual design of a bone supported surgical guide appliance with tripodial screw fixation.

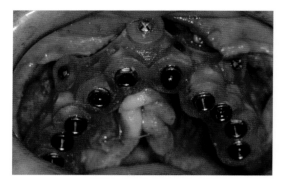

Figure 10.18. Bone-supported surgical guide with tripodial fixation is used to communicate the 3-D implant surgical plan to the grafted maxillary arch.

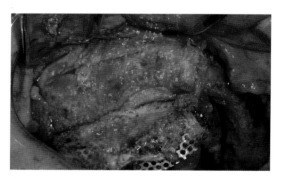

Figure 10.17. Removal of the titanium mesh scaffold matrix reveals definitive graft integration and clinical reconstruction of the virtual augmentation plan.

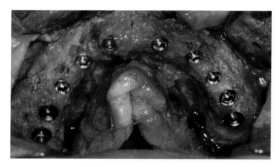

Figure 10.19. Virtual implant planning has been communicated successfully to the clinical surgical setting.

A final bone-supported surgical guide is designed with tripodial screw fixation to accurately communicate the implant plan to the surgical site (Vrielinck et al. 2003) (Fig. 10.16).

Graft Mesh Removal/Guided Implant Surgery

The titanium mesh matrix is removed after 7 months of graft incorporation (Fig. 10.17).

This allows for direct visualization of the 3-D osseous reconstruction that is necessary for seating of the bone-supported surgical guide. Tripodial fixation of the surgical guide is achieved with bone screws (Fig. 10.18).

This permits precision ostectomy preparation. The process accurately communicates the three-dimensional implant orientation from the virtual implant treatment plan to the surgical field. A two-stage implant protocol allows for further maturation of the grafted bone and minimizes forces on the implants in the initial healing period (Fig. 10.19).

Restorative Phase

Implants are exposed after completion of stage I healing and preliminary abutments are

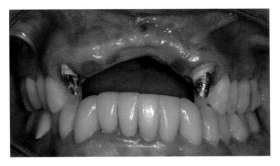

Figure 10.20. Complex 3-D aesthetic zone defect with high smile line prior to loss of canines with insufficient bony ridge height and width for root form implant placement.

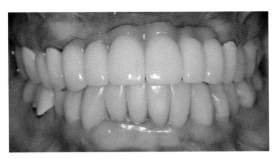

Figure 10.22. Final implant-supported fixed ceramo-metal restoration (6–11) restoring form, function, and aesthetics.

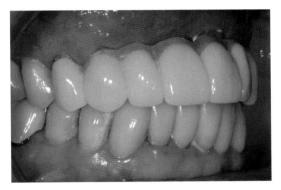

Figure 10.21. Provisional fixed restoration to refine aesthetic, occlusal, and functional parameters and provisionally load the implant-bone complex.

Conclusion

Reverse tissue engineering with Digitally Guided Bone Augmentation is the clinical integration of contemporary biomechanical, surgical, and restorative concepts with the precision of digital rendering and manufacturing technologies. It presents a unique application of three-dimensional CT imaging with interactive digital implant and bone graft planning, and establishes a clinical protocol for predictable regeneration of hard and soft tissue for dental implant reconstruction.

placed to facilitate soft-tissue healing and maturation. The prostheses are relieved and soft relined to accommodate healing abutments and tissue shrinkage. Once tissue healing has occurred, conventional restorative protocols can be implemented to transfer the implant orientation to the laboratory. Custom provisional restorations are fabricated to confirm the plan and refine occlusal, functional, and cosmetic parameters of the final restoration (Spear et al. 2006) (Figs. 10.20, 10.21).

Final ceramometal fixed restorations utilizing milled titanium abutments compose the final restoration and restore form, function, and aesthetics (Fig. 10.22).

References

Elian N, Ehrlich B, Jalbout ZN, Classi AJ, Cho SC, Kamer AR, Froum S, Tarnow DP. 2007. Advanced concepts in implant dentistry: Creating the "aesthetic site foundation." *Dent Clin North Am* 51(2):547–63, xi–xii.

Esposito M, Grusovin MG, Coulthard P, Worthington HV. 2006. The efficacy of various bone augmentation procedures for dental implants: A Cochrane systematic review of randomized controlled clinical trials. *Int J Oral Maxillofac Implants* 21(5):696–710.

Isidor F. 1996. Loss of osseointegration caused by occlusal load of oral implants. A clinical and radiographic study in monkeys. *Clin Oral Implants Res* 7:143–152.

Jensen OT, Pikos MA, Simion M, Vercellotti T. 2004. Bone grafting strategies for vertical alveolar augmentation. In: *Peterson's Principles of Oral and Maxillofacial Surgery,* 2nd ed. Ontario, Canada: BC Decker. 12:223–232.

Marx RE, Carlson ER, Eichstaedt RM, Schimmele SR, Strauss JE, Georgeff KR. 1998. Platelet-rich plasma: Growth factor enhancement for bone grafts. *Oral Surg Oral Med Oral Pathol Oral Radiol Endod* 85(6):638–646.

Misch CE, Bidez MW. 1994. Implant protected occlusion: A biomechanical rationale. *Compend Contin Dent Educ* 15:1330–1343.

O'Keeffe RM, Jr., Riemer BL, Butterfield SL. 1991. Harvesting of autogenous cancellous bone graft from the proximal tibial metaphysis. A review of 230 cases. *J Orthop Trauma* 5(4):469–474.

Pikos MA. 2005. Mandibular block autografts for alveolar ridge augmentation. *Atlas Oral Maxillofac Surg Clin North Am* 13(2):91–107.

Rosenfeld A, Mandelaris G, Tardieu P. 2006. Prosthetically directed implant placement using computer software to insure precise placement and predictable prosthetic outcomes. Part 1: Diagnostics, imaging, and collaborative accountability. *Int J Periodontics Restorative Dent* 26:215–221.

Sarment D, Sukovic P, Clinthorne N. 2003. Accuracy of implant placement with a stereolithographic surgical guide. *Int J Oral Maxillofac Implants* 18:571–577.

Spear FM, Kokich VG, Mathews DP. 2006. Interdisciplinary management of anterior dental esthetics. *J Am Dent Assoc* 137(2):160–169.

Vrielinck L, Politis C, Schepers S, Pauwels M, Naert I. 2003. Image-based planning and clinical validation of zygoma and pterygoid implant placement in patients with severe bone atrophy using customized drill guides. Preliminary results from a prospective follow-up study. *Int J Oral Maxillofac Surg* 32:7–14.

Yokoyama S, Wakabayashi N, Shiota M, Ohyama T. 2004. The influence of implant location and length on stress distribution for three-unit implant-supported posterior cantilever fixed partial dentures. *J Prosthet Dent* 91:234–240.

11
The Implant and Biological Response

THE HEALING BONE-IMPLANT INTERFACE: ROLE OF MICROMOTION AND RELATED STRAIN LEVELS IN TISSUE

John B. Brunski, Jennifer A. Currey, Jill A. Helms, Philipp Leucht, Antonio Nanci, and Rima Wazen

Introduction

Micromotion can be defined as displacement of an implant relative to surrounding bone (Brunski 1988). The literature indicates that osseointegration is favored by implant stability during healing in bone but discouraged by excessive implant micromotion ("relative motion") (Brånemark et al. 1977; Brunski et al. 1979, 2005; Soballe et al. 1992)—a principle that has formed the basis of the well-established delayed loading protocol employed with oral implants *ad modum* Brånemark.

However, with current increased attention to immediate loading (Esposito et al. 2007), there is renewed interest in why certain types of micromotion promote negative outcomes such as interfacial fibrous tissue formation,

while other types of micromotion may lead to positive effects, such as more interfacial bone (De Smet et al. 2005; Rubin and McLeod 1994).

Biomechanically, it is clear that when any implant in bone is loaded—either immediately or after some period of healing—stresses and strains must arise in supporting interfacial tissues. Moreover, due to factors including mismatch of elastic moduli between implant and tissue; the absence of any initial adhesive bond between implant and tissue; and poor initial fit of the implant in its site, the loading will produce implant micromotion to some degree. Our work has hypothesized that the strain distribution in interfacial tissue is a key factor regulating early interfacial cell and tissue response.

Methods

We started to test this hypothesis in a new mouse model (Leucht et al. 2007a, 2007b) that allows control of implant micromotion and interfacial strain fields. The model with CD1 mice consists of a motion device (with externally mounted load cell and LVDT) that allows either stabilization or displacement-control of 0.5 mm diameter implants installed through one cortex of the tibia and extending into the medullary canal (Fig. 11.1).

To produce known strain fields during healing, we designed specially shaped pin and screw-shaped implants for installation in two different types of interface: (1) a bone-implant-gap interface (BIGI), and (2) a direct-bone-implant-interface (DBII). Formed by placing a 0.5 mm diameter implant in a 0.8 mm hole, the BIGI consisted of an initial interface in which a moving implant would produce known strain fields in the early healing regenerate. Alternatively, the DBII

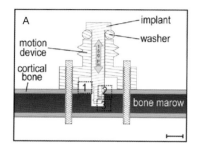

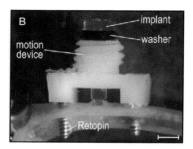

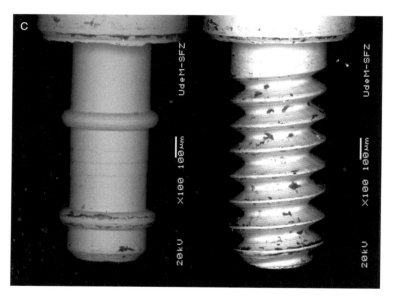

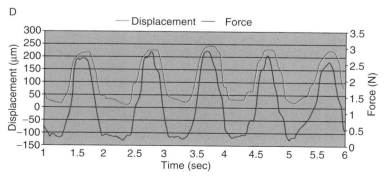

Figure 11.1. a. Schematic diagram of motion device (scale bar = 1 mm). b. Device mounted on excised mouse tibia. c. Pin and screw-shaped implants (OD = 0.5 mm). d. Example traces of motion (red) and force (blue) from a 150 μm motion protocol in vivo.

was designed to resemble a more conventional type of interface; a 0.5 mm diameter screw was inserted into a 0.4 mm tapped hole. All implants were made of 70% L-lactide/30% D,L-lactide (grade LR706, Midwest Plastics, St. Paul, Minnesota, and Medical Micro Machining, Inc., Simi Valley, California) to allow optimal micro-CT imaging and strain analyses. (Current work is also done using titanium implants.)

In experiments A and B of this series, we tested pin and screw implants, respectively, in the BIGI; starting on the day of surgery, pin or screw implants were displaced axially by 150 μm 60 times per day at 1 Hz for 7 days total. In experiment C, we placed 0.5 mm diameter screws in 0.40 mm tapped holes to form a DBII interface on the day of surgery, and applied 150 μm axial micromotion 60 times per day for 7 days. In experiment D we followed the same protocol as in experiment C but displaced the screw in the DBII by only 17–70 μm (ave. 43.5 μm). Implants stabilized in the BIGI and DBII served as controls.

To assess interfacial strain fields, we used machine vision photogrammetry (DISMAP) to analyze pairs of micro-CT images of the interface (Currey and Brunski 2006; Nicolella et al. 2001). We also validated and used an axisymmetric finite element analysis (ABAQUS) of the interface as an adjunct to the experimental strain analyses (Fig. 11.2).

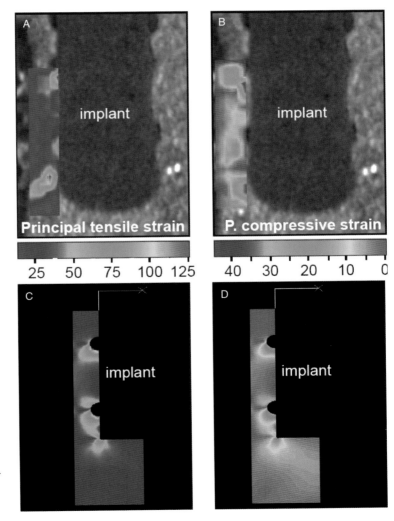

Figure 11.2.   a and b. Contours of principal tensile and compressive strains around a pin-type implant as determined experimentally in a mock interface using DISMAP. c and d. Axisymmetric finite element simulations of cases a and b above.

Decalcified and undecalcified longitudinal sections (Goldner's stain) through the mid-plane of implants in the tibia allowed measurement of the distance between implant surface and first hit of mineralized bone (bone-implant distance, BID). The mean BID over the entire implant periphery was based on data taken from ~30 points around the periphery of each implant. In some cases we also measured BID values at specific local regions of the interface (e.g., at the base of an implant). Statistical tests for differences in distributions of BID for control versus motion interfaces were conducted using Kolmogorov-Smirnov (KS) or Wilcoxon two sample tests.

Results

Our previous work (Leucht et al. 2007a) showed that for pins moving 150 μm in the BIGI (experiment A), the local BID at high strain regions (circumferential ridges and base of the pin implants) was statistically larger than at the lower strain regions (smooth sides of the pin) of the same pin. These results were consistent with the assertion that principal strain magnitudes greater than about 30% disrupted interfacial bone regeneration, while strains below this level permitted bone regeneration. Data from experiments B, C, and D also supported that view, as follows. With

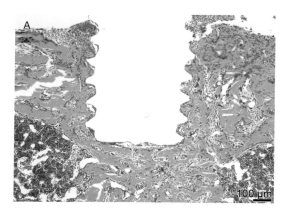
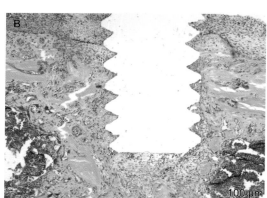
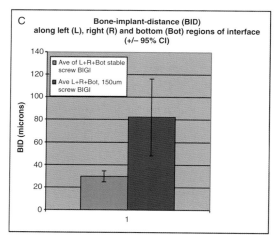
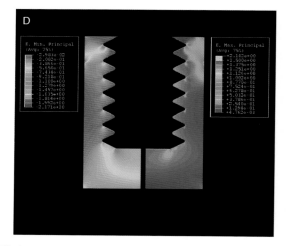

Figure 11.3. Experiment B results: a. Stable screw in BIGI. b. 150 μm motion screw in BIGI for 7 days. c. Mean bone-implant distances (BID) for stable and motion case. d. Finite element predictions of interfacial principal tensile and compressive strains.

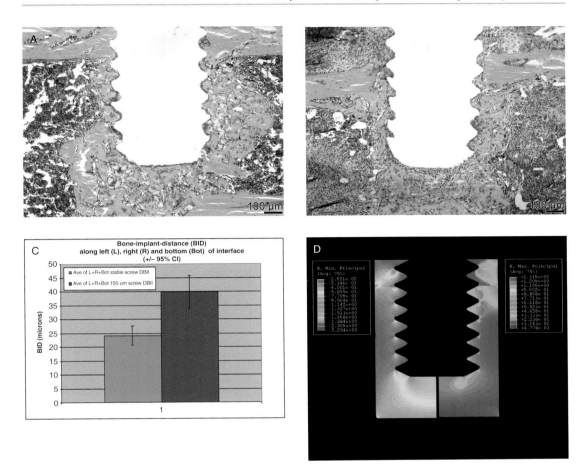

Figure 11.4. Experiment C results: a. Stable screw in DBII. b. 150 μm motion screw in DBII for 7 days. c. Mean bone-implant distances (BID) for stable and motion case. d. Finite element predictions of interfacial principal tensile and compressive strains.

stable screws versus screws moving 150 μm in the BIGI (experiment B), there was a significantly larger BID in the motion cases at 7 days, and these large BIDs co-localized with regions of large (i.e., 30–100%) tensile and compressive principal strains at the tips of the screw threads and beneath the screw (Fig. 11.3).

Likewise, in experiment C with stable screws versus screws moving 150 μm in the DBII interface, there was a significantly larger BID for motion cases, which correlated with the very large (i.e., 30–100%) tensile and compressive principal strain values at screw thread tips and beneath the screw in this DBII (Fig. 11.4).

On the other hand, in experiment D, where screws moved axially by only 17–70 μm in the DBII, there was no difference in the BID values for stable versus motion cases, which correlated with small values of the principal strains at the interfaces of the implants subjected to motion (i.e., less than about 0.0003%) (Fig. 11.5).

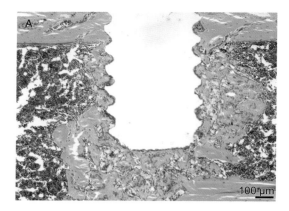
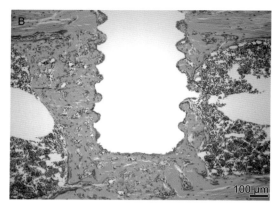
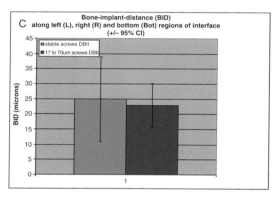
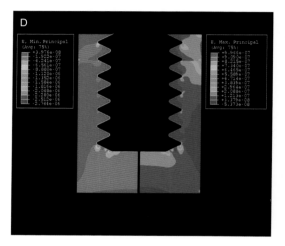

Figure 11.5. Experiment D results: a. Stable screw in DBII. b. 17–70 μm motion screw in DBII for 7 days. c. Mean bone-implant distances (BID) for stable and motion case. d. Finite element predictions of interfacial principal tensile and compressive strains.

Discussion and Conclusions

The largest BIDs (mean values ranging from 40–80 μm) occurred for interfaces of motion implants having high (i.e., >30%) interfacial principal strains over nearly the entire interface, that is, experiments B and C. Also, in experiments B and C thin undecalcified sections showed cellular debris, red blood cells, and other features consistent with localized damage at high strain regions. On the other hand, nearly direct bone-implant apposition (small BID) occurred in the motion cases of experiment D (17–70 μm motion in DBII), which also had very small interfacial princi-

pal strains (<0.0003%). In experiment D, the mean BID was 20–30 μm for the motion implants, which did not statistically differ from the mean BID for stable implants in the DBII.

These experiments did not pinpoint an exact threshold value of principal tensile or compressive strain beyond which bone regeneration was prevented in the interface. However, the data were consistent with the existence of such a strain threshold; for example, in experiment A bone regeneration was disrupted in high strain regions but not low strain regions of the *same* interface. To a first approximation, our results support the notion that principal tensile and/or compressive strains exceeding 30% in the early healing period cause problems with bone regeneration. Interestingly, this proposed 30% threshold is consistent with work in fracture healing, where it has been suggested that dynamic axial strains at a healing fracture site of about 10% permit bone regeneration but strains above 30–40% do not (Claes et al. 2002). Likewise with oral implants, it has been suggested (Simmons et al. 2001) that strains of 8% or less were conducive to appositional bone formation.

A conclusion from this work so far is that while implant micromotion per se is important, it is the interfacial strain field associated with the micromotion that appears to influence the interfacial mechanobiology.

Acknowledgments

NIH R01-EB000504-4.

References

Brånemark PI, Hansson BO, et al. 1977. Osseointegrated implants in the treatment of the edentulous jaw. Experience from a 10-year period. *Scand J Plast Reconstr Surg* (Suppl) 16:1–132.

Brunski J. 1988. The influence of force, motion, and related quantities on the response of bone to implants. In: *Non Cemented Total Hip Arthroplasty*. R. Fitzgerald (ed.). New York: Raven Press. 43.

Brunski J, Glantz P-O, Helms JA, Nanci A. 2005. Transfer of mechanical load across the interface. In: *Osseointegration Book*. PI Brånemark (ed.). Berlin: Quintessenz. 209–249.

Brunski, JB, Moccia AF, Jr., et al. 1979. The influence of functional use of endosseous dental implants on the tissue-implant interface. I: Histological aspects. *J Dent Res* 58(10):1953–1969.

Claes L, Eckert-Hubner K, et al. 2002. The effect of mechanical stability on local vascularization and tissue differentiation in callus healing. *J Orthop Res* 20(5):1099–1105.

Currey JA, Brunski JB. 2006. Characterization of the mechanical environment at an implant interface: An in vitro study. 2006 Summer Bioengineering Conference (Proceedings of BIO2006), Amelia Island, FL, American Society of Mechanical Engineers.

De Smet E, Jaecques S, et al. 2005. Positive effect of early loading on implant stability in the bi-cortical guinea-pig model. *Clin Oral Implants Res* 16(4):402–407.

Esposito M, Grusovin MG, et al. 2007. The effectiveness of immediate, early, and conventional loading of dental implants: A Cochrane systematic review of randomized controlled clinical trials. *Int J Oral Maxillofac Implants* 22(6):893–904.

Leucht P, Kim JB, et al. 2007b. Effect of mechanical stimuli on skeletal regeneration around implants. *Bone* 40(4):919–930.

Leucht P, Kim JB, et al. 2007a. FAK-Mediated mechanotransduction in skeletal regeneration. *PLoS ONE* 2(4):e390.

Nicolella DP, Nicholls AE, et al. 2001. Machine vision photogrammetry: A technique for measurement of microstructural strain in cortical bone. *J Biomech* 34(1):135–139.

Rubin CT, McLeod KJ. 1994. Promotion of bony ingrowth by frequency-specific, low-amplitude mechanical strain. *Clin Orthop Relat Res* 298:165–174.

Simmons CA, Meguid SA, et al. 2001. Mechanical regulation of localized and appositional bone formation around bone-interfacing implants. *J Biomed Mater Res* 55(1):63–71.

Soballe K, Brockstedt-Rasmussen H, et al. 1992. Hydroxyapatite coating modifies implant membrane formation. Controlled micromotion studied in dogs. *Acta Orthop Scand* 63(2):128–140.

The Implant Surface and Biological Response

THE CHANGING INTERFACE

John E. Davies, Peter Schüpbach, and
Lyndon Cooper

Introduction

Over a quarter of a century has passed since the first osseointegration meeting in Toronto. During this time there have been major advances in our understanding of basic biology and a revolution in the treatment modalities available to us in clinical practice, which have been supported by an equally important revolution in technology and communications in general. The human genome project was initiated in 1986 and has had a profound effect on our approach to modern medicine, as have other breakthroughs such as the first liver transplant in 1989; the first self-contained artificial heart in 2001; and the emergence of positron emission tomography and magnetic resonance imaging as routine methods in the detection and diagnosis of disease. All this and much more has been concomitant with technological advances that include, importantly in the context of this chapter, the routine employment of field-emission microscopy in biology, and that otherwise range from the emergence of lithium batteries and supercomputers, to the discovery of buckyballs, quarks, and leptons and the invention of the World Wide Web.

Given these huge and radical changes in technology and medicine over the last quarter of a century, it is not at all surprising that there have also been radical changes in our level of understanding of the basic biology concerning peri-implant healing in both hard and soft tissues. While the 1982 Toronto Osseointegration Conference represented the first North American overture of a revolution in dental implant treatment that had started in Europe in 1969, there have since been very significant advances in both our understanding of peri-implant biology and the role that the material surface plays in orchestrating the pattern of healing. From a clinical perspective this is clearly witnessed by our now being able to successfully place implants in predominantly trabecular rather than cortical bone and our increasingly successful use of immediate dental implant placement strategies. Importantly, these changes have come about as a result of our understanding of the role of micro- and nano-textured surfaces in implant design.

It is salutary to note that, as three independent authors and active researchers, we have each been closely involved with different implant manufacturers, yet we are united in the view that our ongoing exploration of the basic science of the interface between biology and materials science will continue to drive clinical success in this increasingly important area of dental therapy. For this reason we have combined in this chapter a brief synopsis of the understanding of the tissue implant interface at the time of the first osseointegration meeting in 1982; we have chosen to exemplify some of the important characteristics of our current understanding of this interface through examples of our own individual research; and we provide a glimpse into what we feel are some important aspects that require continued research efforts as we advance through the next decades.

The Basic Science Status Quo in 1982

It is now universally accepted that the development of the tissue-implant interface is a complex series of cascades of cellular activity that are preceded by both ionic exchange events and protein adsorption. This wisdom is based on early pioneering work undertaken to understand the biocompatibility of implant materials (reviewed in Williams 1981), the atomic and molecular events occurring at the inorganic implant surface/tissue fluid interface (reviewed in Kasemo and Lausmaa 1988), and the recognition of competitive protein adsorption as a hierarchical series of collision, adsorption, and exchange processes (reviewed in Bamford et al. 1992). Nevertheless, in 1982, our understanding of the tissue interface with dental implant surfaces was still quite rudimentary. Thus while it was recognized that blood clotted around a newly placed implant it was simply stated that "the hematoma becomes transformed into new bone" (Brånemark 1985). At this time, the majority of implants were placed successfully in areas of high volumes of cortical bone, which necessitated long, submerged healing times. Indeed, the creation of a robust interface was best achieved when there was close apposition of both bone and soft tissues to the implant surface, as is illustrated in Figure 12.1, but there was little apposition of new bone in cancellous compartments that led to the misguided designation of the bone in the posterior maxilla as that of "poor quality."

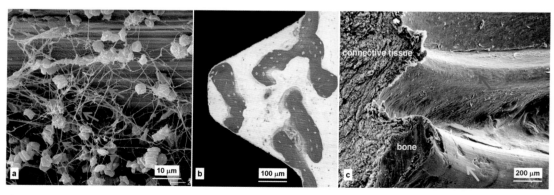

Figure 12.1. Examples of our understanding of the implant interface in 1982. a. The fibrin meshwork (red arrows) of the peri-implant blot clot detached from a machined surface. b. In trabecular bone healing, bone formation was by distance osteogenesis. c. The smooth interfaces between bone and connective tissue and the implant surface indicated an approximation of the tissues to the surface rather than intimate cell/surface interactions.

The Hard-Tissue Interface

We now realize the initial blood contact with the implant surface creates a dynamic state of cellular activity, starting with the activation of platelets and leukocytes in the peri-implant hematoma and the attachment of transitory structural proteins, such as fibrin, to the implant surface. The retention of these proteins by the implant surface is dependent upon the surface topography of the latter, and it is through this three-dimensional biological architecture that putative osteogenic cells migrate to the implant surface. The anchorage of these early proteins to a machined or "turned" titanium-based surface was quite poor (Fig. 12.2a) but has been radically improved with the employment of microtextured-surfaced implants (Fig. 12.2b).

However, with surfaces that facilitate such contact osteogenesis there is also an opportunity, either directly or indirectly, to effect fundamental cell-making processes that drive

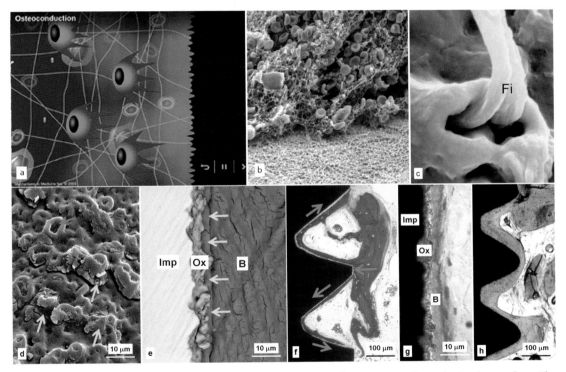

Figure 12.2. a. Osteoconduction is the recruitment and migration of osteogenic cells to the implant surface. The mechanisms are explained in this animation, which is available at http://www.ecf.utoronto.ca/~bonehead/. b. SEM micrograph of a blood clot on an implant surface. The clot (above) can be seen to contain many red blood cells within a rich fibrin matrix that is anchored to the implant surface (below). c. Competitive cellular activity at the implant surface can lead to osteogenic cells that come in contact with the implant surface, as can be seen in this SEM micrograph of a filopodium (Fi) anchored in an open pore of the oxidized surface. d. Apatite deposits in the pores (red arrows) or around the volcano-like elevations of the anodically roughened surface (yellow arrows). e. Cement line (yellow arrows) interposed between the oxidized implant surface (Ox) and the body of the implant (Imp). f. Osteoconductive bone formation outgoing from a contact point between a bone trabeculum and the implant and following the implant surface (red arrows). g. Initially formed woven bone on the crystalline oxidized layer. h. Lamellar bone following in a wallpaper-like configuration the contour of the threads.

reparative mesenchymal cell lineage differentiation, or specifically target the anabolic activity of the osteoblast. Knowing the details of these biological reactions allows us to distinguish between the sequelae of contact and distance osteogenesis and the important effect that implant surface microtopography has on driving the former phenomenon.

Thus, while the importance of platelets and their activation on the implant surface has now been robustly demonstrated experimentally, and has not only been shown to be a product of implant surface microtopography but also that such implant-driven platelet activation can result in increases in leukocyte activation, what is less well understood is the competition for the implant surface by macrophages and cells of the mesenchymal lineages within the peri-implant healing area. It is only through this competitive cellular activity that one can anticipate a putative osteogenic cell being able to occupy the implant surface and beginning to secrete extracellular matrix directly on the implant surface as we now know to occur in the phenomenon of contact osteogenesis (Figs. 12.2c–12.2h).

Indeed, in vitro assays designed to investigate the effects of implant surfaces on cells of the osteoblastic lineage (Cooper et al. 1998) acquire new relevance with the recognition of cellular competition for the implant surface. While the recruitment and migration of such cells to the implant surface in the endosseous compartment still remains a subject to be explored, and is discussed again below, overwhelming evidence has emerged in the last two decades to support the view that microtopographically complex surfaces can significantly increase the degree of bone-to-implant contact compared to relatively smooth surfaces. This has been exhaustively shown in many studies in the dental field but has been equally well understood in the orthopedic field for many years. Thus it is now clear that surfaces with less microtopographical features are likely to exhibit distance osteogenesis, whereas more microtopographically complex surfaces are more likely to exhibit contact osteogenesis. However, it should also be noted that all surfaces are heterogeneous and thus a nominally machined or turned commercially pure titanium implant will have many microtopographical features formed as imperfections in the surface (whereas the harder Ti6Al4V alloy will show fewer such features and therefore appear smoother). Chemical treatment of these metals to render them more microtopographically complex may reverse this differential between cpTi and alloy and, as a result, titanium alloy can be shown to outperform cpTi in rigorous biological assays.

Clearly, in contact osteogenesis, osteogenic differentiation has to occur in addition to cell migration to the implant surface, and there has been a recent explosion of knowledge that has illuminated the molecular switches that control osteoinduction. At least three signalling pathways are critical in the regulation of osteogenesis (Komori 2008; Marie 2008). One pathway leads to the activation of RUNX2, a transcription factor necessary and sufficient for osteoinduction. A second leads to the activation of Osterix, a second transcription factor needed for robust osteoinduction and osteogenesis. When either of these genes is rendered non-functional in mice, the total absence of osteoblasts is observed. A third pathway involves a signalling molecule called beta-catenin that mediates Wnt signalling. Loss of beta-catenin function leads to marked loss of osteoblastic activity. These key regulators may represent targets for engineering of the endosseous implant surface.

However, there are many ways in which a metallic implant surface can be modified to exhibit micro- and nano-scale surface features. One is illustrated by the thickening of the surface oxide layer on titanium by the process of anodic oxidation (Hall and Lausmaa 2000). The thickened oxide layer is highly crystalline, containing anatase and rutile, which are the most common crystalline forms of titanium oxide (Schüpbach et al. 2005), and results in surface pores within volcano-like elevations with diameters in the lower micrometer range into which cell processes may invaginate (Fig. 12.2c). These pores also provide recipient sites for cement line deposition by differentiating osteogenic cells (Fig. 12.2d), which builds up to form an intact layer on the implant surface (Fig. 12.2e). The result of this contact osteogenesis is the establishment of a seam of new bone directly deposited on the implant surface (Figs. 12.2e–12.2h), which matures in contact with the implant surface (Figs. 12.2g, 12.2h) to create stable anchorage in the trabecular compartment (Fig. 12.2h). In this manner, metal oxides can be as effective as traditional plasma-sprayed calcium phosphate–coated implants (Zechner et al. 2003). Other nano-scale modifications are illustrated in Figures 12.3a–12.3f in the surfaces of cpTi treated with hydrofluoric acid (Cooper et al. 2006), zirconia treated with calcium phosphate (Schubach 2008 unpublished), and Ti6Al4V (Mendes et al. 2007).

The biological effects of these scales of modifications have been demonstrated using a bone marrow derived adult mesenchymal stem cell culture system (Cooper et al. 2006; Guo et al. 2007). As illustrated in Figure 12.4, cells adherent to a nano-scale surface displayed higher levels of RUNX2, Osterix, and BSP, which would suggest that superimposition of nano-scale topography on a cpTi surface promotes osteoinductive signalling in the adherent cell.

The Soft-Tissue Interface

Far less attention has been paid to the soft-tissue interface with endosseous implants, but we do know that the primary function of the periodontal tissues is gingival protection. Specifically, the soft tissues provide a seal against the contaminated environment of the oral cavity, they withstand the frictional forces of mastication, and they actively defend the hard-/soft-tissue interface with an immunologic peripheral defense system (Bosshardt and Lang 2005; Schroeder and Listgarten 1997). We also now know that the same is true for the human peri-implant soft tissues, which are in many ways analogous to those

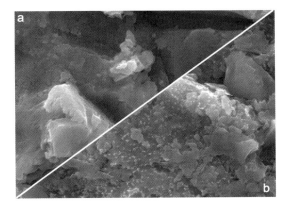
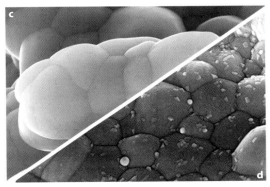
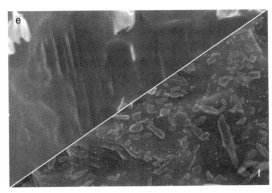

Figure 12.3. Three examples of nanoscale modifications of implant surfaces. (a) Grit-blasted titanium oxide treated with (b) hydrofluoric acid; (c) a zirconia ceramic surface treated with (d) calcium phosphate; and (e) an acid-etched titanium alloy surface treated with (f) nanoscale individual crystals of hydroxyapatite. Each surface modification renders the original more osteoconductive. In the case of (f), the implant surface also exhibits bone bonding. (Field widths = 23.8, 2.5, and 2.5 microns, respectively.)

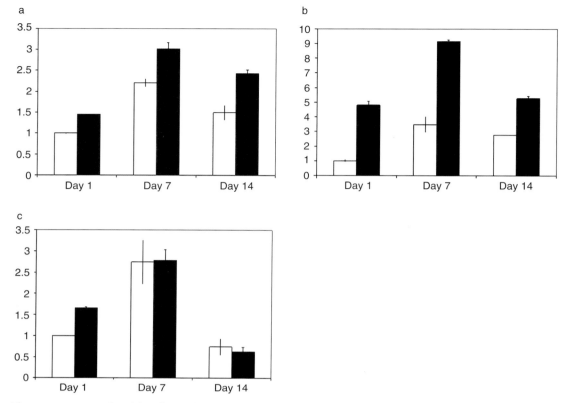

Figure 12.4. Examples of the effects of nano-scale topography on the levels of adherent cell osteoinductive and osteogenic protein gene expression. (a) RUNX-2 mRNA, (b) Osterix mRNA levels, and (c) BSP mRNA levels after 3, 7, and 14 days of culture of osteoprogenitor cells on grit-blasted (open bars) or grit-blasted and HF-treated (closed bars) cp titanium disks. (Ordinates in arbitrary units; adapted from Guo et al. 2007.)

of the natural dentition (for review, see Rompen et al. 2006). The seal is provided by the junctional epithelium directly attached to the implant surface or the abutment via a basal lamina and the formation of hemidesmosomes (Bosshardt and Lang 2005). The junctional epithelium is also the compartment of the peripheral defense (Schüpbach and Glauser 2007), whereas the stability of the peri-implant mucosa is given by the peri-implant connective tissue (Fig. 12.5a).

The influence of surface modifications on interactions between the implant surface and both junctional epithelial cells and connective tissue extracellular matrix was recently evaluated in a human study using one-piece mini-implants with anodically roughened,

acid-etched, or machined surfaces (Glauser et al. 2005; Schüpbach and Glauser 2007).

With machined and acid-etched implants the adherence of the junctional epithelium to the implant surface was characterized by a basal lamina and numerous hemidesmosomes (Fig. 12.5b).

But the interface between connective tissue and the machined and acid-etched implants was smooth, indicating a poor mechanical resistance (Fig. 12.5c), with the collagen fibers running a course more or less parallel to the implant surface (Figs. 12.5d, 12.5e, and 12.5i).

On the other hand, with a microtopographically complex oxidized implant surface, the junctional epithelium showed attachment by

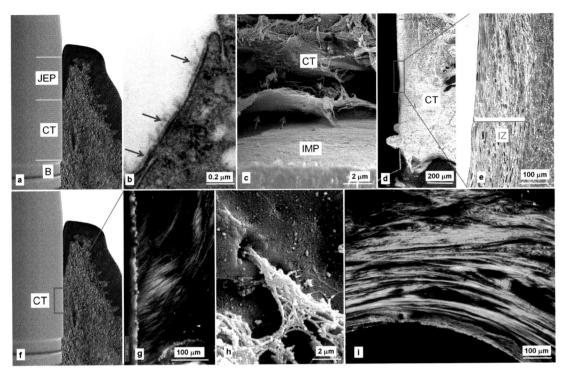

Figure 12.5.   a. Schematic diagram illustrating the junctional epithelium (JEP), the connective tissue (CT), and the alveolar bone crest (B). b. TEM micrograph demonstrating hemidesmosome/basal lamina complexes (red arrows) at the interface to a machined implant surface as seen following removal of the implant. c. SEM micrograph showing adaptation of connective tissue (CT) toward a machined implant (IMP) surface (red arrows). d and e. Orientation of the collagen matrix and fibroblasts parallel to a machined implant surface. Note the avascular scar tissue-like fiber rich zone (IZ). f. Schematic diagram illustrating the connective tissue (CT) compartment. g. Polarized light microscopic image showing functionally oriented collagen fibrils directed toward an oxidized titanium surface. h. SEM image showing connective tissue fibers ending in a pore. i. Polarized view of the circumferentially oriented dense fiber bundles around an implant. Adapted from Schüpbach and Glauser 2007; permission granted by Elsevier Mosby.

hemidesmosomes together with mechanical interdigitation of the innermost cell layer with the open pores or the implant surface, indicating the presence of a less vulnerable seal toward the oral cavity (Schüpbach and Glauser 2007) (Fig. 12.5f). The connective tissue compartment also exhibited collagen functionally oriented toward the implant surface (Figs. 12.5g, 12.5h) in the form of a pseudo-gomphosis.

Thus substantial structural analogies can be demonstrated between gingiva and peri-implant mucosa in humans. In each case, these tissues provide protection of the underlying soft tissue and bone. Several specific antimicrobial defense mechanisms exist in the junctional epithelium (Bosshardt and Lang 2005; Pollanen et al. 2003). As seen around teeth, leukocytes migrate through the junctional epithelium and comprise the most important defense mechanism around implants (Schüpbach and Glauser 2007).

A Glimpse into the Future

We now realize that micro- and nano-textured implant surfaces can recapitulate the bony interface created in natural bone

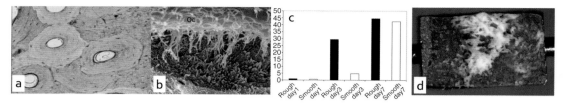

Figure 12.6. Natural bone remodelling (a) is created by the coordinated activities of both osteoclasts and osteoblasts, and results in a robust interface between new and old bone. The surface left by the resorbing osteoclast (b) is now mimicked by some implant surfaces. Indeed, the microtopography of an implant surface can have a profound effect on osteoprotegerin (OPG) levels expressed by implant adherent cells in vivo (from rat tibia after 3 and 7 days) (c), and thus may contribute to suppression of peri-implant osteoclastogenesis. Micro- and nano-topographical features of the implant surface can also permit bone to bond to the implant surface (d) as is seen in natural remodelling (see text for references).

remodelling (Fig. 12.6) and that the mechanically robust interface found at remodeling sites can be achieved with bone-bonding implant surfaces.

However, it is equally clear that we still have much to learn about the biological mechanisms that occur at such interfaces, since bone loss attributable to osteoclastogenesis and osteoclast function (Teitelbaum 2007) can also occur in the peri-implant healing compartment. Indeed, we know that osteoclast and osteoblast activities are coupled to provide physiologic control of bone mass. Osteoclasts are derived from circulating monocytes and are recruited to sites of bone turnover by inflammatory and mechanical (or traumatic) signals (Takayanagi 2005). Over the past three decades, many fundamental aspects of osteoclast regulation have been discovered, not least of which is the identification of the key inducing ligand RANKL (Receptor Activating NF-kappa-B Ligand) and its physiologic inhibitor OPG (osteoprotegrin). One important question is whether implant surface topography can affect the process of osteoclastogenesis at or near the implant surface. Implant surface topography has been shown to alter the expression of OPG by adherent MG63 cells (Lossdörfer et al. 2004). Indeed, we have shown that cultured human mesenchymal stem cells (hMSCs) expressed higher levels of OPG in contact with micro-topographically complex surfaces. To explore this effect in vivo, we implanted

grit-blasted and HCl-etched titanium implants in rat tibiae for 24 and 72 hours and measured OPG mRNA expression in implant-adherent cells (Fig. 12.6c), which was profoundly increased in those samples from the more micro-topographically complex implant group. This work suggests that an implant surface topography may affect the number and activity of osteoclasts in the peri-implant tissue, and is a focus of our ongoing investigations.

These different observations contribute to a body of evidence demonstrating that progenitor cell populations are influenced by the implant surface. Thus in the future it may be possible not only to further enhance osteogenesis at the endosseous dental implant surface and have the bone matrix bonding to the implant surface, but also to influence the osteoclastogenesis that occurs in the surrounding bone. Given that the process of bone adaptation and maturation are critical features of the long-term success of osseointegration, continued attention to the molecular processes underlying these events may create new biological design criteria for implant surface design. This will be particularly important in the coronal regions of implants where crestal bone loss clearly involves a complex interplay between the reactions of both hard and soft peri-implant tissues, and the biomechanical influences on the molecular mechanisms of cell/matrix/implant interactions. With the advent of a myriad

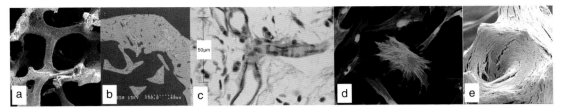

Figure 12.7.   Peri-implant bone regeneration is often clinically enhanced using bone filling materials. New generations of such materials are now becoming available that are fully biodegradable in clinically relevant time frames (a), osteoconductive (b), and can be employed as delivery vehicles for either biologically active molecules or stem cells. The later mesenchymal stem cells, known to be present throughout the body as pericytes (c—seen here surrounding a capillary), can be isolated (d) and grown on biodegradable scaffolds (e), offering new opportunities for bone regeneration therapies (see text for references).

of "immediate" implant placement regimes, many of which involve the use of peri-implant bone-filling materials, balancing materials design with the interactions of both osteoblast and osteoclasts is becoming ever more important (Figs. 12.7a, 12.7b).

Another problem to solve is the provenance of the cells themselves. While it is now generally agreed that mesenchymal stem cells reside in all tissues as pericytes (Fig. 12.7c), little is understood about how these cells are recruited to the implant surface. This is complicated by the fact that we also know that mesenchymal cells can "home" to sites of injury (Schenk et al. 2007), but nothing is currently known about the balance between homing to, and local cell invasion into, the wound site.

Nevertheless, there are currently over 30 clinical trials being undertaken worldwide using mesenchymal stem cells in a wide variety of regenerative therapies (see http://www.clinicaltrials.gov/). As it is now possible to employ either autogenous or allogeneic populations of mesenchymal stem cells as treatment modalities in dental implantology, understanding how these cells survive and function during wound healing becomes critically important to designing realistic cell-based therapies for the future. Of course, in the majority of currently selected dental implant patients, these issues may not be of importance. However, for those increasing populations of prospective implant patients with systemic disease, or who have received chemo-/irradiation therapy, or who are suffering from new pathologies associated with the chronic administration of bone-affecting pharmaceuticals, the advent of either mesenchymal stem cell and/or tissue-engineering strategies to augment implant therapy may critically affect the success of their putative regenerative treatment.

Concluding Remarks

Great progress has been made in our understanding of the role of the implant surface in peri-implant healing, for both hard and soft tissues, since the Toronto Osseointegration Conference in 1982. Due to changes in implant design, implants can now routinely be placed in bone of predominantly trabecular architecture, and we understand the biology of this success. We also now realize how important nano-scale surface features are to the phenomena of osteoconduction and bone bonding, and recent findings suggest that implant surfaces may drive molecular mechanisms in peri-implant cells in both hard- and soft-tissue compartments. This new level of biological understanding will continue to drive improvements in implant surface design but will also lead to the emergence of new materials and cell-based therapies to enhance peri-implant healing in general.

References

Bamford CH, Cooper SL, Tsuruta T (eds.). 1992. *The Vroman Effect: Festschrift in Honour of the 75th Birthday of Dr. Leo Vroman.* Utrecht, The Netherlands: Brill.

Bosshardt DD, Lang NP. 2005. The junctional epithelium: From health to disease. *J Dent Res* 84:9–20.

Brånemark PI. 1985. Introduction to osseointegration. In: *Tissue-Integrated Prostheses: Osseointegration in Clinical Dentistry.* PI Brånemark, GA Zarb, T Albrektsson (eds.). Chicago: Quintessence.

Cooper LF, Masuda T, Yliheikkilä PK, Felton DA. 1998. Generalizations regarding the process and phenomenon of osseointegration. Part II: In vitro studies. *Int J Oral Maxillofac Implants* 13:163–174.

Cooper LF, Zhou Y, Takebe J, Guo J, Abron A, Holmén A, Ellingsen JE. 2006. Fluoride modification effects on osteoblast behavior and bone formation at TiO2 grit-blasted c.p. titanium endosseous implants. *Biomaterials* 27:926–936.

Davies JE. 1998. Mechanisms of endosseous integration. *Int J Prosthodont* 11(5): 391–401.

———. 2003. Understanding peri-implant endosseous healing. *J Dent Educ* 67(8): 932–949. Review. (Reprinted color edition available at http://www.ecf.utoronto.ca/~bonehead/.)

———. 2007. Bone bonding at natural and biomaterial surfaces. *Biomaterials* 28(34):5058–5067.

Feighan JE, Goldberg VM, Davy D, Parr JA, Stevenson S. 1995. The influence of surface-blasting on the incorporation of titanium-alloy implants in a rabbit intramedullary model. *J Bone Joint Surg Am* 77: 1380–1395.

Glauser R, Schüpbach P, Gottlow J, Hammerle CH. 2005. Peri-implant soft tissue barrier at experimental one-piece mini-implants with different surface topography in humans: A light-microscopic overview and histometric analysis. *Clin Implant Dent Relat Res* 7(Suppl 1):S44–S51.

Guo J, Padilla RJ, Ambrose W, De Kok IJ, Cooper LF. 2007. The effect of hydrofluoric acid treatment of TiO2 grit blasted titanium implants on adherent osteoblast gene expression in vitro and in vivo. *Biomaterials* 28:5418–5425.

Hall J, Lausmaa J. 2000. Properties of a new porous oxide surface on titanium implants. *Appl Osseointegration Res* 1:5–8.

Kasemo B, Lausmaa J. 1988. Biomaterials and implant surfaces: A surface science approach. *Int J Oral Maxillofacial Implants* 3:247–259.

Komori T. 2008. Regulation of bone development and maintenance by Runx2. *Front Biosci* 13:898–903. Review.

Lossdörfer S, Schwartz Z, Wang L, Lohmann CH, Turner JD, Wieland M, Cochran DL, Boyan BD. 2004. Microrough implant surface topographies increase osteogenesis by reducing osteoclast formation and activity. *J Biomed Mater Res A* 70:361–369.

Marie PJ. 2008. Transcription factors controlling osteoblastogenesis. *Arch Biochem Biophys* 473(2):98–105.

Masuda T, Salvi GE, Offenbacher S, Felton DA, Cooper LF. 1997. Cell and matrix reactions at titanium implants in surgically prepared rat tibiae. *Int J Oral Maxillofac Implants* 12:472–485.

Mendes VC, Moineddin R, Davies JE. 2007. The effect of discrete calcium phosphate nanocrystals on bone-bonding to titanium surfaces. *Biomaterials* 28(32):4748–4755.

Pawley J. 1997. The development of field-emission scanning electron microscopy for imaging biological surfaces. *Scanning* 19:324–336.

Pollanen MT, Salonen JI, Uitto VJ. 2003. Structure and function of the tooth-epithelial interface in health and disease. *Periodontol 2000* 31:12–31.

Rompen E, Domken O, Degidi M, Pontes AEF, Piatelli A. 2006. The effect of material characteristics, of surface topography and of implant components and connections on soft tissue integration: A literature review.

Clin Oral Implants Res 17(Suppl 2):55–67.

Schenk S, Mal N, Finan A, Zhang M, Kiedrowski M, Popovic Z, McCarthy PM, Penn MS. 2007. Monocyte chemotactic protein-3 is a myocardial mesenchymal stem cell homing factor. *Stem Cells* 25(1):245–251.

Schroeder HE, Listgarten M. 1997. The gingival tissues: The architecture of periodontal protection. *Periodontol 2000* 13:21–31.

Schüpbach P, Glauser R. 2007. The defense architecture of the human peri implant mucosa: A histological study. *J Prosth Dent* 97:S15–S25.

Schüpbach P, Glauser R, Rocci A, Martignoni M, Sennerby L, Lundgren A, Gottlow J. 2005. The human bone-oxidized titanium implant interface: A light microscopic, scanning electron microscopic, back-scatter scanning electron microscopic, and energy-dispersive X-ray study of clinically retrieved implants. *Clin Implant Dent Relat Res* 7(Suppl 1):S36–S43.

Takayanagi H. 2005. Inflammatory bone destruction and osteoimmunology. *J Periodontal Res* 40:287–293. Review.

Teitelbaum SL. 2007. Osteoclasts: What do they do and how do they do it? *Am J Pathol* 170:427–435.

Williams DF (ed.). 1981. *Fundamental Aspects of Biocompatibility*, 2 vols. Boca Raton, FL: CRC Press.

Zechner W, Tangl S, Fuerst G, Tepper G, Thams U, Mailath G, Watzek G. 2003. Osseous healing characteristics of three different implant types. A histologic and histomorphometric study in mini-pigs. *Clin Oral Implants Res* 14:150–157.

The Implant Design and Biological Response

INFLUENCES OF IMPLANT DESIGN AND SURFACE PROPERTIES ON OSSEOINTEGRATION AND IMPLANT STABILITY

Jan Gottlow

Osseointegration

Osseointegration is a prerequisite for successful implant treatment. The term was defined by Brånemark (1985) as "a direct structural and functional connection between ordered, living bone and the surface of a load-carrying implant".

Primary Stability

The primary, or initial, stability is the stability of the implant achieved at insertion in the bone. The primary stability is a result of a biomechanical interlocking of the implant and the surrounding bone. The stability is dependent on the bone quality and quantity, the surgical technique, and the design of the implant.

Bone Quality—Bone Density

The stiffness of cortical bone is 10 to 20 times higher than that of trabecular bone due to its content of dense, mineralized lamellae. This means that the more compact bone in relation to trabecular bone there is, the higher primary stability. The term "bone quality" is slightly misleading. Soft bone is often referred to as poor bone quality. However, there is nothing biologically wrong with the soft bone, although the biomechanical strength is lower. Hence, it would be better to talk about bone density (e.g., soft bone and dense bone).

Surgical Technique

O'Sullivan (2001) found that primary stability was influenced by drill diameter and whether pretapping was used or not. In essence, thinner drill diameters and omitting pretapping resulted in a higher primary stability.

225

Implant Design

The implant itself has impact on stability depending on its geometrical features. In a human cadaver study, O'Sullivan et al. (2000) evaluated the stability of different implant geometries in various bone densities using resonance frequency analysis (RFA). The use of a slightly tapered implant design placed in a site with parallel prepared walls, for example, the Brånemark System Mk IV implant (Nobel Biocare AB, Sweden), increased the stability as compared to a parallel walled implant. Another study in rabbits confirmed the finding of better primary stability when using a one degree taper compared to the standard Brånemark design (O'Sullivan et al. 2004). The micro-geometry of the implant design, for example, the surface texture and roughness, on the other hand, has not been shown to influence the primary stability (Rompen et al. 2000).

Secondary Stability

After implant placement the bone tissue will respond to the surgical trauma, which with time results in a change of the cortical/trabecular bone ratio and an increasing degree of bone-implant contact. The bone formation and remodelling process may continue up to 12–18 months after surgery (Roberts et al. 1984), but the term "secondary stability" usually refers to the stability achieved at second-stage surgery. The conventional healing period of 3–6 months, as proposed by Prof. Brånemark, was based on empirics rather than biology, since high success rates had been demonstrated when utilizing these healing periods (Brånemark 1977).

The bone remodelling and formation process seems to be influenced by the bone density in that the development of the secondary stability differs between implants placed in dense and soft bone. Friberg et al. (1999a) found that with time the stability of implants

placed in soft bone will equal that of implants placed in dense bone. This is most likely due to a change of the trabecular bone to more cortical bone in the close vicinity of the implant. In dense bone, on the contrary, implant stability slightly decreased over time (Friberg et al. 1999b). This finding supports the application of an immediate loading protocol in good bone qualities since, in these cases, the secondary stability will not be superior to the stability achieved already at implant insertion. The decrease in stability is probably due to a slight resorption of the marginal bone, thus decreasing the amount of supporting cortical bone.

The ability to maintain and to increase the primary implant stability is also determined by the healing and remodelling capacity, which in turn is influenced by endogenous and exogenous factors such as health, the use of drugs, smoking, irradiation, and so forth (Sennerby and Roos 1998).

The Machined/Turned Implant Surface

The first generation of osseointegrated implants had a relatively smooth machined (turned) surface (Brånemark et al. 1969). Good long-term clinical outcomes have been reported on all indications when used in bone of high density and using a two-stage procedure (Albrektsson and Sennerby 1991). In more challenging situations such as low bone densities, grafted bone, and immediate loading, increased failure rates have been reported (Becktor et al. 2004; Friberg et al. 1991; Glauser et al. 2001).

Surface Modified Implants

Surface modification is one way of improving implant integration and stability, as shown in numerous experimental studies (for review see Albrektsson and Wennerberg 2004). Davies (2003) proposed that surface irregularities ensure a firm contact with the blood clot in which primitive cells can migrate to the interface, differentiate to osteoblasts, and form bone directly on the surface ("contact osteogenesis"). In contrast, at a smooth implant surface, shrinkage of the blood clot will create a gap at the interface and cells cannot reach the surface. The new bone will form on the old bone of the osteotomy only ("distance osteogenesis"). Therefore, it will take a longer time to achieve osseointegration. Thus, implants with a moderately rough surface integrate more rapidly and with more bone contacts than smooth surfaced implants (e.g., Ivanoff et al. 2001, 2003; Zechner et al. 2003).

Surface Topography and Chemistry

Micrometer Surface Topography

During the last decade research and product development have focused on implant surface topography at the micrometer level. Minimally rough implant surfaces, for example, 3i Osseotite™, have a roughness below 1.0 µm (S_a value). Moderately roughened surfaces have an average height deviation (S_a value) of 1–2 µm and include implants such as Astra Tech TiOblast™, Nobel Biocare TiUnite®, and Straumann SLA™ (Albrektsson and Wennerberg 2004). The topography of these implants has been created by different processes. The Osseotite™ surface is created through dual acid etching. The TiOblast surface is created through blasting by grains of titanium dioxide. The TiUnite surface is oxidized via an electro-chemical process (anodic oxidation). The SLA surface is sandblasted followed by acid etching. The texture of the etching procedure is superimposed on the rougher topography made by the sandblasting. The resulting surfaces show very different textures (Fig. 13.1).

These implants have been extensively documented in vivo, including long-term clinical studies and histological evaluation in humans (e.g. Cochran et al. 2007; Glauser et al. 2005; Ivanoff et al. 2001, 2003; Rasmusson et al. 2005; Rocci et al. 2003b; Schüpbach et al. 2005; Testori et al. 2001; Trisi et al. 2003).

Rocci et al. (2003a) evaluated and retrieved immediately and early loaded oxidized implants after 5–9 months of loading in the posterior mandible. The implants showed a very high bone-to-implant contact (mean value 84.2%) and bone area values (mean value 79.1%). The two immediately loaded implants had a mean bone-to-implant contact of 92.9% and a mean bone area of 84.9% (Fig. 13.2). The study demonstrated that excellent osseointegration of oxidized implants could be accomplished despite the fact that the implants were subjected to immediate or early loading.

Glauser et al. (2003) reported a survival rate of 97.1% for 102 Brånemark System Mk IV TiUnite® implants in 38 patients subjected to immediate loading. The implants were predominantly placed in the posterior regions and in soft bone. Three implants were removed (in the same patient) after 8 weeks of healing due to an infection in the adjacent area of a simultaneous guided bone regeneration procedure. The mean marginal bone resorption after 1 year was 1.2 mm. The outcome is in contrast to a previous study by the same research group (Glauser et al. 2001), where the Brånemark System Mk IV implant with a machined surface was subjected to immediate loading. The study involved 127 implants in 41 patients. A total of 22 implants were lost in 13 patients, resulting in a survival rate of 82.7%.

It can be speculated that the different outcomes of the two studies above are due to the use of a surface modified implant. This is supported by the findings of Rocci et al. (2003b) following immediate loading in the posterior mandible using oxidized and machined implants (randomized). They found a 10% higher success rate using the oxidized implants.

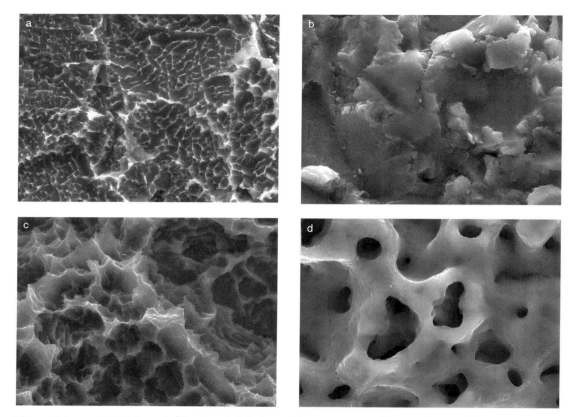

Figure 13.1.   a. SEM of Osseotite™ surface (original magnification × 5,000). b. SEM of TiOblast™ surface (original magnification × 5,000). c. SEM of SLA™ surface (original magnification × 5,000). d. SEM of TiUnite® surface (original magnification × 5,000).

Nanometer Surface Topography and Surface Chemistry

The buzz word of today is surface modifications at the nanometer level and/or claims of direct bone bonding due to changed surface chemistry. Are these "new developments" really new? It's obvious that all existing implant surfaces already possess a nanotopography in addition to the microtopography. But, the nanotopography has not been characterized by the implant producer due to technical difficulties and/or unawareness of the biological (or marketing) value. It should also be realized that it is not easy to document in vivo if a certain biological response to a surface modification is due to the micro-

topography, the nanotopography, or changed surface chemistry. It's also difficult to modify one of the parameters without changing the two others.

The latest surface by Biomet 3i™ is Nano-Tite™. The company claims bone bonding due to "discrete crystalline deposition" of nano-scale calcium phosphate (Mendes et al. 2007).

Histological evaluation of experimental implants placed in the posterior maxilla in humans showed significantly more bone-to-implant contact at modified implants after 4 and 8 weeks of unloaded healing (Goené et al. 2007).

The OsseoSpeed™ surface by Astra Tech is a fluoride modification of the TiOblast™

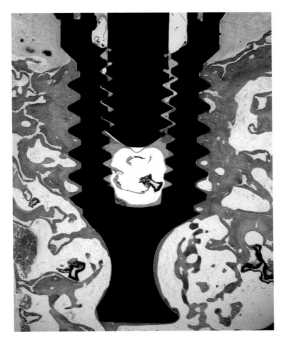

Figure 13.2. Microphotograph of an immediately loaded implant after 9 months in function. The histological evaluation showed a bone-to-implant contact of 93% and a densification of the surrounding bone. The marginal bone level is coronal to the first implant thread.

surface, which improves the affinity to react with phosphates, which in turn will make the surface attractive to calcium phosphate nucleation. Thus calcification and bone growth can start soon after implantation. Significantly more bone-to-implant contact and significantly higher removal torque values were seen for the fluoride modified implant compared to the non-modified control after 1–3 months of healing in rabbit tibial bone (Ellingsen et al. 2004). Increased bone-to-implant contact to the fluoride modified implant was also reported after 2 weeks of healing in a dog model (Berglundh et al. 2007). Clinical documentation is limited to short-term interim reports (e.g., Stanford et al. 2006).

The SLActive™ surface (Straumann) shows hydrophilic properties, whereas the conventional SLA surface is hydrophobic. The increased wettability is accomplished by storing the implants in glass ampoules containing isotonic NaCl solution following the acid-etching procedure. The purpose is to protect the pure Ti surface from contamination with carbonates and organic components occurring in the atmosphere and thus maintain a chemically clean and reactive surface. Buser et al. (2004) found increased bone-to-implant contact during early healing (2–4 weeks) in mini-pigs when comparing the SLActive™ surface to that of SLA. Test and control implants had the same microtopography. An immunohistochemical study in dogs (Schwartz et al. 2007) also found significantly more bone-to-implant contact at SLActive™ implants during early healing (1–28 days). A removal torque study in mini-pigs (Ferguson et al. 2006) showed that the SLActive™ surface was more effective in enhancing the interfacial shear strength of implants in comparison with the conventional SLA surface during early stages of bone healing (2–8 weeks).

Originally, the TiUnite® implants were packed in glass ampoules and the implant surface had hydrophilic properties. Later, the package was changed and the surface became hydrophobic. It should be noted that all oxidized study implants used in the cited references above (Glauser et al. 2003; Rocci et al. 2003a, 2003b; Schüpbach et al. 2005) were packed in glass ampoules and had hydrophilic properties.

The Neoss Bimodal™ surface is created through blasting in two steps. First, the threaded portion is blasted with ZrO_2 particles (100–300 μm). Then the full length of the implant is blasted with Ti-based particles (75–150 μm). The implants are delivered in glass ampoules. The surface shows hydrophilic properties. Sennerby et al. (2008) found bone formation directly on the bimodal surface after 3 and 6 weeks of healing in rabbits. Andersson et al. (2008) reported a survival rate of 98.1% for 102 Neoss implants in 44 consecutively treated patients (two-stage procedure) with a mean bone loss of 0.7 mm after 1 year in function.

Thus, it's obvious that a lot of interesting research and product development is going on based on refined surface modifications and surface chemistry. The question remains if the outcomes are yet of clinical significance or if they, presently, rather serve as marketing tools for the industry. Nevertheless, I am convinced that future research *will*, sooner or later, give us improvements of the biological response that also are of true clinical significance.

IMPLANT SURFACE DESIGN AND LOCAL STRESS FIELDS— EFFECTS ON PERI-IMPLANT BONE FORMATION AND RETENTION WITH "SHORT" POROUS-SURFACED IMPLANTS

Robert M. Pilliar

Summary

Where Were We in 1982?

The principle of osseointegration of a screw-shaped titanium implant with a machined surface was acknowledged. The implants were loaded after a submerged healing period of 3–6 months.

Where Are We Now?

Numerous studies have documented successful treatment of fully edentulous, partially edentulous, and single-tooth replacements in all areas of the mouth and in various bone densities. Surface modifications have shortened the healing time. Treatment protocols of early loading and immediate loading have been established.

Where Are We Going?

Development of bioactive implant surfaces will further speed up the osseointegration process as well as improve the quality and strength of the bone/implant interface. This will increase the predictability of treatment in soft bone densities and in compromised patients. It will also increase the possibility and predictability of early/immediate loading.

Introduction

Porous-surfaced implants formed by sintering Ti alloy powders over intended bone-interfacing regions of machined Ti alloy substrates display remarkable performance as "short" (≤7 mm) implants. Figure 13.3 shows the structure of Endopore® dental implants, so formed based on our early studies of this concept (Deporter et al. 1988). The porous surface region is approximately 0.3 mm thick and consists of two or three "layers" of sintered Ti6Al4V alloy powders securely bonded to the underlying solid substrate. Pore size and the volume percent porosity (~35%) allow uninhibited bone ingrowth. Notable features of the porous region are its mechanical integrity, open-pored structure suitable for bone ingrowth, uniform pore distribution throughout, and sub-micron-sized surface features over the sintered Ti alloy particles.

Based on observations from human clinical and animal studies, these characteristics appear to contribute to two significant features, namely reliable osseointegration of "short" implants (≤7 mm) and rapid bone ingrowth (osteoconductivity). The mechanical stress fields generated in peri-implant tissues during healing and following osseointegration next to the porous surface region appear significant in this regard as discussed below. A brief summary of clinical performance of "short" Endopore® implants follows.

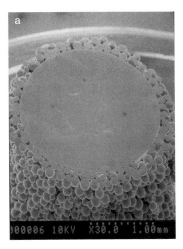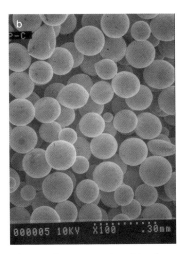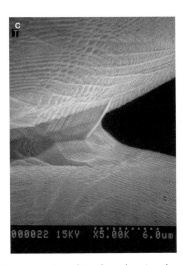

Figure 13.3. Scanning electron images of sintered porous-surfaced implants: (a) cross-sectioned implant showing the 300 micron thick sintered porous Ti alloy particles bonded to the machined Ti alloy substrate; (b) surface view of porous-surfaced region; (c) higher magnification image showing a sinter neck region (particle-particle bonding) and thermal etch lines forming a sub-micron scale texture on the particle surfaces.

Clinical Experience with "Short" Porous-Surfaced Implants

Porous-surfaced implants have been in clinical use since the early 1990s with 7–10 mm long implants being used initially for overdenture stabilization in edentulous mandibles. The longest of these have now been in function for over 16 years. (The 10-year results were reported in a 2002 publication; Deporter et al. 2002). Porous-surfaced implants of 7, 9, and 12 mm length have been used with equal success for supporting fixed partial dentures and as free-standing implants (Rokni et al. 2005). The success, particularly with 7 mm long implants, led to the introduction of even shorter 5 mm long wide-body implants (5 mm diameter) for use in the highly resorbed posterior mandible (Deporter et al. 2008). Significant crestal bone loss is especially unacceptable with "short" implants where loss of 1–2 mm of bone along the length of the implant region intended for osseointegration can be critical to long-term implant stability and survival. This is considered the major reason for the relatively poor performance of conventional threaded implants of lengths ≤8 mm (Naert et al. 2002; Tawil and Younan 2003).

Crestal bone loss with all implant designs is attributable to one or more of the following factors: establishment of "biologic width" (reduced somewhat by use of "platform switching") (Lazzara and Porter 2006), infection resulting in peri-implantitis, and biomechanics as discussed below (either overloading or stress shielding resulting in bone loss due to disuse atrophy).

Biomechanical Causes of Peri-Implant Bone Loss

For threaded implant designs, regions of high stress concentration develop in bone during implant loading especially adjacent to the superior-most threads. This can lead to bone microfracture and resorption of the damaged bone and inhibition of new bone formation preventing the re-establishment of osseointegration. Rather, fibrous tissue forms if local distortional strains are greater than a critical level (Carter and Giori 1991). Continued implant loading can result in progressive bone microfracture and resorption along the length of the implant, resulting in implant loosening. Only if firm fixation is able to develop early on next to more inferior implant regions where lower peri-implant stresses and strains are expected will such an interface "unzipping" process be prevented. For "short" threaded implants this is less likely, which probably explains the low success rates of threaded implants of length ≤8 mm.

A strategy that has been applied to threaded implant design to potentially reduce this local overstressing effect is modification of the coronal implant region by introducing "microgrooves" (Hansson 1999). The microgrooves are intended to allow partial force transfer at these more coronal regions, resulting in the distribution of forces over a greater peri-implant bone volume, thereby lowering stresses next to the regular threads.

An alternative strategy for achieving lower peak peri-implant bone stresses is to design implants that allow efficient force transfer over a greater portion of the bone-interfacing implant surface. Designs that result in 3-D interfacial interlock of bone and implant do this by allowing transfer of tensile as well as shear and compressive forces across this interface. Porous-surfaced Endopore® implants represent such a design.

The different peri-implant stress distributions resulting during functional loading of porous-surfaced versus threaded implants are depicted in Figure 13.4.

As a result of the ability to transfer tensile forces across the interface (the interlocking of bone with the porous structure "tethers" the bone to the implant), peri-implant stresses act over a larger bone volume with porous-surfaced implants. The result is a reduction in peak stress within peri-implant tissues for this design compared with the threaded implant. A recent finite element model (FEM) study of porous-surfaced and threaded implants used

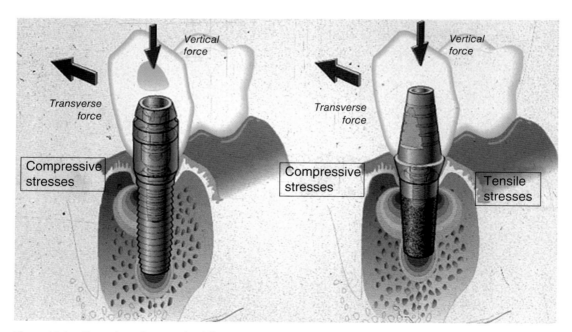

Figure 13.4. Illustrations showing the different compressive and tensile stress distributions in peri-implant bone for threaded and porous-surfaced implants resulting from the applied forces. Peri-implant shear stresses would also be present for both designs.

as anchorage units during orthodontic (transverse) traction force application in dogs predicted a more uniform stress pattern with lower peak stresses with the porous-surfaced design (Pilliar et al. 2006).

Thus, less crestal bone loss as a result of overloading was predicted next to the porous-surfaced implants, a conclusion that appeared to be validated by results of the animal study on which the FEM was based (Oyonarte et al. 2005). The observed success of "short" free-standing dental implants used in humans also appears to validate the FEM prediction (Deporter et al. 2000, 2002b, 2005, 2008; Rokni et al. 2005).

Crestal bone loss can also result from understressing of bone next to implants (so-called "stress shielding"). This occurs in regions of bone that force bypasses during implant loading. This can happen next to the "smooth" machined collar region of all implant designs including porous-surfaced implants (assuming secure fixation occurs more apically). This has been observed both in animal studies (Deporter et al. 1988; Pilliar et al. 1991) and in human clinical studies with porous-surfaced implants (Deporter et al. 2002a). However, in virtually all these studies, crestal bone loss appears limited to the smooth (non-porous) coronal region of the implants where lower stresses are expected (Vaillancourt et al. 1995). Provided that the peri-implant region remains infection-free and notwithstanding the extent of bone loss due to "biologic width" development, bone ingrowth and secure implant fixation are maintained virtually to the smooth-to-porous-surfaced junction with this design.

Implant Design and Rate of Osseointegration

Avoidance of (1) excessive relative movement at the implant-host bone interface during healing (e.g., due to inadvertent forces acting), and (2) establishment of a biofilm prior to connective tissue (preferably bone) formation

over the implant surface positioned within bone are two necessary conditions for osseointegration to develop with any implant design. The faster that osseointegration can occur, the less likely are such undesirable consequences. Thus, increasing the rate of osseointegration (either by bone ingrowth or bone ongrowth) is important for increasing the probability of successful implant performance. Peri-implant stress fields as influenced by implant surface design appear to significantly influence the rate of bone formation and hence osseointegration potential of implants.

We developed an animal model for investigating the early healing response of press-fit implants placed in primarily cancellous bone (simulating dental implant placement in the maxilla and posterior mandible sites, for example). The model involved placing implants transversely within the rabbit femoral condyle in primarily cancellous bone with a thin cortical shell (Simmons et al. 1999). The initial study compared porous-surfaced versus plasma spray-coated Ti implants following 4-, 8-, and 16-day implantation periods. Implant fixation was assessed by mechanical pull-out testing (to determine interface stiffness and shear strength) and interface structure assessment (by histology and scanning electron microscopy). The relatively short implantation periods used allowed a comparison of early healing events at the implant-tissue interface region leading to eventual implant osseointegration. The plasma spray-coated design was selected as representative of implants prepared with textured surfaces for comparison to the 3-D interlocking surfaces presented by the sintered porous surface structure.

The results indicated significantly faster rates of osseointegration with the porous-surfaced design reflected by both the pull-out tests and structural assessments. Bone formation was observed within the pores of the sintered porous surface zone by day 8, indicating significantly faster osseointegration with the porous-surfaced design. A finite element model study indicated that this faster rate of bone formation with the porous-surfaced design was attributable to differences in stress/strain fields in tissues apposing the implants for the two designs (Simmons et al. 2001). Lower distortional strains were predicted within the porous region that, according to the tissue differentiation hypothesis proposed by Carter et al. (1991), represents a more osteogenic environment leading to earlier bone formation. This was consistent with the observations made in the animal study. This model was used subsequently to investigate surface modification of porous-surfaced implants for further enhancing their "osseointegration potential" through the addition of a thin calcium phosphate film (a sol-gel-formed carbonated hydroxyapatite film) (Gan et al. 2004; Taché et al. 2004). The rabbit studies suggested that this could shorten the time for bone ingrowth and osseointegration by about one-third.

Summary

The success of "short" porous-surfaced endosseous dental implants is attributable to the structural characteristics of the porous region with which tissues can interlock to form a 3-D tissue-implant interpenetrating structure. The resulting peri-implant stress field next to porous-surfaced implants favors both rapid osseointegration and its maintenance for the long term following osseointegration. These properties are particularly significant for the success of "short" (≤7 mm) implants as evidenced by over 15 years of clinical use.

Acknowledgements

The clinical findings referred to in this article are due primarily to literature contributions by Dr. D.A. Deporter and colleagues whose clinical experiences with the Endopore® implant system have demonstrated the successful use in humans of "short" porous-surfaced implants in challenging sites of limited bone volume and density.

References

Abrahamsson I, Berglundh T, Linder E, Lang NP, Lindhe J. 2004. Early bone formation adjacent to rough and turned endosseous implant surfaces. An experimental study in the dog. *Clin Oral Implants Res* 15(4): 381–392.

Albrektsson T, Brånemark PI, Hansson HA, Lindström J. 1981. Osseointegrated titanium implants: Requirements for ensuring a long-lasting, direct bone to implant anchorage in man. *Acta Orthop Scand* 52: 155–170.

Albrektsson T, Sennerby L. 1991. State of the art in oral implants. *J Clin Periodontol* 18(6):474–481.

Albrektsson T, Wennerberg A. 2004. Oral implant surfaces: Part 1: Review focusing on topographic and chemical properties of different surfaces and in vivo responses to them. *Int J Prosthodont* 17(5):536–543.

Andersson P, Verrocchi D, Viinamäki R, Sennerby L. 2008. A one-year clinical, radiographical and RFA study of Neoss implants used in two-stage procedures. *Appl Osseointegration Res* 6:23–26.

Becktor JP, Isaksson S, Sennerby L. 2004. Survival analysis of endosseous implants in grafted and nongrafted edentulous maxillae. *Int J Oral Maxillofac Implants* 19(1): 107–115.

Berglundh T, Abrahamsson I, Albouy JP, Lindhe J. 2007. Bone healing at implants with a fluoride-modified surface: An experimental study in dogs. *Clin Oral Implants Res* 18(2):147–152.

Brånemark PI, Hansson BO, et al. 1977. Osseointegrated implants in the treatment of the edentulous jaw. Experience from a 10-year period. *Scand J Plast Reconstr Surg* (Suppl) 16:1–132.

————. 1985. Introduction to osseointegration. In: *Tissue-Integrated Prosthesis: Osseointegration in Clinical Dentistry.* PI Brånemark, GA Zarb, and T Albrektsson (eds.). Chicago: Quintessence. 11–76.

Brånemark PI, Adell R, Breine U, Hansson BO, Lindström J, Ohlsson A. 1969. Intraosseous anchorage of dental prosthesis. I: Experimental studies. *Scand J Plast Reconstr Surg* 3(2):81–100.

Buser D, Broggini N, Wieland M, Schenk RK, Denzer AJ, Cochran DL, Hoffmann B, Lussi A, Steinemann SG. 2004. Enhanced bone apposition to a chemically modified SLA titanium surface. *J Dent Res* 83(7): 529–533.

Carter DR, Giori NJ. 1991. Effect of mechanical stress on tissue differentiation in the bony implant bed. In: *The Bone-Biomaterial Interface.* JE Davies (ed.) Toronto: University of Toronto Press. 367–376.

Cochran D, Oates T, Morton D, Jones A, Buser D, Peters F. 2007. Clinical field trial examining an implant with a sand-blasted, acid-etched surface. *J Periodontol* 78(6): 974–982.

Davies JE. 2003. Understanding peri-implant endosseous healing. *J Dent Educ* 67:932–949.

Deporter DA, Caudry S, Kermalli J, Adegbembo A. 2005. Further data on the predictability of the indirect sinus elevation procedure used with short, sintered porous-surfaced dental implants. *Int J Periodontics Restorative Dent* 25:585–593.

Deporter DA, Ogiso B, Sohn D-S, Ruljancich K, Pharoah M. 2008. Use of an "ultrashort" sintered surface dental implant to replace posterior teeth. A case series report. *J Periodont.* In press.

Deporter DA, Todescan R, Caudry S. 2000. Simplifying management of the posterior maxilla using short, porous-surfaced dental implants and simultaneous indirect sinus elevation. *Int J Periodontics Restorative Dent* 20:477–485.

Deporter DA, Todescan R, Riley N. 2002a. Porous-surfaced dental implants in the partially edentulous maxilla. Assessment of subclinical mobility. *Int J Periodontics Restorative Dent* 22:184–192.

Deporter DA, Watson P, Pharoah M, Todescan R, Tomlinson G. 2002b. Ten-year results of a post-operative study using porous-surfaced dental implants and a mandibular overdenture. *Clin Implant Dent Rel Res* 4:183–189.

Deporter DA, Watson PA, Pilliar RM, Howley TP, Winslow J, Hansel P, Parisien K. 1988. A histological evaluation of a functional endosseous, porous-surfaced, titanium alloy dental implant system. *J Dent Res* 67(9):1190–1195.

Ellingsen JE, Johansson C, Wennerberg A, Holmen A. 2004. Improved retention and bone-to-implant contact with fluoride-modified titanium implants. *Int J Maxillofac Implants* 19(5):659–666.

Ferguson SJ, Broggini N, Wieland M, de Wild M, Rupp F, Geis-Gerstorfer J, Cochran DL, Buser D. 2006. Biomechanical evaluation of the interfacial strength of a chemically modified sandblasted and acid-etched titanium surface. *J Biomed Mater Res* 78A(2):291–297.

Friberg B, Jemt T, Lekholm U. 1991. Early failures in 4,641 consecutively placed Brånemark dental implants: A study from stage 1 surgery to the connection of completed prostheses. *Int J Maxillofac Implants* 6(2):142–146.

Friberg B, Sennerby L, Linden B, Gröndahl K, Lekholm U. 1999b. Stability measurements of one-stage Brånemark implants during healing in mandibles. A clinical resonance frequency study. *Int J Oral Maxillofac Surg* 28:266–272.

Friberg B, Sennerby L, Meredith N, Lekholm U. 1999a. A comparison between cutting torque and resonance frequency measurements of maxillary implants. A 20-month clinical study. *Int J Oral Maxillofac Surg* 28:297–303.

Gan L, Wang J, Tache A, Valiquette N, Deporter D, Pilliar R. 2004. Calcium phosphate sol-gel-derived thin films on porous-surfaced implants for enhanced osteoconductivity. Part II: Short-term in vivo studies. *Biomaterials* 25:5313–5321.

Glauser R, Lundgren AK, Gottlow J, Sennerby L, Portmann M, Ruhstaller P, Hämmerle CHF. 2003. Immediate occlusal loading of Brånemark TiUnite® implants placed predominantly in soft bone: 1-year results of a prospective, clinical study. *Clin Implant Dent Relat Res* 5(Suppl 1):47–56.

Glauser R, Rée A, Lundgren AK, Gottlow J, Hämmerle C, Schärer P. 2001. Immediate occlusal loading of Brånemark implants applied in various jawbone regions: A prospective, 1-year clinical study. *Clin Impl Dent Rel Res* 3:204–213.

Glauser R, Ruhstaller P, Windisch S, Zembic A, Lundgren AK, Gottlow J, Hämmerle C. 2005. Immediate occlusal loading of Brånemark System® TiUnite® implants placed predominantly in soft bone: 4-year results of a prospective, clinical study. *Clin Implant Dent Relat Res* 7(Suppl 1):52–59.

Goené RJ, Testori T, Trisi P. 2007. Influence of a nanometer-scale enhancement on de novo bone formation on titanium implants: A histomorphometric study in human maxillae. *Int J Periodontics Restorative Dent* 27(3):211–219.

Hansson S. 1999. The implant neck: Smooth or provided with retention elements—a biomechanical approach. *Clin Oral Implants Res* 10:394–405.

Ivanoff CJ, Hallgren C, Widmark G, Sennerby L, Wennerberg A. 2001. Histologic evaluation of the bone integration of TiO$_2$ blasted and turned titanium microimplants in humans. *Clin Oral Implants Res* 12(2):128–134.

Ivanoff CJ, Widmark G, Johansson C, Wennerberg A. 2003. Histologic evaluation of bone response to oxidized and turned titanium micro-implants in human jawbone. *Int J Oral Maxillofac Implants* 18(3):341–348.

Lazzara RJ, Porter SS. 2006. Platform switching: A new concept in implant dentistry for controlling post-restorative crestal bone levels. *Int J Periodontics Restorative Dent* 26:9–17.

Mendes VC, Moineddin R, Davies JE. 2007. The effect of discrete calcium nanocrystals on bone-bonding to titanium surfaces. *Biomaterials* 28(32):4748–4755.

Naert I, Koutsiskakis G, Duyck J, Quirynen M, Jacobs R, Van Steenberghe D. 2002. Biological outcome of implant-supported restorations in the treatment of partial edentulism. Part I: A longitudinal clinical evaluation. *Clin Oral Implants Res* 13:381–389.

O'Sullivan D. 2001. Factors of importance for primary stability of dental implants. University of Bristol, Bristol, UK. Thesis.

O'Sullivan D, Sennerby L, Meredith N. 2000. Measurements comparing the initial stability of five designs of dental implants: A human cadaver study. *Clin Implant Dent Rel Res* 2(2):85–92.

O'Sullivan D, Sennerby L, Meredith N. 2004. Influence of implant taper on the primary and secondary stability of osseointegrated titanium implants. *Clin Oral Implants Res* 15(4):474–480.

Oyonarte R, Deporter D, Pilliar RM, Woodside DG. 2005. Peri-implant response to orthodontic loading: Part 2. Implant surface geometry and its impact on regional bone remodeling. *Am J Orthod Dentofacial Orthop* 128:182–189.

Pilliar RM, Deporter DA, Watson PA, Valiquette N. 1991. Dental implant design—effect on bone remodeling. *J Biomed Mater Res* 25:467–483.

Pilliar RM, Sagals G, Meguid SA, Oyonarte R, Deporter DA. 2006. Threaded versus porous-surfaced implants as anchorage units for orthodontic treatment: Three-dimensional finite element analysis of peri-implant bone tissue stresses. *Int J Oral Maxillofac Impl* 21:879–889.

Rasmusson L, Roos J, Bystedt H. 2005. A 10-year follow-up study of titanium dioxide-blasted implants. *Clin Implant Dent Relat Res* 7(1):36–42.

Roberts WE, Smith RK, Zilberman Y, Mozsary PG, Smith RS. 1984. Osseous adaptation to continuous loading of rigid endosseous implants. *Am J Orthod* 86(2):30–42.

Rocci A, Martignoni M, Burgos P, Gottlow J, Sennerby L. 2003a. Histology of retrieved immediately and early loaded oxidized implants. Light microscopic observations after 5 to 9 months of loading in the posterior mandible of 5 cases. *Clin Implant Dent Relat Res* 5(Suppl 1):88–98.

Rocci A, Martignoni M, Gottlow J. 2003b. Immediate loading of Brånemark System with TiUnite and machined surfaces in the posterior mandible: A randomised, open-ended trial. *Clin Implant Dent Relat Res* 5(Suppl 1):57–63.

Rokni S, Todescan R, Watson P, Pharoah M, Adegbembo AO, Deporter DA. 2005. An assessment of crown-to-root ratios with short sintered porous-surfaced implants supporting prostheses in partially edentulous patients. *Int J Oral Maxillofac Impl* 20:69–76.

Rompen E, DaSilva D, Lundgren AK, Gottlow J, Sennerby L. 2000. Stability measurements of a double-threaded titanium implant design with turned or oxidised surface. *Appl Osseointegration Res* 1:18–20.

Schüpbach P, Glauser R, Rocci A, Martignoni M, Sennerby L, Lundgren AK, Gottlow J. 2005. The human bone-oxidized titanium implant interface: A light microscopic, scanning electron microscopic, back-scatter scanning electron microscopic, and energy-dispersive X-ray study of clinically retrieved dental implants. *Clin Implant Dent Relat Res* 7(Suppl 1):36–43.

Schwarz F, Ferrari D, Herten M, Mihatovic I, Wieland M, Sager M, Becker J. 2007. Effects of hydrophilicity and microtopography on early stages of soft and hard tissue integration at non-submerged titanium implants: An immunohistochemical study in dogs. *J Periodontol* 78(11):2171–2184.

Sennerby L, Gottlow J, Engman F, Meredith N. 2008. Histological and biomechanical aspects of surface topography and geometry of Neoss implants. A study in rabbits. *Appl Osseointegration Res* 6:18–22.

Sennerby L, Roos J. 1998. Surgical determinants of clinical success of osseointegrated oral implants: A review of the literature. *Int J Prosthodont* 11(5):408–420.

Simmons CA, Meguid SA, Pilliar RM. 2001. Mechanical regulation of localized and appositional bone formation around bone-interfacing implants. *J Biomed Mater Res* 55:63–71.

Simmons CA, Valiquette N, Pilliar RM. 1999. Osseointegration of sintered porous-surfaced and plasma spray-coated implants: An animal model study of early post-implantation healing response and mechanical stability. *J Biomed Mater Res* 47:127–138.

Stanford CM, Johnson GK, Fakhry A, Gartton D, Mellonig JT, Wagner W. 2006. Outcomes of a fluoride modified implant one year after loading in the posterior-maxilla when placed with the osteotome surgical technique. *Appl Osseointegration Res* 5:50–55.

Taché A, Gan L, Deporter D, Pilliar R. 2004. Effect of surface chemistry on the rate of osseointegration of sintered porous-surfaced Ti-6Al-4V implants. *Int J Oral Maxillofac Impl* 19:19–29.

Tawil G, Younan R. 2003. Clinical evaluation of short machined surface implants followed for 12 to 96 months. *Int J Oral Maxillofac Implants* 18:894–901.

Testori T, Wiseman L, Woolfe S, Porter SS. 2001. A prospective multicenter clinical study of the Osseotite implant: Four-year interim report. *Int J Maxillofac Implants* 16(2):193–200.

Trisi P, Lazzara R, Rebaudi A, Rao W, Testori T, Porter SS. 2003. Bone-implant contact on machined and dual acid-etched surfaces after 2 months of healing in the human maxilla. *J Periodontol* 74(7):945–956.

Vaillancourt H, Pilliar RM, McCammond D. 1995. Finite element analysis of bone remodeling around porous-coated dental implants. *J Applied Biomater* 6:267–282.

Zechner W, Tangl S, Fürst G, Tepper G, Thams U, Mailath G, Watzek G. 2003. Osseous healing characteristics of three different implant types. A histologic and histomorphometric study in mini-pigs. *Clin Oral Impl Res* 14(2):150–157.

Loading Protocols and Biological Response

Peter K. Moy, Georgios E. Romanos, and Mario Roccuzzo

Current loading protocols have clearly changed from the first published, scientifically established clinical protocol by Brånemark and collaborators (1977). Data presented by this group showed treatment outcomes of 235 edentulous jaws with observation periods of 9 months to 8 years obtaining 85% success with all prosthetic suprastructures delivered. This original protocol recommended strict adherence to surgical and prosthodontic techniques. More importantly, the protocol recommended a "non-disturbed" healing period of 3–6 months. After this healing period, an abutment connection surgery was performed, and the suprastructure prosthesis was fabricated and screw-retained to the implant (Zarb and Jansson 1985). This remarkable procedure to treat the completely edentulous patient and long-term clinical results were introduced by Brånemark and colleagues during the initial Toronto Conference in 1982. Subsequent long-term follow-up studies for edentulous jaws (Adell et al. 1990; Lindquist et al. 1996) and partially dentated jaws (Lekholm et al. 1994, 1999) showed high predictability of implant treatment is achievable when the original loading protocol is adhered to. Since this original delayed loading protocol was

introduced, several authors (Becker et al. 2003; Ericsson et al. 2000; Payne et al. 2002; Tawse-Smith et al. 2002) have evaluated early loading protocols and found high success and survival rates comparable to the conventional loading protocol. Today clinicians are placing loading or non-loading forces on implants earlier and in some instances immediately. However, the clinician often carries out these early and immediate loading protocols without understanding the science or evidence-based principles to support the clinical decisions.

The first area of variability to understand is the terminology used for loading protocols. Does the clinician know what constitutes immediate, early, or delayed loading? Immediate loading represents a prosthesis connected to the implant(s) within the first 48 hours. Early loading requires the insertion of the prosthesis after the first 48 hours but prior to 3 months. Delayed loading would constitute placement of a prosthesis after the initial 3 months of healing, which follows the original protocol. Other variables that should be considered by the clinician in his or her decision-making process are patient variables, especially with medically compromised patients, implant design variables, and surgical and prosthodontic protocol variables.

The implant patient will present with a variety of medical and clinical findings that will alter the clinician's decision whether to provide immediate, early, or delayed loading for his or her patient. The scientific literature has reported that patients presenting with specific medical compromises may experience a higher failure rate with implants using conventional loading techniques (Moy et al. 2005). These medical risk factors include smoking, diabetes, and radiation therapy to the head and neck region, as well as post-menopause in women. It appears that these medical conditions may be associated with an impaired healing process and the rate of healing in these patients. Due to these impairments, immediate loading or even early loading may be a relative contraindication for patients presenting with these medical findings.

Another patient-specific factor that would affect the clinician's decision to provide immediate loading is the quantity and quality of bone. The presence of dense bone and adequate volume would provide the clinician with the ability to establish adequate primary stability, once the implant is placed. Jaffin and Berman (1991) showed increased implant failures in areas with loose trabecular bone (type D4). Some authors recommended avoiding the use of a tap in the recipient sites that demonstrated poor bone quality (Romanos 2004; Salama et al. 1995; Schnitman et al. 1990, 1997). When the implant is placed into this non-tapped site, it simulates a condensation technique and improves the mechanical stability of the implants during insertion. Even though the focus has been on establishing this initial stability during placement, there are a variety of other factors that play a role in providing the surgeon with the ability to establish initial retention of the implant. Implant length, as determined by available bone quantity, also plays a role in establishing primary stability. Micromovements along the interface have a tolerance limit of 50–150 μm (Brunski 1993; Cameron et al. 1972, 1973).

Micromotion beyond these limits will result in connective tissue encapsulation of the implant body, resembling the periodontal ligament of teeth (Pilliar et al. 1986; Szmukler-Moncler et al. 1998). This has led several authors to recommend a minimum implant length of 10 mm (Babbush et al. 1986; Chiapasco et al. 1997; Jaffin et al. 2000; Ledermann 1996; Tarnow et al. 1997).

The implant design plays a significant role in establishing initial stability. Degidi and Piattelli (2003) studied the prognosis of 646 immediately loaded implants placed in 152 patients. Only six failures were reported in the first 6 months of loading. Soft diet was recommended for the initial stages of the healing. Different implant systems with various geometries were used. The authors presented different survival rates depending on the implant site. Specifically, the survival rate was very high in the anterior part of the mandible and in the full-arch restoration of the lower jaw, as well as in the posterior part of the maxilla (100%). Significantly lower survival rates were found with the posterior part of the mandible (91%), the complete restoration of the maxilla (98.5%), or the anterior maxillary region (87.5%) (Figs. 14.1a–14.1f).

The geometry of the implant (macrointerlocking) influences the micromotion and initial retention of the implant in the recipient bone bed. The various design characteristics have transformed initially from blade-shaped implants to hollow baskets to cylindrical forms, and finally to the solid screw. These designs were also available in one-piece or two-piece designs for immediate loading. In general, screw-designed implants should be used for immediate loading, as their mechanical retention may be better immediately after implant placement (Brunski 1992). This was confirmed in anatomical (Bade et al. 2000) and photoelastic (Nentwig et al. 1992) studies using an implant with progressive thread geometry. From a purely mechanical standpoint, the screw-shaped body provides the optimal design to establish the initial stability, a prerequisite for immediate loading.

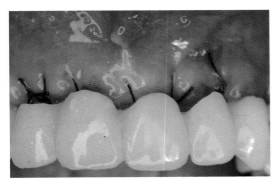

Figure 14.6c. Provisional restoration in place immediately after implant placement for immediate loading.

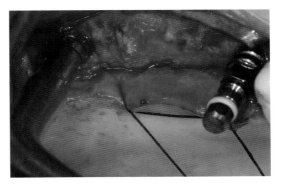

Figure 14.7. Site preparation with osteotome in the maxillary molar area, where the bone is extremely soft.

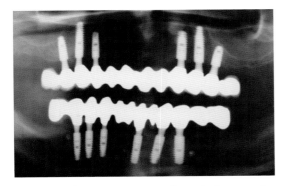

Figure 14.6d. Postoperative radiograph 5 years after immediate loading in the maxilla and the mandible presenting no crestal bone loss.

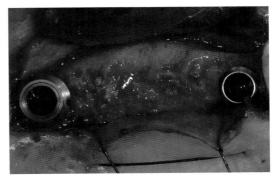

Figure 14.8. Implant positioning with primary stability.

investigation on implants with porous surfaces found that the implants may be loaded successfully after only 6 weeks if two implants are splinted together (Deporter et al. 1988). Another study in monkeys that looked at TPS-coated single implants loaded 30 days after placement compared to non-loaded implants found no significant difference with bone levels between the two groups (Piatteli et al. 1993). The role of implant surface roughness on immediately loaded implants comparing the maxilla versus mandible was also evaluated (Jaffin et al. 2000). Lower success rates were found with smooth-surface implants compared to roughened surfaces, especially in poor quality bone sites. Finally, when dealing with alveolar ridges demon-

strating poor quality bone, several authors have recommended against tapping the recipient sites (Romanos 2004; Salama et al. 1995; Schnitman et al. 1990, 1997), underpreparing (Cannizzaro and Leone 2003), or using an osteotome technique (Roccuzzo and Wilson 2001) to prepare areas with poor bone density as a condensation technique to improve the mechanical stability of the implants during insertion (Figs. 14.7–14.13).

The partially dentated and single-missing-tooth patient presents the clinician with a different set of problems and issues from an immediate loading standpoint. Cross-arch splinting is not possible in many of the partially dentated situations and with all

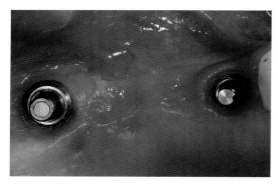

Figure 14.9.   Soft-tissue healing at 3 weeks post-op.

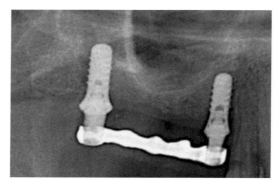

Figure 14.12.   Radiograph of the implant after loading with provisional bridge.

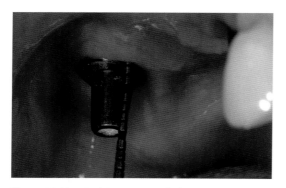

Figure 14.10.   Probing at time of abutment connection at 35Ncm for final restoration.

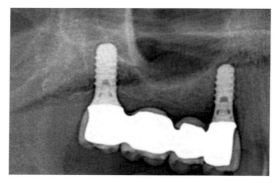

Figure 14.13.   Radiograph at 1 year follow-up in the posterior maxilla (18 early loaded implant).

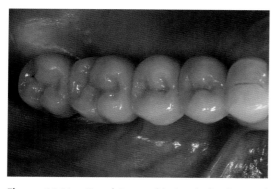

Figure 14.11.   Porcelain-to-gold fused fixed partial denture.

single-tooth situations, the implant must provide all of the support for any functional loading generated by the crown placed onto the implant (Figs. 14.14–14.16).

So what factors play a major role in these clinical situations and what are the success rates for immediate loading in the partially dentated and single-missing-tooth patients? In general, risks are higher for immediate loading in these patients due to bending movements applied on fewer implants during occlusal loading. Rocci and co-workers (2003) have evaluated an immediate loading protocol using Brånemark implants, comparing two surfaces (machined vs. TiUnite®). The authors noted 10% higher success rates with implants coated with TiUnite® versus machined-smooth surface implants.

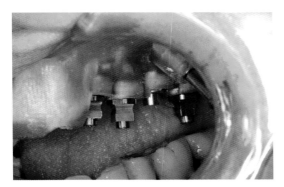

Figure 14.14. A NobelGuide® surgical template used in flapless, guided surgery for placement of implants in partially dentated patients.

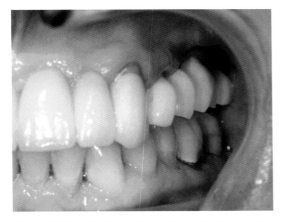

Figure 14.15. The immediate delivery of a fixed partial denture for immediate loading showing a small horizontal cantilever from the width of the pontics.

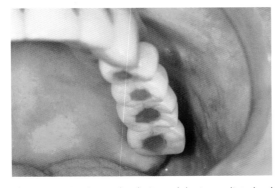

Figure 14.16. An occlusal view of the immediate load prosthesis and the splinting effect from the four units of the fixed partial denture.

Calandriello and co-workers (2003) restored Brånemark machined-smooth surface implants placed in the posterior portion of the jaw, using the implants to support single molar crowns. A 98% survival rate after 1 year of full occlusal loading was reported. Certain criteria were followed: high primary stability was established with insertion torque values of 40 Ncm, light occlusal contact with no contacts in lateral movements, no cantilevering moments were permitted, and patients were instructed to stay on a soft diet for 1 month. The cumulative success rate after 18 months of functional loading was 98%. Other authors (Testori et al. 2003) looked at the concept of immediate non-occlusal loading in partially dentated jaws, comparing 52 implants with immediate non-occlusal loading with implants receiving early loading. The cumulative survival rate after 19 months of loading was almost 96%.

In the single-missing-tooth situation, studies of immediate loading on these patients have been performed and reported by different groups using various implant systems (Ericsson et al. 2000; Malo et al. 2000; Wöhrle 1998). Ericsson and co-workers (2000) used immediate functional loading of Brånemark implants placed anterior to the molars by placing provisional crowns for 6 months. The definitive restoration was delivered after this period. Using this protocol, the authors found 2 implants failed out of 14 placed, for an 86% survival rate. They also noted minimal bone changes after a mean loading period of 18 months. This data was confirmed with a 5-year observation period (Ericsson et al. 2000). Chaushu and co-workers (2001) compared immediate-loaded implants placed into healed sites with implants placed into extraction sockets and found a statistical difference. For implants placed into healed alveolar ridges, the survival rate was 100%, while the implants placed into extraction sockets had a survival rate of 82.4% (Figs. 14.17–14.26).

From the studies and articles referenced, the biological response by the patient to immediate loading is a remarkable one. When the clinician follows the proper loading

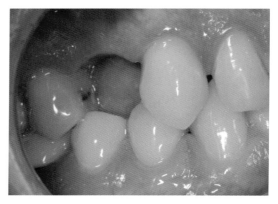

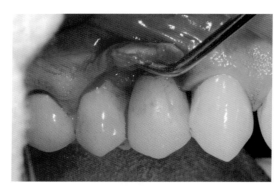

Figure 14.20. The delivery of an immediate loading provisional crown with full occlusal contact.

Figure 14.17. A clinical situation with a single missing tooth. Note the steep inclines of the buccal cusps of the maxillary teeth.

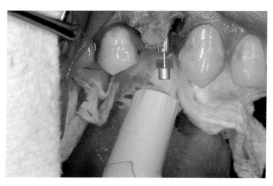

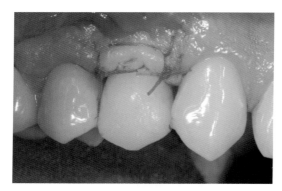

Figure 14.18. After placement of the implant, the stability is checked using RFA (resonance frequency analysis) to measure the ISQ (implant stability quotient).

Figure 14.21. Soft tissue closure around the provisional crown.

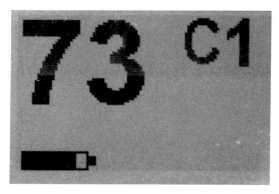

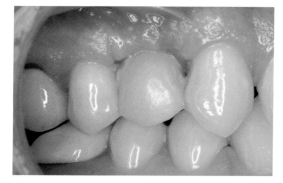

Figure 14.19. An ISQ number greater than 50 indicates a stable implant.

Figure 14.22. One month follow-up with complete soft-tissue healing and stable implant.

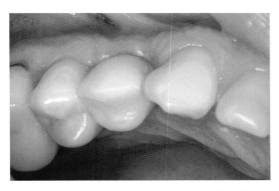

Figure 14.23. Occlusal view indicating a stable clinical situation at 1 month post–immediate loading.

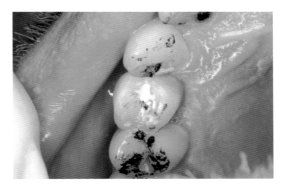

Figure 14.26. Note minimal contact in all planes of movement on the provisional implant restoration.

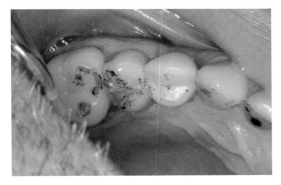

Figure 14.24. Inspection with occlusal articulating paper; light centric contact is seen on the implant restoration and some lateral excursive contact.

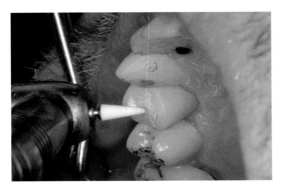

Figure 14.25. Adjusting and removing the contact during lateral excusive movements.

protocol, it is possible to provide patients with immediate functional loading in all clinical situations, from the completely edentulous state to the partially dentated to the single missing tooth. The clinician must realize the importance of following the principles outlined, especially as one moves into the more demanding partially dentated patients. The most critical factors to observe when attempting to provide patients with an immediate-loaded prosthesis are establishing initial rigid stability of the implant immediately after placement; minimal manipulation of the implant-abutment components; splinting of multiple implants using the framework of the prosthesis when possible; careful observation of the occlusal forces with complete removal of lateral excursive contacts; and careful selection of patients, observing the patient-specific factors that affect the integration rate, such as smoking, diabetes, poor quality bone, and parafunctional habits. The clinician following these careful selection criteria and strictly adhering to immediate loading protocols will be able to achieve very high success rates with immediate-loaded implants comparable to, or better than, success rates found with conventional or early loading protocols.

References

Adell R, Eriksson B, Lekholm U, Brånemark PI, Jemt T. 1990. Long-term follow-up study of osseointegrated implants in the treatment of totally edentulous jaw. *Int J Oral Maxillofac Implants* 5:347–359.

Babbush CA, Kent JN, Misiek DJ. 1986. Titanium plasma-sprayed (TPS) screw implants for the reconstruction of the edentulous mandible. *J Oral Maxillofac Surg* 44: 274–282.

Bade H, Günes Y, Koebke J. 2000. Untersuchungen zur Primärstabilität von Dentalimplantaten. *Z Zahnärztl Implantol* 16:33–39.

Becker W, Becker BE, Huffstetler S. 2003. Early functional loading at 5 days for Brånemark implants placed into edentulous mandibles: A prospective, open-ended, longitudinal study. *J Periodontol* 74(5):695–702.

Brånemark PI, Hansson BO, Adell R, Breine U, Lindström J, Hallen O, Ohman A. 1977. Osseointegrated implants in the treatment of the edentulous jaw. Experience from a 10-year period. *Scand J Plast Reconstr Surg* (Suppl) 16:1–132.

Brånemark PI, Zarb GA, Albrektsson T (eds.). 1985. *Tissue-Integrated Prostheses: Osseointegration in Clinical Dentistry.* Chicago: Quintessence. 11–61.

Brunski JB. 1992. Biomechanical factors affecting the bone-dental implant interface. *Clin Mater* 10:153–201.

———. 1993. Avoid pitfalls of overloading and micromotion of intraosseous implants. *Dent Implantol Update* 4:77–81.

Calandriello R, Tomatis M, Vallone R, Rangert B, Gottlow J. 2003. Immediate occlusal loading of single lower molars using Brånemark system wide-platform TiUnite® implants: An interim report of a prospective open-ended clinical multicenter study. *Clin Implant Dent Relat Res* 5(Suppl):74–80.

Cameron H, MacNab I, Pilliar RM. 1972. Porous surfaced Vitallium staples. *S Afr J Surg* 10:63–70.

Cameron HU, Pilliar RM, MacNab I. 1973. The effect of movement on the bonding of porous metal to bone. *J Biomed Mater Res* 7:301–311.

Cannizzaro G, Leone M. 2003. Restoration of partially edentulous patients using dental implants with a microtextured surface: A prospective comparison of delayed and immediate full occlusal loading. *Int J Oral Maxillofac Implants* 18(4):512–522.

Chaushu G, Chaushu S, Tzohar A, Dayan D. 2001. Immediate loading of single-tooth implants: Immediate versus non-immediate implantation. A clinical report. *Int J Oral Maxillofac Implants* 16:267–272.

Chen J, Lu X, Paydar N, Akay HU, Roberts WE. 1994. Mechanical simulation of the human mandible with and without an endosseous implant. *Med Eng Phys* 16:53–61.

Chiapasco M, Gatti C, Rossi E, Haefliger W, Markwalder TH. 1997. Implant-retained mandibular overdentures with immediate loading. A retrospective multicenter study on 226 consecutive cases. *Clin Oral Implants Res* 8:48–57.

Corigliano M, Quaranta M, Scarano A, Piattelli A. 1995. Bone reactions to early loaded plasma-sprayed titanium implants. IADR Abstr. Singapore.

Degidi M, Piattelli A. 2003. Immediate functional and non-functional loading of dental implants: A 2- to 60-month follow-up study of 646 titanium implants. *J Periodontol* 74:225–241.

Deporter DA, Watson PA, Pilliar RM, Howley TP, Winslow J. 1988. A histological evaluation of a functional endosseous, porous-surfaced, titanium alloy dental implant system in the dog. *J Dent Res* 67:1190–1195.

Ericsson I, Randow K, Nilner K, Petersson A. 2000. Early functional loading of Brånemark dental implants. A 5-year follow-up study. *Clin Implant Dent Rel Res* 2:70–77.

Frost HM. 1990. Skeletal structural adaptations to mechanical usage (SATMU). 1: Redefining Wolff's law: The bone modeling problem. *Anat Rec* 226:403–413.

Goodman S, Aspenberg P. 1993. Effects of mechanical stimulation on the differentiation of hard tissues. *Biomaterials* 14: 563–569.

Goodship AE, Kenwright J. 1985. The influence of induced micromovement upon the healing of experimental tibial fractures. *J Bone Joint Surg* 67B:650–655.

Hansson HA, Albrektsson T, Brånemark PI. 1983. Structural aspects of the interface between tissue and titanium implants. *J Prosthet Dent* 50:108–113.

Hert J, Pribylova E, Liskova M. 1972. Reaction of bone to mechanical stimuli. 3: Microstructure of compact bone of rabbit tibia after intermittent loading. *Acta Anat (Basel)* 82:218–230.

Jaffin RA, Berman CL. 1991. The excessive loss of Brånemark fixtures in type IV bone: A 5-year analysis. *J Periodontol* 62:2–4.

Jaffin RA, Kumar A, Berman CL. 2000. Immediate loading of implants in partially and fully edentulous jaws: A series of 27 case reports. *J Periodontol* 71:833–838.

Kan JYK, Rungcharassaeng K, Lozada J. 2003. Immediate placement and provisionalization of maxillary anterior single implants: 1-year prospective study. *Int J Oral Maxillofac Implants* 18:31–39.

Kenwright J, Richardson JB, Cunningham JL, Goodship AE, Adams MA, Magnusson PA, Newmann JM. 1991. Axial movement and tibial fractures. A controlled randomized trial of treatment. *J Bone Joint Surg (Br)* 73B:654–659.

Ledermann PD. 1979. Stegprothetische Versorgung des zahnlosen Unterkiefers mit Hilfe von plasmabeschichteten Titanschraubenimplantaten. *Dtsch Zahnärztl Z* 34:907–911.

———. 1983. Sechsjährige klinische Erfahrung mit dem titanplasmabeschichteten ITI-Schraubenimplantat in der Regio interforaminalis des Unterkiefers. *Schweiz Mschr Zahnheilk* 93:1070–1089.

———. 1996. Über 20jährige Erfahrung mit der sofortigen funktionellen Belastung von Implantatstegen in der Regio interforaminalis. *Z Zahnärztl Implantol* 12:123–136.

Lekholm U, Gunne J, Henry P, Higuchi K, Lindén U, Bergström C, Van Steenberghe D. 1999. Survival of the Brånemark implant in partially edentulous jaws: A 10-year prospective multicenter study. *Int J Oral Maxillofac Implants* 14:639–645.

Lekholm U, Van Steenberghe D, Herrmann I, Bolender C, Folmer T, Gunne J, Henry P, Higuchi K, Laney WR, Lindén U. 1994. Osseointergrated implants in the treatment of partially edentulous jaws: A prospective 5-year multicenter study. *Int J Oral Maxillofac Implants* 9:626–635.

Lindquist LW, Carlsson GE, Jemt T. 1996. A prospective 15-year follow-up study of mandibular fixed prostheses supported by osseointegrated implants. *Clin Oral Implants Res* 7:627–635.

Malo P, Rangert B, Dvarsater L. 2000. Immediate function of Brånemark implants in the esthetic zone: A retrospective clinical study with 6 months to 4 years of follow-up. *Clin Implant Dent Relat Res* 2: 138–146.

Moy PK, Medina D, Shetty V, Aghaloo TL. 2005. Dental implant failure rates and associated risk factors. *Int J Oral Maxillofac Implants* 20:569–577.

Nentwig G-H, Moser W, Knefel T, Ficker E. 1992. Dreidimensionale spannungsoptische Untersuchungen der NM-Implantatgewindeform im Verleich mit herkömmlichen Implantatgewinden. *Z Zahnärztl Implantol* 8:130–135.

Oda J, Sakamoto J, Aoyama K, Sueyoshi Y, Tomita K, Sawaguchi T. 1996. Mechanical stresses and bone formation. In: *Biomechanics: Functional Adaptation and Remodeling*. K Hayashi, A Kamiya, and K Ono (eds.). Tokyo: Springer. 123–140.

Payne AG, Tawse-Smith A, Duncan WD, Kumara R. 2002. Conventional and early loading of unsplinted ITI implants supporting mandibular overdentures. *Clin Oral Implants Res* 13(6):603–609.

Piattelli A, Ruggeri A, Franchi M, Romasco N, Trisi P. 1993. A histologic and histomorphometric study of bone reactions to unloaded and loaded non-submerged single implants in monkeys: A pilot study. *J Oral Implantol* 19:314–320.

Pilliar RM. 1989. Porous surfaced endosseous dental implants-design/tissue response. In: *Oral Implantology and Biomaterials*. H Kawahara (ed.). New York: Elsevier. 151–161.

Pilliar RM, Lee JM, Maniatopoulos C. 1986. Observations on the effect of movement on bone in-growth into porous-surfaced implants. *Clin Orthop* 208:108–113.

Roberts WE, Marshall KJ, Mozsary PG. 1990. Rigid endosseous implant utilized as anchorage to protract molars and close an atrophic extraction site. *Angle Orthod* 60:135–152.

Rocci A, Martignoni M, Gottlow J. 2003. Immediate loading of Brånemark system TiUnite® and machined surface implants in the posterior mandible: A randomized open-ended clinical trial. *Clin Implant Dent Relat Res* 5(Suppl 1):57–63.

Roccuzzo M, Wilson TA. 2001. A prospective study evaluating a protocol for 6 weeks' loading of SLA implants in the posterior maxilla: One-year results. *Clin Oral Implants Res* 13(5):502–507.

Romanos GE. 2004. Surgical and prosthetic concepts for predictable immediate loading of oral implants. *California Dental Assoc J* 32:991–1001.

Romanos GE. 2005. *Immediate Loading of Oral Implants in the Posterior Mandible: Animal and Clinical Studies*. Berlin: Quintessence.

Romanos GE, Damouras M, Veis A, Schwarz F, Parisis N. 2007. Oral implants with different thread designs. A histometrical evaluation. IADR. New Orleans.

Salama H, Rose LF, Salama M, Betts NJ. 1995. Immediate loading of bilaterally splinted titanium root-form implants in fixed prosthodontics. A technique reexamined: Two case reports. *Int J Periodontics Restorative Dent* 15:344–361.

Sarmiento A, Schaeffer JF, Beckermann L, Latta LL, Enis JE. 1977. Fracture healing in rat femora is affected by functional weight-bearing. *J Bone Joint Surg Am* 59:369–375.

Schnitman PA, Wöhrle PS, Rubenstein JE. 1990. Immediate fixed interim prostheses supported by two-stage threaded implants: Methodology and results. *J Oral Implantol* 16:96–105.

Schnitman PA, Wöhrle PS, Rubenstein JE, DaSilva JD, Wang NH. 1997. Ten-year results for Brånemark implants immediately loaded with fixed prostheses at implant placement. *Int J Oral Maxillofac Implants* 12:495–503.

Skalak R. 1983. Biomechanical considerations in osseointegrated prostheses. *J Prosthet Dent* 49:843–848.

Søballe K, Hansen ES, Brockstedt-Rasmussen H, Bünger C. 1992. Tissue ingrowth into titanium and hydroxyapatite coated implants during stable and unstable mechanical conditions. *J Orthopaedic Res* 10:285–299.

Szmukler-Moncler S, Salama H, Reingewirtz Y, Dubruille JH. 1998. Time of loading and effect of micromotion on bone-dental implant interface: Review of experimental literature. *J Biomed Mater Res* 43:192–203.

Tarnow DP, Emtiaz S, Classi A. 1997. Immediate loading of threaded implants at stage 1 surgery in edentulous arches: Ten consecutive case reports with 1- to 5-year data. *Int J Oral Maxillofac Implants* 12:319–324.

Tawse-Smith A, Payne AG, Kumara R, Thomson WM. 2002. Early loading on unsplinted implants supporting mandibular overdentures using a one-stage operative procedure with two different implant systems: A 2-year report. *Clin Implant Dent Rel Res* 4(1):33–42.

Testori T, Bianchi F, Del Fabbro M, Szmukler-Moncler S, Francetti L, Weinstein RL. 2003. Immediate non-occlusal loading vs. early loading in partially edentulous patients. *Pract Proced Aesthet Dent* 15:787–794.

Thomas KA, Cook SD, Renz EA, Anderson RC, Haddad RJ, Jr., Haubold AD, Yapp R.

1985. The effect of surface treatment on the interface mechanics of LTI pyrolytic carbon implants. *J Biomed Mater Res* 19:145–159.

Wöhrle PS. 1998. Single-tooth replacement in the aesthetic zone with immediate provisionalization: Fourteen consecutive case reports. *Pract Periodont Aesthet Dent* 10: 1107–1114.

Zarb GA, Jansson T. 1985. Prosthodontic procedures. In: *Tissue-Integrated Prosthesis*. PI Brånemark, G Zarb, and T Albrektsson (eds.). Chicago: Quintessence. 241–282.

15

Restorative Phase Treatment Planning

INTEGRATION OF BIOLOGICAL PRINCIPLES TO ACHIEVE STABLE AESTHETICS

Clark M. Stanford

Introduction

Since the mid-1960s, research on endosseous dental implants has revolutionized dental care. The clinical success of implants is related to improvements in surgical management combined with greater understanding of biological responses and engineering of dental implants (Stanford and Brand 1999). While high success rates of >95% hold for many anatomic sites in the jaws, the bony response within the thin cortical plates and diminished cancellous bone characterizing the posterior maxilla is less successful with conventional machined surfaced implants (i.e., 65–85%) (Widmark et al. 2001). In a meta-analysis, Lindh et al. (1998) observed that implant success in the posterior maxillae is less than in other regions of the mouth and is highly dependent on adequate bone volume in the area. Strategies to increase the quantity and

quality of osseous tissue at the interface are an important means to provide predictable implant therapy for patients with poor bone quality as well as to provide greater predictability for immediate loading of implants at the time of placement (Stanford 2005).

As a means to develop initial implant stability, different implant designs (lengths, thread features, surface topography) as well as surgical technologies are used to assist the primary stability in poor quality bone (Stanford 2002, 2003). The healing process of conversion from primary to secondary bone has been reviewed elsewhere (Brunski et al. 2000; Stanford 1999, 2002; Stanford and Brand 1999; Stanford and Keller 1991; Stanford and Schneider 2004). Dental implant surface technologies have used various approaches to alter the surface: micro- and nano-topography and recently the surface chemistry of the titanium dioxide surface. Improved bone bonding and accelerated bone formation appear to be possible with roughened surfaces modified with certain acid treatments. Sandblasted and acid-etched surfaces have been demonstrated to enhance bone apposition in histomorphometric and removal torque analyses (Shalabi et al. 2006). These studies indicate that a subtractive surface modification has an osteoconductive effect on bone integration to the implant surface (osseointegration) and suggest a synergistic mechanism to enhance bone formation occurring between the macro-topography (due to blasting procedure) and the microtexture (due to the acid etching) of the implant (Bagno and Di Bello 2004).

Implant Macro-Retentive Features

Implants used in the oral environment have three major types of macro-retentive features: screw threads (tapped or self-tapping), solid body press-fit designs, and/or sintered bead technologies. Each of these approaches is designed to achieve initial implant stability and/or create large volumetric spaces for bone ingrowth. Implant designs incorporate thread-cutting profiles to reduce interfacial shear stress such as a 15° thread profile (ITI/Straumann, Institut Straumann AG, Waldenburg, Switzerland) with a rounded tip to reduce shear forces at the tip of the tread, which maintains bone in a favorable compressive zone beneath the thread profile (Schroeder and Buser 1989; Schroeder et al. 1981, 1996). Other thread designs (Microthread™ Astra Tech AB, Mölndal, Sweden) have focused on reducing the surrounding transcortical shear forces by reducing the height of the thread profile (reducing the contribution of any one thread) with a rounded tip surface, along with an increase in the number of threads per unit area of the implant surface (Hansson 1999). This has the added benefit of increasing the strength of the implant body by increasing the amount of remaining wall thickness of the implant body (Binon 2000). The addition of microthreads to the upper portion of the implant body has been copied by other implant designs on the market (BioLok™/Biohorizon™ and the Groovy™ implant, Nobel BioCare, Goteborg, Sweden). Finally, orthopedic prosthesis (e.g., femoral stems, pelvic acetabular caps, knee

prostheses, etc.) have used various sintering technologies to create mesh or sintered beads as a surface for bone to grow into. The application of this technology to dental implants has involved attempts to improve the success rate of short implants (<10 mm in length), which are associated with the highest failure rates (Lindh et al. 1998).

Implant Micro-Retentive Features

Upon the placement of an implant into a surgical site, there is a cascade of molecular and cellular processes that provides for new bone growth and differentiation along the biomaterial surface. The goal of a number of current strategies is to provide an enhanced osseous stability through micro-/nano-surface mediated events. These strategies can be divided into those that attempt to enhance the inmigration of new bone (e.g., osteoconduction) through changes in surface topography (e.g., surface "roughness") and biological means to manipulate the type of cells that grow onto the surface.

What Is Surface Roughness?

A common means to improve implant success is through alterations to the implant surface topography and surface chemistry. In implant design, it is typically assumed that a greater surface area (per unit of bulk metal surface) will allow a greater area for load transfer of bone against the implant surface (Buser et al. 1991; Hansson 2000; Hansson and Norton 1999; Wennerberg et al. 1997) (Fig. 15.1).

It should be clarified that surface roughness is often a poorly described characteristic of implant surfaces, making comparisons between implant systems difficult (Wennerberg and Albrektsson 2000). One advantage of gentle acid etching is the increase in the roughness of a grit-blasted surface on a

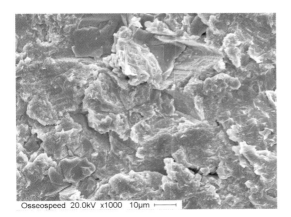

Figure 15.1. Scanning electron micrograph of a fluoride-modified implant surface following gentle etching in a dilute HF solution. The etching process is intended to avoid losing the macroscopic roughening necessary for bone ingrowth onto the implant surface (magnification = 1000×).

nanometer-scale level without losing the macro-retentive areas for bone tissue to grow into (Brunski et al. 2000; Kasemo and Lausmaa 1994).

Various titanium surfaces have utilized surface roughness created by a grit-blasting and etching procedure or blasting of the surface alone under tightly controlled conditions to obtain a pre-defined optimal surface topography. One such optimization criterion has been proposed (Hansson 1999). This criterion suggests an implant surface has an optimal balance between pore size on the surface (pore sizes of 1–5 μm diameter and 1–5 μm depth) and number of pores per unit area (Hansson 2000; Hansson and Norton 1999). This model relates the relative shear strength of bone (τ_s) with a topography of interfacial load-carrying capacity for a surface topographic feature ("pit effectivity factor") combined with a value for the optimal number of pits per unit area of the surface ("pit density factor") (Hansson 1999). These topographic features are then combined with macroscopic implant thread profiles (pitch, angle, and position) to provide a high compressive loading (low shear) implant interface (Hansson and Norton 1999). This surface topography is currently available from one manufacturer

and shows promise by maintaining crestal bone at the level of the head of the implant (Abrahamsson et al. 1999; Arvidson et al. 1998; Astrand et al. 1996; Cooper et al. 1999; Davis and Packer 1999; Isidor 1997; Makkonen et al. 1997; Nordin et al. 1998; Warrer et al. 1993).

Implant Micro-Retentive Features: Surface Roughness by Blasting/Etching

Various studies have also addressed the issue of surface roughness through various means of grit-blasting followed by a surface etching or coating procedure. This has included titanium plasma spray (TPS) (Buser et al. 1991), abrasion (TiO$_2$ blasting or use of soluble abrasives), combinations of blasting and etching (e.g., Al$_2$O$_3$ with H$_2$SO$_4$/HCL) (Buser et al. 1991), thin apatite coating (Vercaigne et al. 1998), or sintered beads (Deporter et al. 1996). Commercially available roughened surfaces using the large grit-blasted and acid-etched surface (ITI/Straumann's SLA surface) have shown both laboratory and clinical evidence of elevated success rates in areas of the posterior maxilla (Buser et al. 1991, 1994, 1996, 2000; Cochran 1999). The role of the roughened surface is complex since the actual strength of bone contact against a titanium oxide surface is low (4 MPa or less); weak enough that without macroscopic surface topography (e.g., resulting from a grit-blasting process) little bone contact occurs (Brunski et al. 2000). Clinically, the combination of large grit-blasted and etched surfaces in a one-stage surgical procedure has documented greater than 10-year cumulative survival rates of 96.2% (Buser et al. 1999). An alternative commercially surface-etched implant design uses a combination of HCL/H$_2$SO$_4$ to create a surface topography (Osseotite™, Biomet 3i Implant Innovations, Palm Beach Gardens, Florida). The application of a roughened surface topography appears to have become the current "state of the art" with multiple implant systems coming out with new or modified products to reflect this increased interest.

Implant Micro-Retentive Features: Alterations of Surface Chemistry

Various attempts have been made to systematically alter the surface topography and/or composition of the oxide surface on commercially pure and Ti-6Al-4V titanium alloy. These approaches have involved techniques to increase the surface oxide thickness, creation of repeated patterns (e.g., through additive or subtractive lithography), or means to control oxide composition through the sterilization techniques used during or following manufacturing. Titanium, being a non-noble metal, spontaneously forms a 3–5 nm thick oxide surface (primarily dioxide and trioxides) upon exposure to air (Stanford and Keller 1991; Wataha 1996). In vitro studies have been performed to characterize changes in the cell and molecular regulation of bone-related matrix proteins as a function of the oxide composition resulting from sterilization procedures (Kasemo and Lausmaa 1988; Kawahara et al. 1996; Keller et al. 1990; Lausmaa et al. 1985; Michaels et al. 1991; Stanford et al. 1994). These studies emphasize the need for implants to be manufactured, packaged, and clinically handled in a very careful manner. This then leads to a provocative question: Can the results of a simple cleaning and sterilization process impact subsequent biological healing?

Interestingly, recent studies on surface sterilization have led to implant surfaces having a relatively enriched oxide content of fluoride. Fluoride appears to play a significant role not only in modulating the physical chemistry of hydroxyapatite formation but also in stimulating new bone growth, matrix expression, and subsequent mineralization (Farley et al. 1991; Jowsey 1977; Mehta et al. 1995; Meunier 1990; Modrowski et al. 1992; Mohr

and Kragstrup 1991; Mundy 1999; Stein and Lian 1993). It is known that fluoride can stimulate the production of new bone, in part by stimulating the proliferation of osteoblasts (Baylink et al. 1995; Bellows et al. 1990; Wergedal et al. 1988). The introduction of fluoride to the oxide surface can be performed by initially grit-blasting the surface with a known diameter of titanium dioxide particles followed by etching in a dilute HF acid solution. The etching step is carefully controlled to create a moderately rough surface with potential biological effects on undifferentiated mesenchymal stem cells that migrate onto the implant surface by way of the fibrin scaffold (Cooper 2003; Ellingsen and Lyngstadaas 2003; Ellingsen et al. 2004; Keller et al. 2003; Schneider et al. 2003, 2004; Stanford et al. 2003). In vivo research has indicated that following a 3-month healing period, fluoride-modified implant surfaces demonstrated significantly higher bone-to-metal contact and retention to bone compared to implants with similar surface roughness (Fig. 15.2) (Ellingsen et al. 2004).

Surface modification of titanium with fluoride changes the surface chemical structures, resulting in an increased affinity to the titanium dioxide surface for calcium and phosphate ions. The capability to adsorb Ca and PO_4 promotes bone formation and the

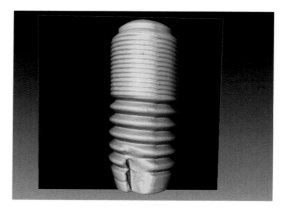

Figure 15.2. Micro-CT 3-D imaging of a fluoride-modified implant at 8 weeks showing uniform adapted bone around the implant surface.

process of bone bonding in vitro and in vivo (Ellingsen et al. 2004; Hanawa and Ota 1991; Yan et al. 1997).

In vitro studies have shown that differences in the microtopography of an implant surface can affect the expression of key bone matrix-related proteins and osteogenic transcription factors that will enhance osteogenesis on implant surfaces (Ogawa et al. 2002; Schneider et al. 2003; Stanford et al. 2003). In a laboratory-based comparison study of the fluoride-modified implant surface (OsseoSpeed™ Astra Tech AB, Mölndal, Sweden) compared to a hydrophilic surface (SLActive™, Institute Straumann, Basel, Switzerland), Masaki et al. (2005) found that the fluoride-modified surface specifically led to the up-regulation of a key transcription factor, RUNX-2/cbfa-1, vital to the differentiation of osteoblasts. These observations were extended by Isa et al. (2006) with an analysis of gene expression coupled with analysis of the changes in the nano-topography on the oxide surface due to the HF exposure. Other laboratory studies (Cooper et al. 2006) have shown effects on the BMP-2 expression as well as effects on the expression of other key genes involved in bone matrix expression (e.g., Bone Sialoprotein).

In order to assess the impact of the fluoride modification on tissue-level response, a series of animal studies were performed. Using a Sprague-Dawley rat tibia model, two different threaded implants (1.5×2 mm) were compared with either a TiO_2 grit-blasted or blasted and treated with a fluoride containing solution. After 21 days, a significantly greater amount of bone contact had occurred on the fluoride-coated surfaces (55.5% vs. 34.2%; P < 0.027) (Abron et al. 2001).

Histomorphometrically, the fluoride-exposed surface demonstrated greater osteo-conductive growth of trabecular bone in the marrow cavity. In a rabbit tibial model, Wennerberg et al. (2000) demonstrated enhanced pull-out strengths (57% increase from 54 to 85 Ncm at 3 months) and a more rapid formation of bone contact on implant

surfaces that were exposed to this fluoride surface treatment. In a rabbit tibia model, Ellingsen et al. (2004) demonstrated greater bone-to-implant (BIC) on the fluoride-modified surface as compared to a titanium dioxide grit-blasted surface at 1 and 3 months. As a measure of the interfacial strength, removal torque and interfacial shear strength values were measured. Whereas the fluoride-modified surface did not result in any difference at 1 month of healing, by 3 months the fluoride-modified surface had a significantly higher removal torque (85 ± 16 Ncm) relative to the titanium dioxide grit-blasted surface (TiOblast) implants (54 ± 12 Ncm) (Ellingsen et al. 2004). In a rat tibia model, Cooper et al. (2006) demonstrated elevated BIC ($55.45 \pm 22.01\%$) relative to the non-modified TiO-blasted implants ($34.21 \pm 12.08\%$) 3 weeks following implantation, a difference considered significant (p < 0.027). In the oral cavity canine dog model, Lee et al. (2007) demonstrated enhanced bone formation around the fluoride-modified implant surface using 3-D micro-CT imaging (Fig. 15.2).

This approach showed greater adaptive bone contact on the walls of the implant surface (osteoconductive properties) and holds the potential for predictable implant outcomes even in patients with genetic malformations (Figs. 15.3a–15.3g).

Conclusion

Dental implant therapy has undergone an explosion in surface technologies and applications of implant designs. These have led to more predictable biology and hold the potential for predictable long-term clinical outcomes. It is important for the clinician to understand how minor changes to surface technology can create the potential for significant changes in bone contact and biomechanical strength that have the potential to allow more rapid clinical function of implants. This can only be validated with rigorous clinical testing and evaluation.

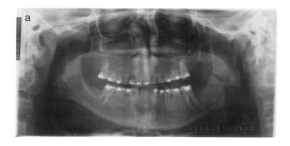

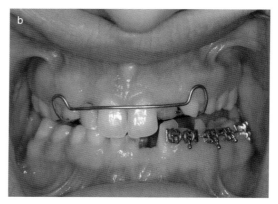

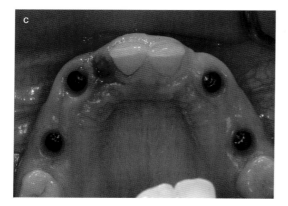

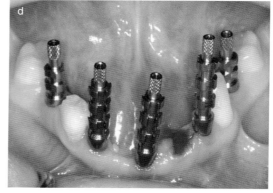

Figures 15.3a–d.   Clinical example of stable implant-supported prosthesis in a patient with Witkops/ED Syndrome. Combination of surface technologies, stable implant abutment connection, and a prosthetic abutment transition contour that allows an integration of biological principles for a predictable outcome. Presenting condition of oligodontia (a and b) managed with implants treatment planned for multiple ceramo-metal fixed partial dentures. Distribution of implant placements and impression copings (c and d).

CHANGING RATIONALES: CONNECTING TEETH WITH IMPLANTS BY A SUPRASTRUCTURE

Paul Weigl

Introduction

Connecting a tooth to an implant sharing a support for a fixed bridge may in specific situations be an advantage in treatment planning in particular cases compared to a full implant-borne bridge. One such situation is when there is inadequate bone quantity adjacent to an already crowned tooth and the patient wants to avoid an augmentation procedure. Combining tooth and implant with a bridge may also be considered when the patient prefers a minimally invasive intervention. However, an implant tooth-supported fixed partial denture presents a biomechanical design problem, because the implant is rigidly anchored by the bone, and the tooth is surrounded by a periodontal ligament that allows some movement. Until recently, therapy guidelines have differed as they have been based on biomechanical considerations and limited clinical data to support or reject the use of tooth-implant-connected bridges.

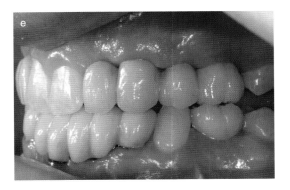

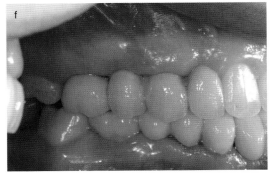

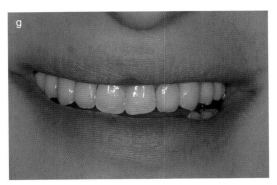

Figures 15.3e–g.   Delivery of fixed reconstruction (e and f) that established satisfactory aesthetics (g).

Recent new knowledge may influence the rationale selecting this particular treatment option.

Biomechanics and Related Theories

Due to the different anchorages of a tooth and an implant their biomechanical behavior under load is quite different. The stiffness between bone and implant surface is higher than a damped anchorage of a tooth root by the periodontal ligament. Therefore, if a one-piece bridge is loaded solely in the region of the abutment tooth, by, for example, chewing hard food at this spot, the bridge will act as a long cantilever supported only by the implant. The cantilever generates a high load at the bone implant interface and causes a moment of torque at the implant itself and especially on the abutment-implant joint in a two- or multi-unit implant system. The tooth, in contrast, is loaded below normal physiological levels. To diminish the cantilever effect and enable a physiological loading of the tooth, one solution was to separate the bridge with a precision attachment, which would ensure a non-rigid connection between the tooth and the implant (Figs. 15.4a, 15.4b).

Another biomechanical model has recently been put forward that may partially explain load transfer from the tooth root into the alveolar bone. This model relates to the high impulse (Newton-seconds) for fracture during the first bite into foods (Dan and Kohyama 2007). When a high impulse acts on a fluid the viscosity is increased, for example, blood in the periodontal ligament. It can therefore be hypothesized that the tooth, due to high-impulse fracturing in first bites, demonstrates viscoelastic properties equivalent to that of an osseointegrated implant.

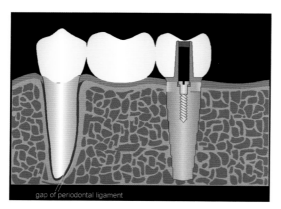

Figure 15.4a. Scheme of tooth-implant connected bridge. The gap of the periodontal ligament allows a damped anchorage.

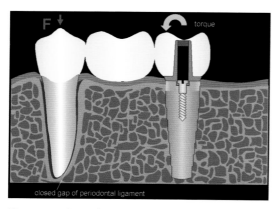

Figure 15.4b. Scheme of tooth-implant connected bridge loaded (F) at the region of the abutment tooth. The closed gap of the periodontal ligament causes a high moment of torque at the implant due to the long cantilever.

General Consensus in 1982

At the time it was believed that the elasticity of a periodontal ligament would preclude the stiff connection of a tooth with a rigid osseointegrated implant by a suprastructure, the consensus arising from the desire to avoid an implant overloading. If the tooth and the implant were splinted by a non-rigid precision attachment, an intrusion of the tooth

was frequently observed. One of the first theories was based on the idea that a lack of normal stimulation of the periodontal ligament produces atrophy of the periodontal ligament and intrusion of the tooth. Thus, a tooth-implant-connected bridge—whether rigid or non-rigid—was not previously an option.

Today's Rationale: Connecting Implants with Teeth

To the surprise of clinicians and biomechanics the tooth-implant-connected bridges after 5 years in function demonstrate a similar estimated survival rate (95.5%) to implant-borne bridges (95.2%), as assessed in a systematic review of the literature (Pjetursson et al. 2007). However, clinical studies show that the risk for an intrusion of a tooth is higher with a non-rigid splinted bridge (Block et al. 2002; Naert et al. 2001) than with a rigid bridge (Nickenig et al. 2006). To explain this phenomenon, debris impaction or microjamming, a ratchet effect related to the use of precision attachments, are discussed as possible causes. In other words, the precision attachments increase the friction or lock completely in an intrusive position relative to the tooth. Both prevent the relocation of the intruded tooth. Therefore, the connection, if made, should be completely rigid to avoid intrusion of abutment teeth (Palmer et al. 2005). It can be easily achieved in a one-piece bridge by aligning a tilted implant abutment to the insertion path of the ground abutment tooth. The bridge has to be cemented on the abutment tooth as well as on the implant-abutment (Figs. 15.5a, 15.5b).

In situations where the periodontal ligament of the abutment tooth may not able to adequately distribute the load into the alveolar socket, almost the whole load is transferred to the implant by the bridge acting as a long cantilever. Due to the large momentum that is created it will seem advantageous to use a mechanically very strong implant to

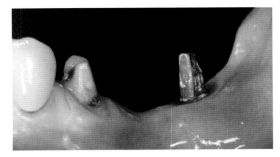

Figure 15.5a. Prepared second left premolar and implant at region left second molar.

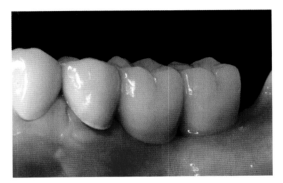

Figure 15.5b. Cemented tooth-implant connected bridge replacing the first left molar. (Source: G. Trimpou.)

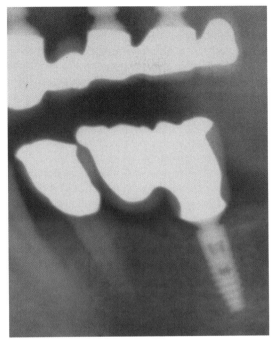

Figure 15.6a. Orthopantomogram-detail of an implant at the region first left molar retaining a molar-crown with a cantilever replacing the second premolar. The crown cemented on the first left premolar is not connected to this implant-borne suprastructure and has therefore not been removed.

prevent technical failure by overload and/or by fatigue. One-piece implants or implant-abutment joints with a lack of dynamic micro-motion at the implant-abutment interface may have benefits in this respect (Meng et al. 2007; University of Frankfurt am Main 2008; Zipprich et al. 2007). Additionally, a combined tooth-implant-supported FDP should be limited to three units, thereby limiting the length of the cantilever as well. All these factors related to a rigid tooth-implant-connected bridge give an opportunity to achieve in the future the same survival summary estimate of implant-implant-supported bridges after 10 years—86.7%—instead of the 77.8% estimated by tooth-implant-supported bridges (Pjetursson et al. 2007).

Another connection between tooth and implant can be easily achieved with a tapered crown removable denture. The integrated abutment teeth show promising clinical long-term behavior without any sign of an intrusion (Krennmair et al. 2007; Weigl and Lauer 2000).

Outlook

Following the osseointegration of an implant the trabecular framework retaining the implant will adapt to the amount and the direction of applied mechanical forces (Huiskes et al. 2000). Consequently the density and strain-related alignment of the three-dimensional trabecular framework adjust to the non-axial forces of the implant as well (Akagawa et al. 2003; Celletti et al.

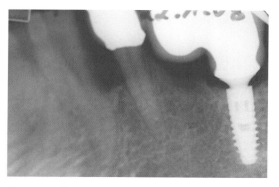

Figure 15.6b. Radiograph after the 1-year follow-up. No sign of biological failure can be recognized.

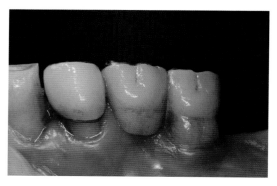

Figure 15.6c. The implant-borne crown with a mesial cantilever after 1 year in function.

1995; Ruimerman et al. 2005). Taking this into account, a three-unit bridge connecting a tooth and an implant could be workable even in the case where the full mastication force is transferred only to the implant. The bridge can be substituted by an implant-borne crown that is connected with a pontic replacing the missing teeth between the implant and the natural abutment tooth. The implant-borne crown and the pontic result in a shorter cantilever than the estimated cantilever of a tooth-implant-connected bridge, in which the abutment tooth cannot transfer any load to the alveolar bone (Figs. 15.6a–15.6c).

Future clinical trials will be able to prove or reject the hypothesis that an implant-borne crown with the one crown-sized cantilever works as well as a rigid, combined tooth-implant-supported FDP. Furthermore, this solution for replacing two missing teeth is cost-saving and in avoiding tooth preparation represents a minimally invasive approach. Also the risk of complications at the abutment tooth, such as caries, apical ostitis, root fracture, and so forth, can be avoided with the solely implant-borne suprastructure (Brägger et al. 2001; Hosny et al. 2000; Naert et al. 2001).

References

Abrahamsson I, Berglundh T, et al. 1999. Peri-implant tissues at submerged and non-submerged titanium implants. *J Clin Periodontol* 26(9):600–607.

Abron A, Kun P, et al. 2001. Fluoride modification effects on bone formation at TiO2-grit blasted cpTitanium endosseous implants. Academy of Osseointegration, Toronto.

Akagawa Y, Sato Y, Teixeira ER, Shindoi N, Wadamoto M. 2003. A mimic osseointegrated implant model for three-dimensional finite element analysis. *J Oral Rehabil* 30(1):41–45.

Arvidson K, Bystedt H, et al. 1998. Five-year prospective follow-up report of the Astra Tech Dental Implant System in the treatment of edentulous mandibles. *Clin Oral Implants Res* 9(4):225–234.

Astrand P, Almfeldt I, et al. 1996. Non-submerged implants in the treatment of the edentulous lower jaw. A 2-year longitudinal study [published erratum appears in *Clin Oral Implants Res* 1997 8(4):342]. *Clin Oral Implants Res* 7(4):337–344.

Bagno A, Di Bello C. 2004. Surface treatments and roughness properties of Ti-based biomaterials. *J Materials Sci-Materials in Medicine* 15(9):935–949.

Baylink DJ, Duane PB, et al. 1983. Monofluorophosphate physiology: The effects of fluoride on bone. *Caries Res* 17(Suppl 1): 56–76.

Baylink DJ, Wergedal JE, et al. 1995. On fluo-ride and bone strength. [Comment]. *Calcified Tissue Int* 56(5):415–418.

Bellows CG, Heersche JN, et al. 1990. Determination of the capacity for proliferation and differentiation of osteoprogenitor cells in the presence and absence of dexamethasone. *Developmental Biology* 140(1):132–138.

Binon PP. 2000. Implants and components: Entering the new millennium. *Int J Oral Maxillofac Implants* 15(1):76–94.

Block MS, Lirette D, Gardiner D, Li L, Finger IM, Hochstedler J, Evans G, Kent JN, Misiek DJ, Mendez AJ, Guerra L, Larsen H, Wood W, Worthington P. 2002. Prospective evaluation of implants connected to teeth. *Int J Oral Maxillofac Implants* 17(4):473–487.

Brägger U, Aeschlimann S, Burgin W, Hammerle CH, Lang NP. 2001. Biological and technical complications and failures with fixed partial dentures (FPD) on implants and teeth after four to five years of function. *Clin Oral Implants Res* 12(1):26–34.

Brunski JB, Puleo DA, et al. 2000. Biomaterials and biomechanics of oral and maxillofacial implants: Current status and future developments. *Int J Oral Maxillofac Implants* 15(1):15–46.

Buser D, Belser UC, et al. 2000. The original one-stage dental implant system and its clinical application. *Periodontology* 17: 106–118.

Buser D, Dula K, et al. 1996. Long-term stability of osseointegrated implants in bone regenerated with the membrane technique. 5-year results of a prospective study with 12 implants. *Clin Oral Implants Res* 7(2): 175–183.

Buser D, Mericske-Stern R, et al. 1999. Clinical experience with one-stage, non-submerged dental implants. *Adv Dent Res* 13:153–161.

Buser D, Schenk RK, et al. 1991. Influence of surface characteristics on bone integration of titanium implants. A histomorphometric study in miniature pigs. *J Biomed Mater Res* 25(7):889–902.

Buser D, Weber HP, et al. 1994. Tissue integration of one-stage implants: Three-year results of a prospective longitudinal study with hollow cylinder and hollow screw implants. *Quintessence Int* 25(10):679–686.

Celletti R, Pameijer CH, Bracchetti G, Donath K, Persichetti G, Visani I. 1995. Histologic evaluation of osseointegrated implants restored in nonaxial functional occlusion with preangled abutments. *Int J Periodontics Restorative Dent* 15(6):562–573.

Cochran DL. 1999. A comparison of endosseous dental implant surfaces. *J Periodontol* 70(12):1523–1539.

Cooper LF. 2003. Cellular interactions at commercially pure titanium implants. In: *Bio-Implant Interface: Improving Biomaterials and Tissue Reactions*. JE Ellingsen and SP Lyngstadaas (eds.). Boca Raton FL: CRC Press. 165–179.

Cooper LF, Scurria MS, et al. 1999. Treatment of edentulism using Astra Tech implants and ball abutments to retain mandibular overdentures. *Int J Oral Maxillofac Implants* 14(5):646–653.

Cooper LF, Zhou Y, Takebe J, Guo J, Abron A, Holmén A, Ellingsen JE. 2006. Fluoride modification effects on osteoblast behavior and bone formation at TiO2 grit-blasted c.p. titanium endosseous implants. *Biomaterials* 27(6):926–936.

Dan H, Kohyama K. 2007. Interactive relationship between the mechanical properties of food and the human response during the first bite. *Archives Oral Biology* 52(5): 455–464.

Davis DM, Packer ME. 1999. Mandibular overdentures stabilized by Astra Tech implants with either ball attachments or magnets: 5-year results. *Int J Prosthodont* 12(3):222–229.

Deporter DA, Watson PA, et al. 1996. Simplifying the treatment of edentulism: A new type of implant. *J Am Dent Assoc* 127(9): 1343–1349.

Ellingsen JE, Johansson CB, et al. 2004. Improved retention and bone-to-implant contact with fluoride-modified titanium implants. *Int J Oral Maxillofac Implants* 19(5):659–666.

Ellingsen JE, Lyngstadaas SP. 2003. Increasing biocompatibility by chemical modification of titanium surfaces. In: *Bio-Implant Interface: Improving Biomaterials and Tissue Reactions*. JE Ellingsen and SP Lyngstadaas (eds.). Boca Raton FL: CRC Press. 323–335.

Farley JR, Hall SL, et al. 1991. Skeletal alkaline phosphatase specific activity is an index of the osteoblastic phenotype in subpopulations of the human osteosarcoma cell line SaOS-2. *Metabolism: Clinical & Experimental* 40(7):664–671.

Hanawa T, Ota M. 1991. Calcium phosphate naturally formed on titanium in electrolyte solution. *Biomaterials* 12(8):767–774.

Hansson S. 1999. The implant neck: Smooth or provided with retention elements—a biomechanical approach. *Clin Oral Implants Res* 10(5):394–405.

———. 2000. Surface roughness parameters as predictors of anchorage strength in bone: A critical analysis. *J Biomechanics* 33(10): 1297–1303.

Hansson S, Norton M. 1999. The relation between surface roughness and interfacial shear strength for bone-anchored implants. A mathematical model. *J Biomechanics* 32(8):829–836.

Hosny M, Duyck J, Van Steenberghe D, Naert I. 2000. Within-subject comparison between connected and non-connected tooth-to-implant fixed partial prostheses: Up to 14-year follow-up study. *Int J Prosthodont* 13(4):340–346.

Huiskes R, Ruimerman R, Harry van Lenthe G, Janssen JD. 2000. Effects of mechanical forces on maintenance and adaptation of form in trabecular bone. *Nature* 405: 704–706.

Isa ZM, Schneider GB, et al. 2006. Effects of fluoride-modified titanium surfaces on osteoblast proliferation and gene expression. *Int J Oral Maxillofac Implants* 21(2):203–211.

Isidor F. 1997. Clinical probing and radiographic assessment in relation to the histologic bone level at oral implants in monkeys. *Clin Oral Implants Res* 8(4): 255–264.

Jowsey J. 1977. Osteoporosis: Dealing with a crippling bone disease of the elderly. *Geriatrics* 32(7):41–50.

Kasemo B, Lausmaa J. 1988. Biomaterial and implant surfaces: A surface science approach. *Int J Oral Maxillofac Implants* 3(4):247–259.

Kasemo B, Lausmaa J. 1994. Material-tissue interfaces: The role of surface properties and processes. *Environmental Health Perspectives* 102(Suppl 5):41–45.

Kawahara D, Ong JL, et al. 1996. Surface characterization of radio-frequency glow discharged and autoclaved titanium surfaces. *Int J Oral Maxillofac Implants* 11(4): 435–442.

Keller JC, Draughn RA, et al. 1990. Characterization of sterilized CP titanium implant surfaces. *Int J Oral Maxillofac Implants* 5(4):360–367.

Keller JC, Schneider GB, et al. 2003. Effects of implant microtopography on osteoblast cell attachment. *Implant Dent* 12(2):175–181.

Krennmair G, Krainhöfner M, Waldenberger O, Piehslinger E. 2007. Dental implants as strategic supplementary abutments for implant-tooth-supported telescopic crown-retained maxillary dentures: A retrospective follow-up study for up to 9 years. *Int J Prosthodont* 20(6):617–622.

Lausmaa J, Kasemo B, et al. 1985. Accelerated oxide growth on titanium implants during autoclaving caused by fluorine contamination. *Biomaterials* 6(1):23–27.

Lee R, Morgan TA, Schroeder N, Krizan K, Sieren J, Stanford CM. 2007. Micro-CT evaluation of bone adaptation to implant surfaces. New Orleans, IADR.

Lindh T, Gunne J, et al. 1998. A meta-analysis of implants in partial edentulism. *Clin Oral Implants Res* 9(2):80–90.

Makkonen TA, Holmberg S, et al. 1997. A 5-year prospective clinical study of Astra Tech dental implants supporting fixed bridges or overdentures in the edentulous mandible. *Clin Oral Implants Res* 8(6): 469–475.

Masaki C, Schneider GB, et al. 2005. Effects of implant surface microtopography on osteoblast gene expression. *Clin Oral Implants Res* 16(6):650–656.

Mehta S, Reed B, et al. 1995. Effects of high levels of fluoride on bone formation: An in vitro model system. *Biomaterials* 16(2): 97–102.

Meng JC, Everts JE, Qian F, Gratton DG. 2007. Influence of connection geometry on dynamic micromotion at the implant-abutment interface. *Int J Prosthodont* 20(6):623–625.

Meunier PJ. 1990. Treatment of vertebral osteoporosis with fluoride and calcium. *Progress in Clin & Biological Res* 332: 221–230.

Michaels CM, Keller JC, et al. 1991. In vitro periodontal ligament fibroblast attachment to plasma-cleaned titanium surfaces. *J Oral Implantol* 17(2):132–139.

Modrowski D, Miravet L, et al. 1992. Effect of fluoride on bone and bone cells in ovariectomized rats. *J Bone Mineral Res* 7(8): 961–969.

Mohr H, Kragstrup J. 1991. A histomorphometric analysis of the effects of fluoride on experimental ectopic bone formation in the rat. *J Dent Res* 70(6):957–960.

Mundy GR. 1999. What can we learn from bone biology for the treatment for osteoporosis? *Osteoporosis Int* 9(Suppl 2): S40–S47.

Naert IE, Duyck JA, Hosny MM, Van Steenberghe D. 2001. Freestanding and tooth-implant connected prostheses in the treatment of partially edentulous patients. Part I: An up to 15-year clinical evaluation. *Clin Oral Implants Res* 12(3): 237–244.

Nickenig HJ, Schäfer C, Spiekermann H. 2006. Survival and complication rates of combined tooth-implant-supported fixed partial dentures. *Clin Oral Implants Res* 17(5):506–511.

Nordin T, Jonsson TG, et al. 1998. The use of a conical fixture design for fixed partial prostheses. A preliminary report. *Clin Oral Implants Res* 9(5):343–347.

Ogawa T, Sukotjo C, et al. 2002. Modulated bone matrix-related gene expression is associated with differences in interfacial strength of different implant surface roughness. *J Prosthodont* 11(4):241–247.

Palmer RM, Howe LC, Palmer PJ. 2005. A prospective 3-year study of fixed bridges linking Astra Tech ST implants to natural teeth. *Clin Oral Implants Res* 16(3): 302–307.

Pjetursson BE, Brägger U, Lang NP, Zwahlen M. 2007. Comparison of survival and complication rates of tooth-supported fixed dental prostheses (FDPs) and implant-supported FDPs and single crowns (SCs). *Clin Oral Implants Res* 18(Suppl 3): 97–113.

Ruimerman R, Hilbers P, Van Rietbergen B, Huiskes R. 2005. A theoretical framework for strain-related trabecular bone maintenance and adaptation. *J Biomechanics* 38(4):931–941.

Schneider GB, Perinpanayagam H, et al. 2003. Implant surface roughness affects osteoblast gene expression. *J Dent Res* 82(5):372–376.

Schneider GB, Zaharias R, et al. 2004. Differentiation of preosteoblasts is affected by implant surface microtopographies. *J Biomed Mater Res Part A* 69(3):462–468.

Schroeder A, Buser DA. 1989. ITI-system. Basic and clinical procedures. *Shigaku—Odontology* 77(SPEC):1267–1288.

Schroeder A, Sutter F, et al. 1996. *Oral Implantology Basics, ITI Hollow Cylinder System.* New York: Thieme Medical Publishers, Inc.

Schroeder A, Van der Zypen E, et al. 1981. The reactions of bone, connective tissue, and epithelium to endosteal implants with titanium-sprayed surfaces. *J Maxillofac Surg* 9(1):15–25.

Shalabi MM, Gortemaker A, et al. 2006. Implant surface roughness and bone healing: A systematic review. *J Dent Res* 85(6):496–500.

Stanford CM. 1999. Biomechanical and functional behavior of implants. *Adv Dent Res* 13:88–92.

———. 2002. Surface modification of implants. In: *Emerging Biomaterials*. JC Keller and MJ Buckley (eds.). Philadelphia: Saunders. 39–52.

———. 2003. Bone quantity and quality: Are they relevant predictors of implant outcomes? *Int J Prosthodont* 16(Suppl): 43–51.

———. 2005. Application of oral implants to the general dental practice. *J Am Dent Assoc* 136(8):1092–1100.

Stanford CM, Brand RA. 1999. Toward an understanding of implant occlusion and strain adaptive bone modeling and remodeling. *J Prosthet Dent* 81(5):553–561.

Stanford CM, Keller JC. 1991. The concept of osseointegration and bone matrix expression. *Crit Rev Oral Biol Med* 2(1):83–101.

Stanford CM, Keller JC, et al. 1994. Bone cell expression on titanium surfaces is altered by sterilization treatments. *J Dent Res* 73(5):1061–1071.

Stanford CM, Schneider GB. 2004. Functional behaviour of bone around dental implants. *Gerodontology* 21(2):71–77.

Stanford CM, Schneider GB, Perinpanayagam H, Keller JC, Midura R. 2003. Biomedical implant surface topography and its effects on osteoblast differentiation, in vitro. In: *Bio-Implant Interface: Improving Biomaterials and Tissue Reactions*. JE Ellingsen and SP Lyngstadaas (eds.). Boca Raton FL: CRC Press. 41–64.

Stein GS, Lian JB. 1993. Molecular mechanisms mediating proliferation/differentiation interrelationships during progressive development of the osteoblast phenotype. *Endocrine Reviews* 14(4):424–442.

University of Frankfurt am Main. 2008. Micromovements at the Implant-Abutment Interface: Measurement, Causes, and Consequences. URL: www.kgu.de/zzmk/werkstoffkunde. Accessed March 15, 2008.

Vercaigne S, Wolke JG, et al. 1998. Bone healing capacity of titanium plasma-sprayed and hydroxylapatite-coated oral implants. *Clin Oral Implants Res* 9(4):261–271.

Warrer K, Karring T, et al. 1993. Periodontal ligament formation around different types of dental titanium implants. I: The self-tapping screw type implant system. *J Periodontol* 64(1):29–34.

Wataha JC. 1996. Materials for endosseous dental implants. *J Oral Rehabil* 23(2): 79–90.

Weigl P, Lauer H-Ch. 2000. Advanced biomaterials used for a new telescopic retainer for removable dentures: Ceramic vs. electroplated gold copings, Part II: Clinical effects. *J Biomed Mater Res* 53(4):337–347.

Wennerberg A, Albrektsson T. 2000. Suggested guidelines for the topographic evaluation of implant surfaces. *Int J Oral Maxillofac Implants* 15(3):331–344.

Wennerberg A, Ektessabi A, et al. 1997. A 1-year follow-up of implants of differing surface roughness placed in rabbit bone. *Int J Oral Maxillofac Implants* 12(4): 486–494.

Wennerberg A, Johansson CB, et al. 2000. Enhanced fixation to bone with flouride modified oral implants. IADR/AADR/CADR, Washington, DC.

Wergedal JE, Lau KH, et al. 1988. Fluoride and bovine bone extract influence cell proliferation and phosphatase activities in human bone cell cultures. *Clinical Orthopaedics Related Res* 233:274–282.

Widmark G, Andersson B, et al. 2001. Rehabilitation of patients with severely resorbed maxillae by means of implants with or without bone grafts: A 3-to 5-year follow-up clinical report. *Int J Oral Maxillofac Implants* 16(1):73–79.

Yan WQ, Nakamura T, et al. 1997. Apatite layer-coated titanium for use as bone bonding implants. *Biomaterials* 18(17): 1185–1190.

Zipprich H, Weigl P, Lange B, Lauer H-C. 2007. Erfassung, Ursachen und Folgen von Mikrobewegungen am Implantat-Abutment-Interface. *Implantologie* 15(1): 31–46.

Restorative Phase Treatment Planning Using Shortened Clinical Protocols

16

STABILITY OF IMPLANT-ABUTMENT CONNECTIONS

Thomas D. Taylor

In 1982 the only abutment interface available on the market for osseointegrated dental implants was the external hexagon design of the Brånemark implant system as marketed by NobelPharma of Sweden. This external hexagon connection was the industry standard for more than 15 years and served more than adequately in most clinical situations. The most common complication associated with this screw-retained connection was screw loosening and occasional screw fracture (Goodacre et al. 2003). Subsequent to 1982 additional implant systems appeared on the market with different implant abutment connections, but the external hexagon was used as the connection of choice by most implant manufacturers during the 1980s and early 1990s.

The mechanics of the external hexagon connection are surprisingly complex. It must first be realized that the external hexagon on the top of the implant was placed there primarily to serve as a wrench-engaging connec-

tion used to insert the implant into the osteotomy site. It is questionable whether the external hexagon functions at all in the pillar of final implant restoration. While the external hexagon may be engaged to resist rotational force, particularly in single tooth restorations, the external hexagon connection is in actuality a flat to flat bolted joint (Fig. 16.1).

Due to the necessary tolerances between parts for ease of assembly, the hexagon is not engaged by the abutment and does not add strength or stability to the joint. Resistance to loosening across this bolted flat to flat joint is focused in the abutment screw. When tightened the screw effectively stretches and creates a clamping force across the joint. This clamping force is termed "preload." The greater the torque applied to the screw during tightening, the greater the preload or clamping force across the joint. It is critical to the stability of the joint that the preload remain at or near its initial level. Micromovement and microabrasion of the bolted joint and the threads of the abutment screw may, over time, cause a gradual relaxation in the preload level.

Non-axial loading of an implant pillar places certain areas of that pillar under

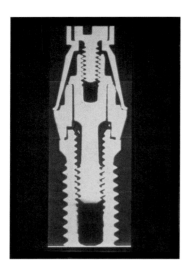

Figure 16.1. Photograph of an external hexed dental implant showing the lack of vertical wall contact between the abutment and the hex of the implant. The hex is utilized as a wrench-engaging interface during implant placement but it is unlikely to provide resistance to dislodgement or bending forces when coupled with an abutment.

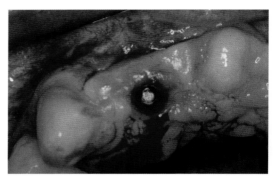

Figure 16.2. Clinical photograph of a fractured abutment screw in an external hex implant pillar. The abutment screw was likely subjected to non-axial bending moments due to the cantilever of the prosthesis anteriorly. The prosthesis had been in place for 7 years.

compression and other areas under tension. In general the side at which the load is being applied (ipsilateral side) is placed under tensile loading and the contralateral side is placed under compression. It is important to realize that the application of non-axial forces to the implant abutment interface will cause a temporary reduction in the ipsilateral preload and simultaneously cause an increase in the contralateral preload. As long as the preload of the abutment screw on the ipsilateral side is not surpassed by the magnitude of the load being applied, no additional strain is being applied to the abutment screw itself and the joint remains stable. If over time the preload has been reduced either from micromotion loosening or by component wear and/or deformation, a non-axial load of the same magnitude as had been applied previously may now surpass the ipsilateral preload. At this point a bending moment is imparted to the body of the abutment screw and flexure begins to occur. Ultimately, failure of the abutment screw will occur through flexure fatigue (Fig. 16.2).

This mode of failure is clearly time dependent and is based upon the assumption that screw preload is not maintained over time. If the screw stays tight, the joint does not become weakened. If preload is lost, flexure fatigue leading to ultimate failure of the screw is a potential result.

Occasional failure of implant-supported restorations by fracture of the abutment screw led some clinicians to seek alternative types of connections that would reduce the potential for abutment screw failure. Numerous manufacturers created alternative designs based primarily on a connection that was internal to the body of the implant and that reduced the dependence on maintaining screw preload across a flat to flat interface. In the late 1990s and into the early 21st century internal connections became very popular and are the connection of choice today.

The advantages of internal connections, particularly those based upon some form of tapered connection, are several. The internal connection relies less on the preload of the abutment screw to keep the joint stable. Contact between the abutment and the wall of the implant reduces the potential for micromotion and loss of preload of the screw, making the initial amount of preload less critical. Internal connections are inherently more resistant to non-axial loading than are flat to flat joints. With most internal connection systems there is minimal rotational misfit or "slop," and they exhibit strong antirotational resistance. It would seem that the complications associated with loose or fractured abutment screws in the flat to flat connection implants have been largely overcome with internal connection implants.

There are several long-term concerns that must be considered with internal connection implant systems. The wall of the implant becomes the load-bearing interface with the forces being directed from inside to out. These externally directed stresses in a cylindrical implant body are termed "hoop stresses" as one would see with outward pressure on the staves of a barrel or similar container. Resistance to hoop stresses becomes critical to the integrity of the implant itself in such internally connected systems, as the walls of the implant must resist these stresses over the lifetime of the structure. Stated another way, with internal connection–type implant systems, if something fails due to fatigue and fracture it is likely to be the body of the implant itself. While broken abutment screws in the original flat to flat configuration can be retrieved and replaced with minimal difficulty, a broken implant wall is a catastrophic failure that compromises the entire pillar or series of pillars of the restoration.

What is the likelihood of implant fracture in routine clinical use? The incidence of implant fracture in the traditional flat to flat type of assembly was minimal with only a small percent of implants fracturing over 10–15 years of follow-up. It cannot be determined at this time what the frequency of implant fracture with the newer internal connections will potentially be. Failure through fatigue loading is time dependent and the risk of failure increases over time. One concern is that implant failure due to hoop stress–induced wall fracture may become a not uncommon problem in the foreseeable future. Stated another way, we haven't been using internal connection implant systems long enough to see the results of long-term loading. It is hoped that failure through implant frac-

ture will remain as a very small percentage of implants placed and that undue concern about failure of these newer designs is unwarranted (Figs. 16.3–16.6).

What other options currently exist that might increase the chances of long-term success of mechanical implant components, particularly in the posterior part of the mouth where forces are usually very high? Increasing the diameter of the implant body and as a result the walls of the internal connection would seem to be one obvious course to take when one is concerned about heavy occlusal

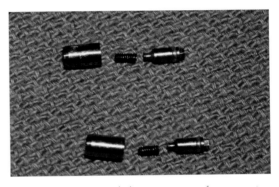

Figure 16.3. Fractured abutment screws from an external hex implant restoration. The cause of failure was most likely fatigue fracture resulting from loss of preload across the bolted implant to abutment joint.

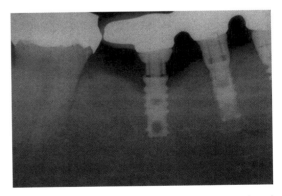

Figure 16.4. Fractured internal connection dental implant. Duration of loading prior to fracture is unknown. Note the associated bone loss adjacent to the implant, which may be due to percolation of debris from the internal aspect of the implant through a crack in the implant wall.

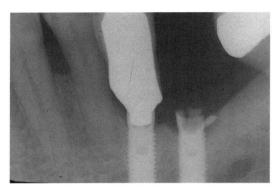

Figure 16.5. Fractured internal connection dental implant. Duration of loading prior to fracture is unknown. Note the unfavorable crown to implant ratio and the proximity of the mental foramen, which is at risk should an attempt be made to remove the broken implant with a trephine.

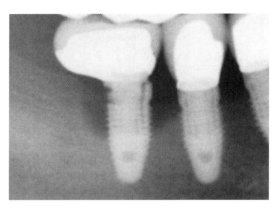

Figure 16.7. Fractured wide-diameter internal connection dental implant. Duration of loading prior to fracture is unknown. Note the associated bone loss and the distal cantilever of the supported crown.

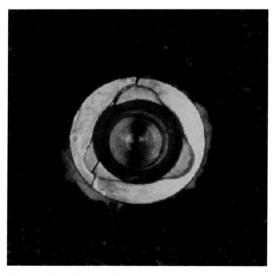

Figure 16.6. Fractured internal connection dental implant that has been removed surgically. Note that the fracture extends through the thinnest areas of the internal connection. (Courtesy Dr. Kenneth Kurtz.)

function or parafunction. Increasing implant radius does not increase strength linearly but rather exponentially (squared) and increases resistance to bending load according to the principle of moment of inertia. Wall thickness similarly controls stress in an exponential manner. So a small increase in diameter and wall thickness may provide substantial improvement in resistance to fatigue overload. But even wide-diameter internal connection implants have been reported to fracture under occlusal loads (Fig. 16.7).

It is certainly appropriate to recommend that reduced-diameter internal connection implants not be placed in posterior areas of the mouth where forces are higher. The introduction of solid one-piece implants may include the advantage of maximized strength for the implant pillar and may be an appropriate rationale for the use of this type of implant in the posterior part of the mouth (Fig. 16.8).

Another design that would likely be more resistant to hoop stress fatigue failure is the single-stage implant design (Fig. 16.9).

With this design occlusal load is transferred through the restoration to the external walls of the implant body rather than through the abutment to the internal connection of the implant. As a result load applied to this design actually places the walls of the implant under compressive force rather than under tensile hoop stress forces as seen with two-stage internal connection implant designs.

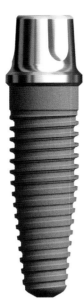

Figure 16.8. A solid one-piece implant in which the abutment is incorporated as part of the implant may provide superior resistance to fatigue fracture in areas of heavy occlusal load.

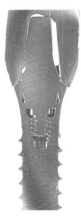

Figure 16.9. A single-stage or transmucosal-type dental implant in cross-section. This is a specimen prepared for laboratory testing and was not used clinically. Note that the crown rests on the external shoulder of the implant body. Load transfer from the occlusal table to the implant is focused on this external shoulder, resulting in inward compressive forces rather than externally directed hoop stresses. This implant design may provide superior resistance to fatigue fracture in areas of heavy occlusal load. This design also provides abutment retrievability and may be used for screw-retained or cement-retained reconstructions.

Conclusion

In conclusion, the implant abutment connection has evolved over the past 25 years and will certainly continue to evolve. The external connection has largely been replaced by the internal connection and the associated problems have changed from loose broken abutment screws to fractured implant walls. The scope of mechanical failure of internal connection implant systems is unknown but is likely to become more commonplace as implants age with use. The alternative of solid one-piece or single-stage implants may prove to be superior in heavy load situations and should be considered as the implant design of choice for posterior sites.

SHORTENED CLINICAL PROTOCOLS: THE (R)EVOLUTION IS STILL ONGOING

Roland Glauser

Introduction

Original protocols for placing and restoring dental implants included a strictly staged approach as the standard modus operandi. Over the years, a myriad of developments have been introduced aimed at simplification and concision without jeopardizing treatment outcomes. A main focus is on a reduction of the number of interventions, the invasiveness of the surgery, and the duration of the treatment. However, past experiences may favor a staged approach in areas with challenging tissue status or in aesthetically demanding areas. Hence, the future is moving toward a differentiation strategy of "when" and "how" to favor shortened surgical and prosthetic protocols and when to follow more traditional staged treatment sequences.

Factors Influencing the Clinical Approach

The original treatment approach included two main prerequisites for proper implant treatment: adequate preoperative examination and thorough pre-treatment planning (Lekholm and Zarb 1985). With regard to time point of implant loading and prosthesis placement, three concepts are currently discussed (Aparicio et al. 2003; Cochran et al. 2004): (1) immediate implant loading/restoration; (2) early implant loading/restoration; and (3) late implant loading/restoration. These categories can be related to biomechanical and histological differences (Szmukler-Moncler et al. 1998). With regard to treatment outcome on a patient rather than per implant basis, current data indicate no statistically significant differences between these three concepts (Esposito et al. 2007). When the feasibility of shortened protocols with early or immediate loading/restoration is discussed, the initial implant anchorage (i.e., primary stability) and the bone quality and quantity at the implant site(s) are most often identified as key for successful osseointegration (Esposito et al. 2007; Szmukler-Moncler et al. 2000). However, for overall treatment success a more comprehensive appraisal at the time of treatment planning is necessary by assessing additional key factors influencing treatment outcome (Table 16.1):

1. *Patient* (general and oral health status, compliance, expectations)
2. *Hard tissues* (healthiness, bone quality and quantity, presence/absence of defects)
3. *Soft tissues* (healthiness, width and volume of keratinized mucosa, texture and scalloping, presence/absence of scars or tattoos)
4. *Prosthetic protocol* (complexity of the prosthetic rehabilitation, potential to pre-manufacture the suprastructure partially or completely)
5. *Team* (skills, routine, timing, and coordination between clinic and lab technician)

Altogether, these five key factors substantially influence whether a shortened protocol can be selected and the likely success of such an approach. However, even if it is possible to successfully load dental implants immediately or early after their placement in selected patients, not all clinicians may achieve optimal results when performing these protocols. In case of doubt, the conventional late loading approach acts as the gold standard and is always a feasible modality.

Patient

Besides general operability and general medical conditions, it is crucial to evaluate oral health status, patient's expectations (realistic vs. unrealistic), and compliance. The more complex and demanding the patient-related factors, the more the treatment adheres to traditional staged sequences with late implant loading/restoration.

Hard Tissues

With regard to timing, the original and general principle has been that the softer the bone the longer the healing period (Brånemark et al. 1977). From the osseointegration point of view, the overall goal is to reach adequate initial implant stability at placement, and to establish a lasting anchorage unit for the prosthetic construction via maintained osseointegration (Sennerby and Rasmusson 2001). It is obvious that some implant sites allow for immediate or early implant loading. Nevertheless, clinicians may consistently select a rather conservative approach with conventional late loading. Nowadays, insistence on selection of such a standard healing period may be considered as resulting in an unjustifiably long waiting time for some patients. With regard to an admissible reduction of the load-free healing period, three main factors influence the decision making:

Table 16.1.

time point of implant loading/restoration

		immediate	early	late

planning level & decision-making unit				
patient	healthy: cooperative/compliant; no occlusal/oral parafunctions			aged patient; reduced wound healing or systemic diseases; smoker;occlusal/oral parafunctions
	patient's demands on treatment outcome are well defined and feasible			esthetically and /or functionally demanding/complex treatment
	low smile line			high smile line
bone	healed bone site		extraction site with mainly good fit of the implant to the bony walls	extraction site with poor fit of the implant to the bony walls
	bone quantity A or B; bone quality I, II or III			reduced bone quantity type C, D or E and/or bone quality type IV
	no peri-implant bone defects directly communicating with implant surface; defect class 0		minor peri-implant bone defects as class 0, I or II and allowing for a transmucosal healing modus	peri-implant bone defects as class III to V and/or sinus lift; defects as class 0, I or II with missing option for a transmucosal healing modus
soft tissue	gingiva morphotype = thick, low scalloped		gingiva morphotype = thin, high scalloped	
	healed soft tissues		extraction site with minor needs for soft tissue grafting and practicable at implant surgery	extraction site with mayor needs for soft tissue grafting
	sufficient amount of soft tissue; sufficient width of keratinized mucosa; no scars or tattoos to be corrected		presence of small-sized soft tissue defects/scars/tattoos where correction is practicable at implant surgery	presence of soft tissue defects with a clear need for correction; presence of scars/tattoos with a need for correction
prosthetics	high diagnostic predictability with regard to design of suprastructure			diagnostic uncertainty of prospective suprastructure
	good control of initial implant load possible (number & length of implants, splinting with suprastructure, infraocclusion)			increased implant loading (reduced number of implants, short implant length, suprastructure unspanned)
	option to produce implant prosthetics fully or at least in part prior to surgery		final prosthetic suprastructure practicable (no provisional necessary)	complex prosthetics; stepwise approach to final design mandatory
team	well established treatment sequences with regard to implant surgery and prosthetics			dental practice/office set-up limited to either surgery or prosthetics
	excellent communication between clinician(s) and dental technician			limitations (distance, frequency) in communication between clinician(s) and dental technician

bone quanitity A-E; bone quality I-IV
according to Lekholm & Zarb 1985

bone defect class D-V
according to Glauser 1999

1. Local bone quality and quantity
2. Number of primary bone-to-implant contacts established with implant placement
3. Speed of new bone formation at the bone-implant interface

Obviously, the more favorable the local hard-tissue conditions, the better the initial stability is maintained over time and the earlier the implant can be functionally loaded (Esposito et al. 2007). On the other hand, implants placed into extraction sockets with remaining bone deficiencies and/or poor bone contact area should be assessed more critically. The larger the fraction of the implant surface without initial bone contact present, the more time is needed until newly formed bone functionally supports the implant in these areas. Nonetheless, due to their morphological configuration some bone defects may allow for faster tissue regeneration (e.g., infrabony defects; class I, Fig. 16.10) and would allow for an early loading approach. In contrast, defect morphologies sparely surrounded by vital bone (class II–V, Fig. 16.10) demand a longer load-free healing period until osseous regeneration is accomplished. Hence, most of the implants presenting with bone defects following placement should be assigned to delayed loading protocols, regardless of technique and/or material used to handle these bone deficiencies (Nkenke and Fenner 2006).

Soft Tissues

It is crucial to evaluate the status of the soft tissues at future implant sites with regard to health, width, and volume of keratinized mucosa, texture and scalloping, and presence/absence of scars or tattoos. Shortened protocols may be selected if the status of the soft tissues can predictably be maintained or corrected at implant installation. With respect to periodontal and morphologic aspects, postoperative soft-tissue reactions at immediately restored implants are comparable with those of conventionally loaded implants (Glauser et al. 2006).

Prosthetic Protocol

At the time of treatment planning it is essential to evaluate whether a prosthetic workflow for an immediate or early implant reconstruction is viable, or if with increasing complexity the prosthetic construction is achieved safely using a stringent stepwise procedure.

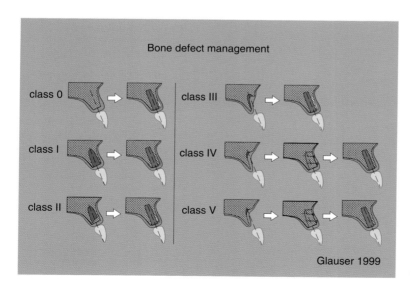

Figure 16.10. Bone defect management according to Glauser 1999. Implants placed in bone defects of class I–V should be assigned to delayed loading protocols, regardless of technique and/or material used to handle these deficiencies.

When considering immediate restoration following implant placement, the suprastructure is preferably pre-manufactured completely or at least in part in order to allow for instant mounting. Thus a critical appraisal of achievement of correct implant position(s), emerging contours, and proper occlusion is mandatory (Van Steenberghe et al. 2005).

When considering a delayed loading protocol, a satisfactory provisional restoration supported by remaining teeth or the mucosa is instrumental in guiding the patient through the longer healing period.

Team

Successful shortening of clinical protocols with application of immediate or early implant restoration is undoubtedly linked to proper diagnostics, treatment planning, and thorough execution. In particular, a close coordination between the treating team (doctor(s), nurses/assistants, lab technicians) is essential. As a *conditio sine qua non*, implant surgery and prosthetics are daily routine and corresponding workflows well established. Immediate implant restoration is often related to time pressure when it comes to finalizing and mounting of the suprastructure. On the other hand, delayed restoration protocols are more related to staged workflows, thereby reducing the time clinicians and technicians are working under pressure. Limited expertise in surgical and/or prosthetic procedures usually favors staged, late protocols where the team can better address technical or clinical issues.

Conclusions

Based on adequate patient selection and thorough treatment planning and execution, success of immediately or early loaded implants may be comparable to that obtained using the traditional approach (Cochran et al. 2004; Nkenke and Fenner 2006). Nevertheless, a more comprehensive appraisal at the time of treatment planning including an assessment of the five key factors is recommended to safely guide the overall rehabilitation to success.

References

Aparicio C, Rangert B, Sennerby L. 2003. Immediate/early loading of dental implants: A report from the Sociedad Española de Implantes World Congress consensus meeting in Barcelona, Spain. *Clin Implant Dent Relat Research* 5:57–60.

Brånemark PI, Hansson BO, Adell R, Breine U, Lindström J, Hallen O, Ohman A. 1977. Osseointegrated implants in the treatment of the edentulous jaw. Experience from a 10-year period. *Scand J Plast Reconstr Surg* (Suppl) 16:1–132.

Cochran DL, Morton D, Weber HP. 2004. Consensus statements and recommended clinical procedures regarding loading protocols for endosseous dental implants. *Int J Oral Maxillofac Implants* 19(Suppl): 109–113.

Esposito M, Grusovin MG, Willings M, Coulthard P, Worthington HV. 2007. The effectiveness of immediate, early, and conventional loading of dental implants: A Cochrane systematic review of randomized controlled clinical trials. *Int J Oral Maxillofac Implants* 22:893–904.

Glauser R, Zembic A, Hämmerle CHF. 2006. A systematic review of marginal soft tissue at implants subjected to immediate loading or immediate restoration. *Clin Oral Implants Res* 17(Suppl 2):82–92.

Goodacre C, Bernal G, Rungcharassaeng K, Kan JYK. 2003. Clinical complications with implants and implant prostheses. *J Prosthet Dent* 90:121–132.

Lekholm U, Zarb GA. 1985. Patient selection. In: *Tissue-Integrated Prostheses: Osseointegration in Clinical Dentistry*. PI Brånemark, GA Zarb, and T Albrektsson (eds.). Chicago: Quintessence. 199–209.

Nkenke E, Fenner M. 2006. Indications for immediate loading of implants and implant success. *Clin Oral Implants Res* 17(Suppl 2):19–34.

Sennerby L, Rasmusson L. 2001. Osseointegration surgery: Host determinants and outcome criteria. In: *Aging, Osteoporosis and Dental Implants.* GA Zarb, U Lekholm, Albrektsson, and H Tennenbaum (eds.). Chicago: Quintessence. 55–66.

Szmukler-Moncler S, Piatelli A, Favero GA, Dubruille JH. 2000. Considerations preliminary to the application of early and immediate loading protocols in dental implantology. *Clin Oral Implants Res* 11:12–25.

Szmukler-Moncler S, Salama H, Reingewirtz Y, Dubruille JH. 1998. Timing of loading and effect of micromotion on bone-dental implant interface: Review of experimental literature. *J Biomater Mater Res* 43:192–203.

Van Steenberghe D, Glauser R, Blombäck U, Andersson M, Schutyser F, Pettersson A, Wendelhag I. 2005. A computed tomographic scan-derived customized surgical template and fixed prosthesis for flapless surgery and immediate loading of implants in fully edentulous maxillae. A prospective multicenter study. *Clin Implant Dent Related Res* 7(Suppl):111–120.

The Transmucosal Component and the Supra-construction Revolution

ABUTMENT DESIGN AND MATERIALS USING CAD/CAM TECHNOLOGY

Steven E. Eckert

History of Abutments Based upon Prosthetic Goals

Early prosthetic designs utilized pre-manufactured transmucosal elements, known as abutments, that connected the endosseous implant to the dental prosthesis. The initial abutments provided by implant manufacturers created an extension from the implant that paralleled the long axis of the implant. These abutments were relatively tall, a minimum of 3 mm in height, and provided little opportunity for a prosthesis to appear to be growing from the implant. Described another way, these implant abutments were highly functional but lacked aesthetic qualities.

Since the most severe functional compromise related to edentulism was associated with the use of mucosal-borne mandibular dentures, endosseous implants were initially applied to the restoration of this jaw only.

Early clinical success led to the extension of the clinical application to the edentulous maxilla. The condition described above whereby a prosthesis is suspended above the soft tissue would be far more problematic in the maxilla than in the mandible. The reason for this is that the orientation of prosthetic teeth to the underlying residual alveolar ridge could affect fluid control and the airflow as the tongue contacts the anterior hard palate or the lingual surfaces of the maxillary anterior teeth.

Recognition that the early parallel-sided abutments failed to provide adequate contours to allow routine restoration of the edentulous maxilla led clinicians to develop other types of transmucosal abutment. At first this was achieved through efforts designed to shorten the abutment, allowing the prosthesis to begin at the crest of the residual ridge. This approach was somewhat beneficial in bringing the superior surface of the implant in closer proximity to the inferior surface of the dental prosthesis, but the configuration of the abutments limited the minimum height to approximately 2 mm.

Other approaches utilized custom-cast abutments that were cemented into the endosseous implant. This approach created a cement line well below the level of the oral mucosa. Debridement of the dental cement was an arduous task that sometimes led to retention of some cement deep beneath the crestal tissue. When cement was retained soft-tissue reactions were observed.

A direct connection between the endosseous implant and the dental prosthesis was then developed. The so-called UCLA abutment provided a cast gold alloy customized abutment design that connected the prosthesis directly to the implant (Lewis et al. 1988, 1989). The earliest generation UCLA abutment used a burnout pattern that was incorporated into the wax pattern for the metal framework of the dental prosthesis. Using a lost wax technique the implant-supported framework was fabricated. Unfortunately the casting accuracy using burnout patterns was not as predictable as one would want. Consequently the rotational freedom between the mating surface of the earliest generation UCLA abutments and the superior surface of the implant was often excessive. This led to a number of screw joint complications and may have also contributed to fracture of some endosseous implants (Eckert and Wollan 1998; Eckert et al. 2000).

With the predictable success of endosseous implants that undergo osseointegration the technique was expanded to situations other than completely edentulous arches. Although the edentulous maxilla and mandible were addressed in somewhat different ways the treatment itself was relatively similar for the two arches. As the treatment expanded to the restoration of partially edentulous arches, new challenges were encountered.

The size differential between implants and the roots being replaced was a formidable problem. With the exception of the mandibular incisor tooth nearly every other natural tooth root is larger in diameter than the implant that would be used to replace that root. Since the prosthesis needs to be a dimension that simulates the tooth, the transition from implant to inferior surface of the prosthesis was often quite abrupt.

The fact that endosseous implants are threaded straight cylinders while natural teeth have crowns that are not in line with the long axis of the root created numerous angulation problems between implants and prostheses. Often the implant was oriented in such a way that the retaining screws passed through the facial aspect of the dental prosthesis. With experience clinicians began to address this situation through the use of restorations that were cemented to custom-cast gold alloy abutments. Once again the use of the UCLA-type abutment proved beneficial for early intervention of techniques in partially edentulous patients.

Unfortunately the clinical performance of the screw joint is affected by the handling of the screw seat. When titanium transmucosal abutments are machined, a very specific surface is created. When a cast gold alloy is used to replace the transmucosal abutment, the surface of this gold alloy differs from that of the traditional titanium abutment. The casting process itself causes roughening of the screw seat, softening of the cast metal, and higher coefficient of friction between the screw seat and the retentive screw (Carr et al. 1996). This situation led to early screw loosening, which was implicated in trauma to the superior surface of the endosseous implant, resulting in an untoward number of fractured implants.

Friction and Its Effect on Screw Joint Integrity

The next generation of direct connection between the endosseous implant and transmucosal abutment utilized machined titanium abutments with gold alloy retaining screws. Since the abutment was machined and the retaining screw was a gold alloy, the coefficient of friction between the two metals was lower than would be experienced with cast gold alloys and gold retaining screws. This led to a higher clamping force, which reduced the number of screw joint complications. Restorations on these abutments were cemented into place, a situation that sometimes led to deep submucosal margins that were difficult to debride. As with the earliest cement-retained abutments, when cement was retained beneath the tissue this led to adverse soft-tissue reactions and may have been implicated in the loss of supporting bone.

Improvements in the biomechanical stability of the abutment-to-implant interface have provided dramatic enhancements in the mechanical stability of restorations and general improvements in the soft- and hard-tissue response around implants. Issues related to the coefficient of friction, use of lubricants in the screw seat, affects of casting and divestment, and configuration of the screw seat all influence biomechanical stability.

In the early era of osseointegration most prostheses were screw-retained. This approach seems logical, as the long-term predictability of implants, although described in the literature as favorable, was not thoroughly understood. With clinical experience it became evident that implants, once osseointegrated, generally maintained stability within bone. The increasing predictability of endosseous implant therapy reduced the emphasis on retrievability of prostheses. This recognition led to an increased popularity in the use of cement-retained restorations. These restorations could be fabricated without considering the screw emergence. Cement-retained restorations therefore provided aesthetic advantages that could not be achieved with screw-retained restorations. The additional factors related to maintenance of the machined screw/screw seat interface led to improved clinical performance with fewer mechanical complications.

Implant manufacturers responded to the need for angulated components by increasing inventory (Sethi et al. 2000). Components could be fabricated with pre-manufactured restorative collars that mimicked the variation seen in soft tissue surrounding a natural tooth. These components could be fabricated in a number of heights, diameters, and cross-sectional configurations. Unfortunately, the myriad of components necessary to address all clinical situations resulted in ever-increasing inventories for the clinicians and the manufacturers. One alternative solution was to use components to which gold alloys could be cast to create favorable contours. This situation, however, resulted in a return to the concerns of damage to the screw/screw seat interface.

Philosophically the ideal treatment approach would be to create a machined transmucosal abutment that possesses an unadulterated screw seat to which an abutment retaining screw of appropriate dimensions and physical properties could be mated. The most logical approach appeared to call for custom fabrication of most transmucosal abutments. Thus was ushered in the era of CAD/CAM.

CAD/CAM

Computer-assisted design, CAD, is a process whereby a clinician or technician can utilize appropriate computer software to design componentry. These designs can be copies of existing components or copies of modified components that are more applicable to a new clinical situation. If designs are copying existing or modified components, these designs must then be imaged in such a way as to allow three-dimensional coordinates to be created and used in the manufacturing process. Alternatively it may be possible to design components virtually. The advantage of virtual design is that it eliminates the process necessary to image the copied design, usually referred to as scanning, and it eliminates the need to create a physical replica of the desired design. When designs can be created virtually there are obvious savings in time and materials. Likewise the need for exceptional skill with the creation and manipulation of the components to be copied is diminished. Virtual design does, however, require strong conceptual understanding of the clinical needs (Figs. 17.1–17.5).

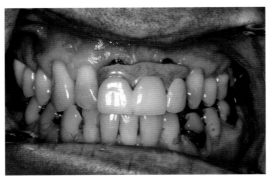

Figure 17.1. Prosthesis fabricated in 1978 retained by pre-manufactured straight abutments that were connected using an infrastructure to which the prosthetic superstructure was luted.

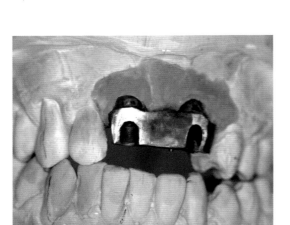

Figure 17.2. Cast infrastructure connects the two implants using straight transmucosal abutments.

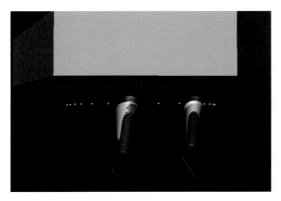

Figure 17.3. Computer-assisted design created entirely in the virtual environment.

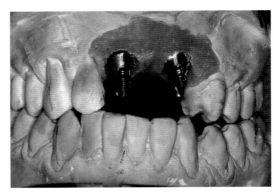

Figure 17.4. Custom abutments fabricated in 2001 using CAD/CAM technology.

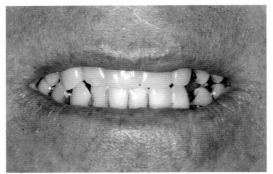

Figure 17.5. Prosthesis in place supported by CAD/CAM abutments.

Computer-assisted manufacturing, CAM, is a process that takes the digital information derived from the physical scans or the virtual designs of the CAD process and manufactures matching componentry from this information. Most of the CAM techniques utilized in dentistry today employ milling processes. When metals are used, such as titanium or titanium alloy, the milling process creates a final product from a block of original material. When ceramic materials are used this situation is somewhat different in that the ceramic material is milled to a certain configuration and then the green state ceramic is treated in a process to create a densely sintered ceramic material. When green state materials are ground and sintered the initial product must be somewhat oversized so that it compensates for the shrinkage of the sintered material (Vigolo et al. 2006).

The advantage of the CAD/CAM approach is that the technical efforts necessary to achieve well-fitting components are no longer the domain of the dental laboratory technician but instead are established by the quality of the scanning equipment, design components, and manufacturing equipment. Once an acceptable level of quality is achieved it is anticipated that this can be repeated ad infinitum. Since implant manufacturers will not be required to stock large volumes of components, the cost associated with the CAD/CAM approach should actually decrease even though every component will be custom made. The clinician and patient benefit from improvements in quality, predictability, and elimination of concerns related to components that are out of stock.

CAD/CAM technology is currently in use for the fabrication of custom abutments and for the fabrication of restorations that fit to these abutments. Restorations using the CAD/CAM design may be made in total or may still require conventional dental laboratory procedures to create the final restoration. When the total restoration is fabricated it is usually done using virtual design technology, whereby the opposing arch is imaged, the transmucosal abutment is imaged, and a restoration is fabricated on the computer using a library of anatomic crown designs. The technician designing such restorations still must make appropriate decisions regarding occlusal and interproximal contacts. The alternative approach, using the CAD/CAM technology only to create a core upon which materials are added, depends upon the laboratory technician to apply materials, traditionally ceramics, to the created core.

Future Directions

Much of the current application of CAD/CAM technology depends upon an amalgamation of traditional technology with CAD/CAM. Most of the work today is done using designs created in wax that are then scanned and duplicated. Virtual designs have been proposed by a number of manufacturers, but the acceptance of these treatment approaches has not been universal. The reasons for this are unclear. It appears that technicians favored the traditional lost wax techniques rather than embracing the time and labor-saving approaches associated with virtual designs. Realistically, given the declining numbers of technical training programs, there is the distinct possibility that the next generation of laboratory technician will be more favorably versed in the approach that is necessary to move into virtual design.

Ultimately the use of traditional impression methods that are designed to create anatomic replicas of implant and tooth positions will be replaced by optical impressions made directly in the oral cavity. This approach already exists for the fabrication of custom-milled restorations, but the general acceptance of this approach remains low. Since endosseous implants demonstrate known geometric configurations, the complications associated with imaging natural tooth preparations will not apply. Images of soft and hard tissue should be relatively easy to develop, thereby eliminating the need for traditional impressions.

Creation of virtual dental casts, transmucosal abutments, opposing arches, and dental restorations is a very real clinical opportunity. A number of manufacturers are currently involved in various phases of this process. It is highly likely that within a relatively short period clinicians will possess the technology to perform all necessary procedures to design and fabricate dental prostheses for most of the conditions encountered in a clinical practice (Figs. 17.6 and 17.7).

Although not the subject of this chapter, it is apparent that there is growing interest in the use of radiographic imaging to guide implant placement. Ultimately the marriage between guided implant placement and pre-fabrication of high-quality, well-fitting dental restorations will allow earlier restorative

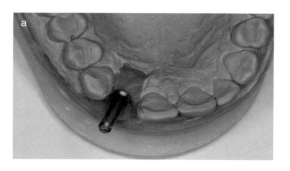
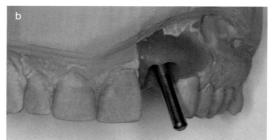
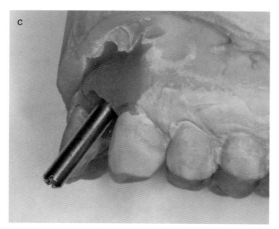

Figures 17.6a–c. Occlusal, facial, and lateral views of the implant analogs in the master cast.

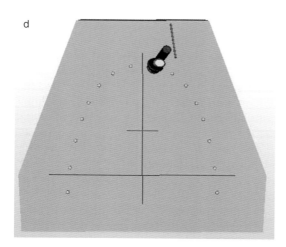
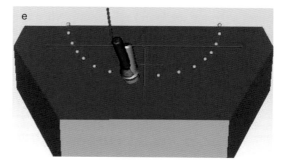
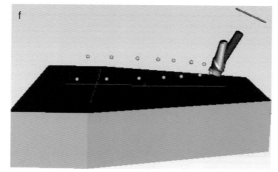

Figures 17.6d–f. Corresponding virtual computer-assisted designs of Figures 17.6a–c for custom abutment.

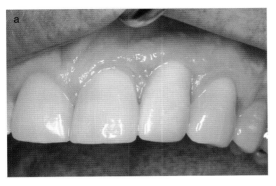
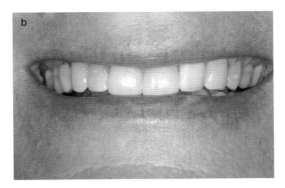

Figures 17.7. Close-up (a) and facial (b) views of the implant-supported lateral incisor crown using custom abutment created through CAD/CAM technology.

intervention at a lower cost and an increased quality.

CAD/CAM IN IMPLANT DENTISTRY

Jörg-R. Strub and Siegbert Witkowski

Introduction

Several fabrication methods are available for implant-retained and -supported restorations. The traditional and most common technique is the framework fabrication using the lost-wax casting technique in combination with dental alloys. However, framework design and construction are demanding in clinical situations with extensive interocclusal distance due to severe bone resorption as well as restoration of jaws with multiple implants and increased width. In these cases large amounts of alloy are required for the fabrication of the abutments and frameworks. Increased costs as well as difficulties in casting and related distortion of the framework bring this technique into question. As a result, non-casting approaches have been developed (Strub et al. 1996). Laser-welded pre-fabricated titanium frameworks (Jemt et al. 2002), laser welded frameworks (Hellden et al. 1999), and carbon/graphite fiber-reinforced poly frameworks (Bergendal et al. 1995) have proven to be a clinically reliable

treatment options. The introduction of CNC (computer numeric control)-milled titanium frameworks in the early 1990s provided a technology that managed to reduce significantly the risk and range of misfit on the working model. This approach was continuously improved and can be considered as a valid alternative to conventional casting procedures (Witkowski 2005). From the outset improvements have been made in the fabrication of screw-retained frameworks designed for individual veneering, bar-types for implant-retained dentures, and custom implant abutments. Milling a framework or abutment out of an industrial pre-fabricated one-piece block is less dependent on manual laboratory procedures in comparison to the conventional lost-wax casting technique. Current CAD/CAM systems with a complete digital workflow process from intraoral scans to CAD/CAM fabrication of abutments and implant frameworks are not available (Strub et al. 2006). Several manufacturers are attempting to develop intraoral scans. However, today conventional impression-taking and pouring for working models (master casts) are still essential, especially when multiple implant restorations are to be fabricated. Thus the precision of the working model remains a major key factor for a excellent clinical fit of implant-supported restorations. With CAD/CAM systems, framework deformation during veneering procedures, suppositional correct framework dimensions,

Table 17.1. Workflow of possible techniques (I, II, III, IV) for digital assisted fabrication of implant connected restorations.

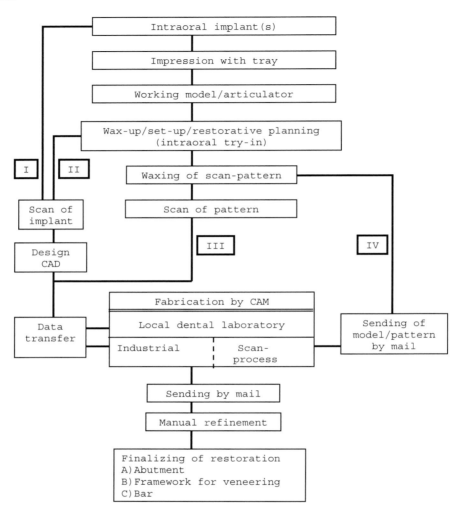

and design seem to be of minor clinical importance.

Table 17.1 provides an overview of various restorative systems available on the market using digital support to process implant prosthodontics in multiple steps. Only a few companies use CAD/CAM for implant-supported frameworks to replace conventional lost-wax processing.

Table 17.2 shows the names of the restorative systems, the possible implant systems, and the available materials and clinical indications. The aim of this section of the chapter is to describe the present state of fabrication techniques applying computer-assisted technology for custom-made abutments, bars, and frameworks for a direct implant connection.

Materials Applied and Clinical Experiences

Titanium and zirconia can be used for the production of CAD/CAM components such as abutments, bars, and frameworks and are available for some implant systems.

Table 17.2. Materials, indications, and names of restorative systems using CAD/CAM technology (Ti = titanium; Zr = zirconia ceramics) for direct implant connection.

Indications		Name of Restorative System			
		Atlantis	Procera	CARES	ARCHITECH PSR
	Manufacturers	Astra Tech, Mölndal, Sweden www.atlantiscomp.com	Nobel Biocare, Zürich, Switzerland www.nobelbiocare.com	Straumann, Basel, Switzerland www.etkon.de	Biomet 3i, Palm Beach Gardens, FL, www.biomet3i.com
	Implant Systems	Astra Biomed 3i BioHorizons Lifecore Nobel Biocare Straumann Zimmer External hex 3.75	Nobel Biocare Camlog Astra Ankylos Straumann External hex 3.75	Straumann	Biomet 3i Astra Straumann Dentsply Innova Nobel Biocare Camlog Biohorizons Zimmer
	Abutment single-unit	Ti/Zr	Ti/Zr	Ti/Zr	Ti
	FPD framework multi-unit		Ti/Zr		
	Bar				Ti

Titanium (grade 2) as an alternative for gold alloy has been discussed in implant dentistry since the early 1990s. The main advantages, especially for extended frameworks application, are the reduced weight and costs in comparison to noble metals, as well as the good biocompatibility. Titanium is therefore widely accepted, and clinical experience with the material is comparable to conventional cast frameworks made of noble alloys (Tschernitschek et al. 2005). Pre-fabricated industrial abutments of titanium are used successfully in various indications on many implant systems. However, titanium frameworks made by casting or milling with ceramic veneering have never become popular and no clinical studies are available in implant dentistry. In the early 1990s the poor customized contour of the CNC-milled frameworks and bonding problems between titanium and ceramics were reported (ADA Council on Scientific Affairs 2003). These factors made the use of acrylic resin and composite as veneering material more popular. Örtorp et al. (2003) showed that CNC-milled titanium implant frameworks (Procera, Nobel Biocare) veneered with acrylic resin teeth can be used as an alternative to conventionally casted gold alloy frameworks in the edentulous jaw.

Yttrium-stabilized zirconia ceramics (Y-TZP, Yttrium-stabilized Tetragonal Zirconia Polycrystals) were introduced in 2003 for the fabrication of custom-made abutments

(Procera Abutments Zirconia) and in 2007 for implant-supported screw-retained restoration frameworks (Procera Implant Bridge Zirconia) (Chevalier 2006; Raigrodski 2004; Witkowski 2008). Y-TZP frameworks are milled as enlarged constructions out of pre-sintered zirconia ceramic blanks, then sintered to full density and shrunk to the desired final dimensions. The final sintering process is, however, sensitive and deformation of the framework and marginal distortion, especially with long-span frameworks, have been observed (Komine et al. 2005). Since zirconia is an opaque ceramic, Y-TZP implant-supported crowns and fixed partial denture frameworks need to be veneered with compatible porcelain materials by using built-up layering by hand, sintering, or lost-wax press techniques. Positive clinical results using pre-fabricated zirconia abutments that can be customized were published by Glauser et al. (2004). They showed no failures after 4 years using zirconia abutments with cemented Empress (Vivadent-Ivoclar, Schaan, Lichtenstein) crowns. Larsson et al. (2006) reported no fractures of the zirconia frameworks (Denzir, Decim AB, Skelleftea, Sweden) of FPDs cemented on titanium abutments after 1 year. Presently there are no clinical studies available on zirconia CAD/CAM-fabricated abutments or cement- and screw-retained FPDs (Kohal et al. 2008).

Applied CAD/CAM Technology

CAD/CAM systems have three functional components: data capture (scanning) to record the surface (implants, abutments, adjacent teeth, occlusal surfaces, and tooth geometry); CAD to design implant abutments or restoration frameworks; and CAM to fabricate the abutment or restoration framework. Available CAD/CAM systems capture data of single and multiple implant units from working models, using mechanical or optical digitizers of various types. The Cerec system (Sirona, Bensheim, Germany) is a recent solution that scans single implants intraorally using a hand-scan unit. 3-D volume data of the restoration or abutment can be created by either a semi-automatic, knowledge-based design with CAD on a digitized surface, or by using reverse engineering by scanning and re-digitizing a wax-up pattern of the final restoration contour. The latter method is also known as "double scan" due to the necessity for a second scan process. The first scan captures the surface and implant position and the second scan captures the pre-waxed form of the final restoration, which has to be fabricated. The software is able to match (overlay) the two sets of data on top of each other and creates a perfectly fitting virtual restoration on the implant of the model (lab analogs). Unlike the CAD design, the processing method of reverse engineering has the advantage of reproducing the exact contour of the pre-planned and waxed restorations. Adjacent teeth, occlusal surfaces, and teeth geometries are registered by an additional scan of an intraoral bite registration. However, some CAD/CAM systems are limited within extreme clinical situations, for example, large implant inclinations. The restorations can be designed but not fabricated by the milling unit. In addition, creation of the path of insertion for multiple abutments or splinted restorations is not always possible in CAD. Depending on the system used, CAD design options reveal significant differences in technical handling and in the variety of design tools.

The most commonly applied CAM technology in manufacturing abutments and frameworks for FPDs connected to implants is the cutting of the contour of the designed restoration out of an industrially pre-fabricated, solid block using burs and diamonds. Modified CNC-milling/-grinding machines that operate with 5 degrees of freedom are able to fit the framework to the implant. Highly sophisticated machines are required for the reproduction of complex multiple implant frameworks with an occlusal screw implant connection or for restorations with complex morphologies of anatomical topographies and coronal abutment contours. Smaller CAM machines or in–dental office systems with restricted degrees of freedom are limited to single abutment fabrication and smaller FPDs without occlusal screw holes.

3-D data of the finished design of a restoration can also be sent by the dental laboratory via the Internet to a production center where the information is converted into appropriate commands to drive the connected CAM system. The outsourcing of the fabrication to milling centers allows in particular small dental laboratories access to sophisticated machining and fabrication facilities. However, data acquisition systems and the software programs cannot be independently transferred between different CAD/CAM systems.

Systems and Indications

Table 17.2 shows the present range of materials, indications, and possible implant systems of each individual system. The first available CAD/CAM-fabricated implant-supported restoration was the Procera Implant Bridge Titanium (formerly All-in-One; Nobel Biocare, Gothenburg, Sweden) and was introduced to the market in 1998. With this system, long-span titanium frameworks with a direct implant connection using occlusal screws could be fabricated. Initially the FPDs were designed for veneering with acrylic resin and denture teeth (Figs. 17.8–17.10).

Since 1994 individual reproduction of a pre-waxed customized framework and abutments has been possible. The working model and the wax pattern had to be sent to the production center in Sweden. In 2006 scanners for working models and wax patterns using the Forte (Procera) scanner were introduced and are located in numerous laboratories (Salinas et al. 2007). In this system the production of the framework is outsourced by the dental laboratory. The connection of the frameworks is offered for several implant

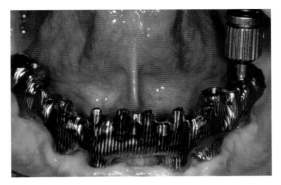

Figure 17.8. Titanium framework (Procera Implant Bridge) on the working model after milling in a production center. Supported on six Brånemark implants (Nobel Biocare, Gothenburg, Sweden).

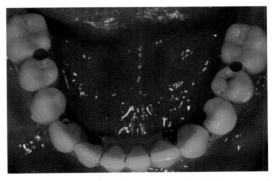

Figure 17.9. Final implant-supported FPD veneered with pre-fabricated resin denture teeth directly connected to the external hexes of the six implants.

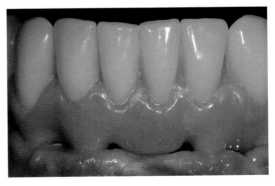

Figure 17.10. Frontal view of the resin veneered titanium framework in place.

systems beside those of Nobel Biocare. From 2003, Y-TZP ceramics could be applied for custom-made abutments (Figs. 17.11 and 17.12) and since 2007 for directly connected FPD frameworks (Van Dooren 2007). The Procera software allows for abutments and frameworks, a CAD design, and a direct scan of a pattern.

In 2005 the CARES (Computer Aided Restoration Service) system, which combines the Cerec InLab (Sirona, Bensheim, Germany) with the Straumann implant system (Basel, Switzerland), was introduced to the market. The Cerec InLab as well as the Etkon scanner (es1 Evolution etkon AG, Munich, Germany; with Straumann since 2007) can be used for digitizing working models with the implant analogs. In a production center operated by Straumann in Basel, digital custom-made abutments can be created by a CAD process on the digitized working model, on-screen, or by scanning of a wax-up of the restoration. Titanium and zirconia are available as abutment materials (Zöller and Benthaus 2006). In 2007 intraoral scans using hand-scan units (Sirona) became available. The captured data can be transferred to the Cerec InLab software. So far, only single-unit abutments can be designed on-screen based on intraoral scan data.

In 2007, Drago and Peterson introduced the ARCHITECH PSR (Biomed 3i) system. It covers the processing of a wide range of abutments (Encode) and restorations that are connected directly to multiple implants of various (ten brands) manufacturers. Bars in three designs (CAM StructSURE; Harder or Dolder or custom zero degree) can be fabricated for implant-retained overdentures. Figures 17.13-17.16 show an edentulous patient who was restored in the maxilla and mandible with implant bar-retained overdentures using this system. CAD/CAM frameworks can be designed for veneering with pre-fabricated denture teeth or for individually anatomical veneering connecting to several implant systems. A scan of the model with the implants and a set-up of teeth in wax or wax pattern (copy milling) is made. In addition, custom-

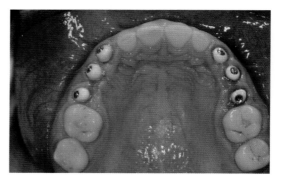

Figure 17.11.   Six screw-retained custom-made Procera Zirconia abutments on implants 4, 5, 6, 11, 12, 13.

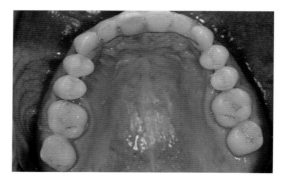

Figure 17.12.   Six cemented Procera Zirconia crowns on Procera Zirconia abutments 4, 5, 6, 11, 12, 13.

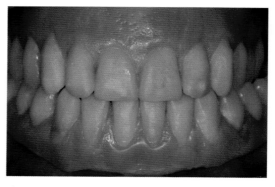

Figure 17.13.   Try-in of diagnostic set-up of acrylic denture teeth in the maxilla and mandible to specify aesthetics, phonetics, and functional aspects.

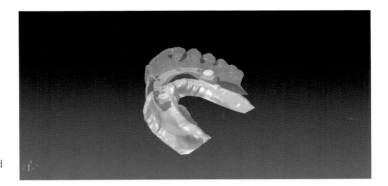

Figure 17.14. CAD view (CAM StructSURE, Biomed 3i) of virtual maxillary bar, soft tissue contour, and the diagnostic set-up of the teeth.

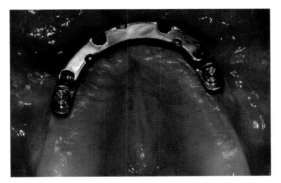

Figure 17.15. Titanium bar screw connected to the four implants; two attachments (Locator, Biomed 3i) are located at the distal extensions of the bar.

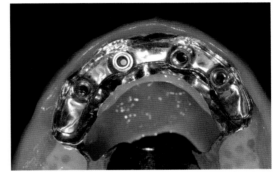

Figure 17.16. Bar milled of a one-piece block of titanium with direct implant connection. Overdenture on the parallel bar (Harder type) reinforced with a non-precious metal alloy. The connection between the bar and framework is casted in type 3 gold.

made titanium healing abutments can be designed with this system (Encode Healing Abutments) (Drago and Peterson 2007).

Atlantis Components Inc. was founded in 1996 to develop CAD/CAM-made custom implant prosthetic components. Titanium (since 2006) (Kerstein and Osorio 2007) and zirconia (since 2007) can be applied for custom-fabricated abutments. Atlantis abutments are processed in production centers in Cambridge, Massachusetts, and Mölndal, Sweden, according to send-in models and wax patterns.

Summary

Up until now the use of CAD/CAM technology has not changed the restorative concept in implant prosthodontics. The digitally supported fabrication of abutments, bars, and frameworks out of industrially pre-fabricated blocks could increase the predictability of implant-supported restorations. Distortion of the framework, especially observed in metal restorations fabricated using the conventional casting techniques, is not an issue with the CAD/CAM technique, resulting in better overall precision of the restorations. Since intraoral scanners for multiple implants are not available, the quality of impressions and working models still remains a key factor for CAD/CAM-fabricated restorations. Outsourcing the fabrication of implant-retained or -supported restorations to milling centers allows for high standardization of the fabrication process and increases the accessibility of CAD/CAM techniques to small dental laboratories. Clinical studies using zirconia CAD/CAM-fabricated abutments and cement and screw-retained FPDs must be available before these treatment procedures can be recommended for daily private practice.

Acknowledgements

Photographs (17.8–17.10 and 17.13–17.16) courtesy of Dr. Marquard (University Hospital Freiburg, School of Dentistry, Department of Prosthodontics); Peter Zech, MDT (patient 17.13–17.16; Zahnlabor Freiburg), Freiburg, Germany; and Jörg Richter, MDT (patient 17.11–17.12; Zahnwerkstatt), Bötzingen, Germany.

References

ADA Council on Scientific Affairs. 2003. Titanium application in dentistry. *J Am Dent Assoc* 134:347–349.

Adell R. 1983. Clinical results of osseointegrated implants supporting fixed prostheses in edentulous jaws. *J Prosthet Dent* 50(2):251–254.

Adell R, Hansson BO, et al. 1970. Intraosseous anchorage of dental prostheses. II: Review of clinical approaches. *Scand J Plast Reconstr Surg* 4(1):19–34.

Adell R, Lekholm U, et al. 1981. A 15-year study of osseointegrated implants in the treatment of the edentulous jaw. *Int J Oral Surg* 10(6):387–416.

Bergendal T, Ekstrand K, Karlsson U. 1995. Evaluation of implant-supported carbon/graphite fiber-reinforced poly (methyl methacrylate) prostheses. A longitudinal multicenter study. *Clin Oral Implants Res* 6(12):246–253.

Brånemark PI, Adell R, et al. 1969. Intraosseous anchorage of dental prostheses. I: Experimental studies. *Scand J Plastic Reconstr Surg* 3(2):81–100.

Brånemark PI, Adell R, et al. 1984. An experimental and clinical study of osseointegrated implants penetrating the nasal cavity and maxillary sinus. *J Oral Maxillofac Surg* 42(8):497–505.

Carr AB, Brunski JB, et al. 1996. Effects of fabrication, finishing, and polishing procedures on preload in prostheses using conventional gold and plastic cylinders. *Int J Oral Maxillofac Implants* 11(5):589–598.

Chevalier J. 2006. What future for zirconia as a biomaterial? *Biomaterials* 27(4):535–543.

Drago CJ, Peterson T. 2007. Treatment of an edentulous patient with CAD/CAM technology: A clinical report. *J Prosthodont* 16(3):200–208.

Eckert SE, Laney WR. 1989. Patient evaluation and prosthodontic treatment planning for osseointegrated implants. *Dental Clinics of North America* 33(4):599–618.

Eckert SE, Meraw SJ, et al. 2000. Analysis of incidence and associated factors with fractured implants: A retrospective study. *Int J Oral Maxillofac Implants* 15(5):662–667.

Eckert SE, Wollan PC. 1998. Retrospective review of 1170 endosseous implants placed in partially edentulous jaws. *J Prosthet Dent* 79(4):415–421.

Glauser R, Sailer I, Wohlwend A, Studer S, Schibli M, Schärer P. 2004. Experimental zirconia abutments for implant-supported single-tooth restorations in esthetically demanding regions: 4-year results of a prospective clinical study. *Int J Prosthodont* 17(3):285–290.

Hellden LB, Derand T, Johansson CB, Lindberg A. 1999. The CrescoTi Precision method: Description of a simplified method to fabricate titanium superstructures with passive fit to osseointegrated implants. *J Prosthet Dent* 82(4):487–491.

Jemt T, Bergendal B, Arvidson K, Bergendal T, Karlsson U, Linden B, Rundcrantz T, Wendelhag I. 2002. Implant-supported welded titanium frameworks in the edentulous maxilla: A 5-year prospective multicenter study. *Int J Prosthodont* 15(6):544–548.

Keller EE, Desjardins RP, et al. 1986. Reconstruction of the severely resorbed mandibular ridge using the tissue-integrated prosthesis. *Int J Oral Maxillofac Implants* 1(2):101–109.

Kerstein RB, Osorio J. 2007. Utilizing computer-generated duplicate titanium custom abutments to facilitate intraoral and laboratory implant prosthesis fabrication. *PPAD* 15(4):311–314.

Kohal RJ, Att W, Bächle M, Butz F. 2008. Ceramic abutments and ceramic dental implants. An update. *Periodontology 2000* 47:224–243.

Komine F, Gerds T, Witkowski S, Strub JR. 2005. Influence of framework configuration on the marginal adaptation of zirconium dioxide ceramic anterior four-unit frameworks. *Acta Odontol Scand* 63(6): 361–366.

Laney WR. 1986. Selecting edentulous patients for tissue-integrated prostheses. *Int J Oral Maxillofac Implants* 1(2):129–138.

Laney WR, Tolman DE, et al. 1986. Dental implants: Tissue-integrated prosthesis utilizing the osseointegration concept. *Mayo Clinic Proceedings* 61(2):91–97.

Lang NP, Wilson TG, et al. 2000. Biological complications with dental implants: Their prevention, diagnosis and treatment. *Clin Oral Implants Res* 11(Suppl 1):146–155.

Larsson C, Van Steyern P, Sunzel B, Nilner K. 2006. All-ceramic two- to five-unit implant-supported reconstructions. A randomized, prospective clinical trial. *Swedish Dent J* 30(2):45–53.

Lewis S, Avera S, et al. 1989. The restoration of improperly inclined osseointegrated implants. *Int J Oral Maxillofac Implants* 4(2):147–152.

Lewis S, Beumer J, 3rd, et al. 1988. The UCLA abutment. *Int J Oral Maxillofac Implants* 3(3):183–189.

Meffert RM. 1993. Periodontitis and periimplantitis: One and the same? *Pract Periodont Aesthet Dent* 5(9):79–80, 82.

National Institute of Health. 1988. Dental implants. *Natl Inst Health Consens Dev Conf Consens Statement* 7(3):1–7.

Örtorp A, Jemt T, Bäck T, Jälevik T. 2003. Comparisons of precision of fit between cast and CNC-milled titanium implant frameworks for the edentulous mandible. *Int J Prosthodont* 16(2):194–200.

Raigrodski AJ. 2004. Contemporary all-ceramic fixed partial dentures: A review. *Dent Clin N Am* 48:531–544.

Salinas TJ, Desa V, Vasilic M. 2007. CAD/CAM multiple-implant screw-retained restorations: Illustration of a technique. *Quintessence Dent Technol* 30(Yearbook 2007): 215–224.

Sethi A, Kaus T, et al. 2000. The use of angulated abutments in implant dentistry: Five-year clinical results of an ongoing prospective study. *Int J Oral Maxillofac Implants* 15(6):801–810.

Strub JR, Rekow, ED, Witkowski S. 2006. Computer-aided design and fabrication of dental restorations—current systems and future possibilities. *J Am Dent Assoc* 137(9):1289–1296.

Strub JR, Witkowski S, Einsele, F. 1996. Prosthodontic aspects of implantology. In: *Prosthodontic Aspects of Implantology.* G Watzek (ed.). Chicago: Quintessence. 319–407.

Tschernitschek H, Borchers L, Guertsen, W. 2005. Nonalloyed titanium as a bioinert metal: A review. *Quintessence Int* 36(6/7): 523–530.

Van Dooren E. 2007. Using zirconia in esthetic implant restorations. *Quintessence Dent Technol* 30(Yearbook 2007):119–128.

Vigolo P, Fonzi F, et al. 2006. An in vitro evaluation of titanium, zirconia, and alumina procera abutments with hexagonal connection. *Int J Oral Maxillofac Implants* 21(4):575–580.

Witkowski S. 2005. (CAD-)/CAM in dental technology. *Quintessence Dent Technol* 28(Yearbook 2005):169–184.

———. 2008. High-tech bioceramics—history and present state. *Quintessence J Dent Technol* 6:8–18.

Zarb GA. 1983. A status report on dental implants. *J Can Dent Assoc* 49(12):841–843.

Zöller A, Benthaus K. 2006. CEREC labside implant restorations: Custom made abutments. In: *CEREC Labside Implant Restorations: Custom Made Abutments*. WH Mörmann (ed.). Berlin: Quintessence. 163–171.

18

The Implant Design and Clinical Outcomes

CONTEMPORARY DENTAL IMPLANTS AND CLINICAL PERFORMANCE

John K. Schulte and Shadi Daher

Modification of the shape and surface texture of smooth screw-shaped implants has been shown to improve clinical performance; however, no specific shape or surface texture has proven to be superior (Kasemo and Gold 1999; Lee et al. 2005; Van Staden et al. 2006; Wagner 1992).

Clinical performance of dental implants can be evaluated by many methods. Two of the most commonly used methods are survival analysis and evaluation of crestal bone levels. Implant survival over a specific time period has been used for many years as a means of documenting implant performance (Adell 1983; Zarb and Symington 1983). Removal or loss of the implant is the primary response variable associated with survival studies. Crestal bone level, a continuous variable, provides information on the current status or health of an implant prior to failure (Elkhoury et al. 2005). Changes in bone levels around the neck of the implant can adversely

affect aesthetics by altering soft-tissue contours, and for this reason crestal bone loss is an important indicator of clinical performance.

Three subjects of clinical relevance serve as the focus of this section:

1. Crestal bone levels associated with implants that are in close proximity to each other and natural teeth.
2. Survival and crestal bone levels of 6 mm length implants.
3. Crown-to-implant ratio and its relationship to implant survival and crestal bone levels.

A brief review of the literature will accompany each of the subjects along with the results of retrospective case series studies designed to measure the clinical performance of the Bicon (Bicon, Boston, Massachusetts) dental implant (Fig. 18.1).

The Bicon dental implant is a plateau-designed, textured-surface implant that has a sloping shoulder and utilizes a locking taper abutment. The Bicon implant is a good example of a contemporary dental implant. Undergraduate and graduate students from the Harvard School of Dental Medicine and

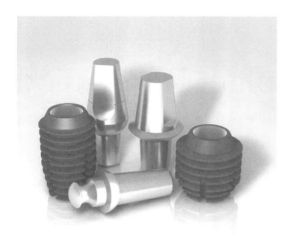

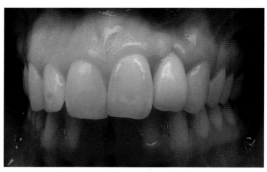

Figure 18.2. The gingival cleft located on the labial surface of the maxillary left lateral incisor developed 1 and a half years after the placement of the crown. Early crestal bone loss is partially responsible for the formation of this cleft.

Figure 18.1. Bicon dental implants illustrated with locking taper abutments. The Bicon implant is a plateau-designed, textured-surface, sloping shoulder, press-fit implant.

the University of Minnesota School of Dentistry conducted these studies. The materials and methods used in these studies are similar and have been published previously (Gentile et al. 2005).

Crestal Bone Levels Associated with Implants That Are in Close Proximity to Each Other and Natural Teeth

Brånemark was one of the first to document crestal bone loss (Brånemark et al. 1977). In this classic paper he stated that crestal bone loss of 1.5 mm during the first year of function could be anticipated. This is followed by a "steady state" in which bone loss of .2 mm per year can be expected. Tarnow et al. (2002) established that in addition to vertical bone loss, horizontal bone loss of 1.5 mm is possible during the early years of function. This may result in loss of the bone crest between two implants that are in close proximity. This study supports the guideline that in order to

minimize vertical crestal bone loss implants should not be placed closer than 3 mm to one another. Esposito et al. (1993) conducted a study where they radiographically evaluated the marginal bone loss at the tooth surface adjacent to single implants. Average bone loss associated with anterior teeth was 1.4 ± 1.5 mm. This study supports the guideline that implants should not be placed closer to a tooth than 1.5 mm. Additional studies that support these guidelines can be found in the literature (Gastaldo et al. 2004; Hatley et al. 2001; Krennmair et al. 2003; Saadoun et al. 2004). A clinical example of soft-tissue changes resulting from crestal bone loss is illustrated in Figure 18.2.

A retrospective case series study was designed and conducted to determine crestal bone levels associated with the Bicon dental implant. Crestal bone levels were determined by direct measurement of standardized radiographs and mathematically corrected for distortion. One of the objectives of this study was to determine crestal bone levels of implant surfaces that violated the guidelines for implant spacing. Therefore only implant surfaces that were less than 3 mm apart or closer than 1.5 mm to a natural tooth were included in this part of the study. Measurements that were recorded are illustrated in Figure 18.3.

Changes in bone levels associated with natural teeth were determined by comparing the bone level at the time of implant placement with the last available radiograph. Twenty-six implant surfaces were adjacent to an edentulous area and served as a control. Fifty-two implant surfaces were adjacent to a tooth and 122 surfaces were adjacent to another implant. The average length of time

the implants were in function was 3.2 ± 2.3 years. The 52 implant surfaces were 1.0 ± 0.5 mm from a natural tooth. The bone level on the implant surfaces that were adjacent to a tooth was -0.4 ± 0.8 mm from the top of the implant. Pre-treatment bone levels on the natural tooth from the cementoenamel junction were -2.4 ± 1.4 mm. Post-treatment bone levels were -2.7 ± 1.4 mm. There is no significant difference between pre-treatment bone levels and post-treatment bone levels. The 122 implant surfaces that were adjacent to each other were separated by 1.5 ± 0.8 mm. The bone levels on the sloping shoulder were -0.8 ± 0.8 mm from the top of the implant. The bone crest between implants was $+0.8 \pm 1.0$ mm above a line connecting the top of adjacent implants. Bone levels of the control group were -0.6 ± 0.6 mm from the top of the implant. There was no significant difference between test and control groups.

The results of this study show that the crestal bone loss associated with the Bicon dental implant is less than previously published values. The clinical significance of this study is that Bicon implants can be placed in close proximity to each other and a natural tooth without experiencing soft-tissue changes due to bone loss (Figs. 18.4 and 18.5).

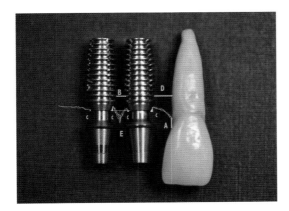

Figure 18.3. Measurements obtained from standardized radiographs. a. Distance of bone crest from cementoenamel junction. b. Distance between implant surfaces. c. Distance of bone contact from the top of the implant. d. Distance of implant surface from natural tooth. e. Vertical distance of bone crest from a line connecting the top of the implants.

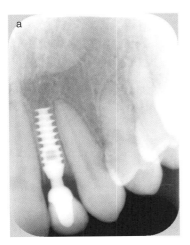
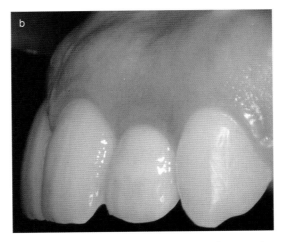

Figures 18.4a and b. Radiograph (a) and clinical photograph (b) of an implant-supported lateral incisor, in which the implant is in close proximity to the adjacent teeth. This 12-year post-insertion image displays good bone levels on the adjacent teeth.

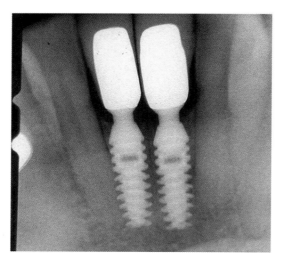

Figure 18.5. Two implants separated by .75 mm. The distance was determined by measurement of the space between the two analogs after placing them in the impression. The bone level between the implants is located at the top of the sloping shoulder.

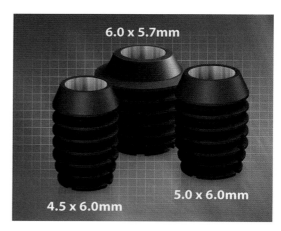

Figure 18.6. Bicon short implants. The 5 × 6 mm implant is the focus of an ongoing clinical trial.

Survival and Crestal Bone Levels of 6 mm Length Implants

Goodacre et al. (2003) cited 13 publications that reported survival data of implants in a paper reviewing complications with implants and implant prostheses. A 10% failure rate was reported for implants that were 10 mm or less in length compared to a 3% failure rate for implants longer than 10 mm. Historically, the use of short implants (6–9 mm) has been associated with higher failure rates than those for longer implants (Bahat 1993; Herrmann et al. 2005; Jemt 1991; Jemt and Lekholm 1995; Naert et al. 2002; Weng et al. 2003; Winkler et al. 2000; Wyatt and Zarb 1998). Recently, clinical studies have shown that short implants have a similar failure rate to implants of longer lengths (Goene et al. 2005; Hagi et al. 2004; Nedir et al. 2004). Renouard and Nisand (2006) made reference to 12 clinical studies that reported poor survival of short implants and noted that 11 of the 12 studies utilized a machined smooth-surface implant. They also made reference to

13 clinical studies that reported good survival of short implants and noted that 11 of the 13 utilized a textured-surface implant. Feldman et al. (2004) conducted one of the few studies that directly compared the survival of machined smooth-surface implants to textured-surface implants. They reported higher survival rates for the textured-surface implants. The literature supports the belief that textured-surface implants have improved the survival of short implants; however, it must not be assumed that all textured-surface implants will experience a high survival rate (Albrektsson and Wennerberg 2004).

Bicon dental implants are manufactured in 5.7, 6, 8, and 11 mm lengths. Gentile et al. (2005) have shown that the 6 mm wide, 5.7 mm length implant has the same survival as the longer length implants. A 5 mm wide, 6 mm length implant has recently been included in the selection of implants for clinical use. A retrospective case series study was conducted to determine preliminary results on the survival of the 5 × 6 mm implant (Fig. 18.6).

Five hundred and forty-two single tooth-supported implants were placed in 324 patients between January 2005 and August 2006. The average length of time the implants were in function was 13 ± 8.4 months. Thirty-three failures occurred for a short-term survival of

94%. Forty-two percent (226) of the implants were placed in the posterior maxilla and experienced a lower survival rate of 92.5%. Twenty-eight percent (151) of the implants were placed in type 4 bone and experienced a survival rate of 91.5%. Expected higher failure rates occurred in the posterior maxilla, which typically has the poorest quality bone. This study was conducted at a private practice facility (Implant Dentistry Centre, Boston, Massachusetts) and included all patients who received a 5 × 6 mm implant between January 2005 and August 2006. No attempt was made to exclude patients who may have had risk factors associated with implant failure. All restorations were unsplinted single tooth. These factors are important when comparing the results of survival studies. The methods used to select patients and provide implant therapy may differ to such a degree that a comparison is not possible or advised (Malo et al. 2007; Romeo et al. 2006; Ten Bruggenkate et al. 1998).

Determining crestal bone levels by evaluation of radiographs is a common practice used by clinicians to judge the current status or health of an implant. A retrospective case series study was conducted to determine the crestal bone levels of the 5.7 and 6 mm length Bicon dental implants. Measurements of mesial and distal bone levels on standardized periapical radiographs were used to determine bone levels. All radiographs were mathematically corrected for distortion. All 5.7 and 6 mm length implants placed between February 1997 and December 2005 were included in the study. The length of time the implants were in function was established by calculating the time between loading of the implant and most current radiograph. Five hundred and thirty-four implants were placed in 314 patients. The mean time the implants were in function was 15.8 months. The mean crestal bone levels on the mesial surfaces were −0.2 ± 0.7 mm and −0.2 ± 0.9 mm on the distal surfaces. No statistically significant differences could be found regarding implant width, maxillary versus mandibular, or anterior versus posterior.

The results of this study are impressive when compared to what we consider normal crestal bone loss during the first years of function. What is surprising is that the bone levels on the 5.7 and 6 mm length Bicon implants appear to be better than the bone levels on the Bicon implants of greater length.

A few studies related to crestal bone levels associated with short implants can be found in the literature. Friberg et al. (2000) found mean bone loss of 0.5 ± 0.6 mm during the first year of function and losses of 0.7 ± 0.8 mm at 5 years and 0.9 ± 0.6 mm at 10 years. Tawil and Younan (2003) recorded mean crestal bone loss of 0.7 ± 0.65 mm in their study. Renouard and Nisand (2005) found a mean crestal bone loss of 0.4 ± 0.5 mm after 2 years of function. The results of these studies are superior to what has been accepted as normal. Additional studies will be required to validate the trend that is developing with regard to short implants and crestal bone levels.

Crown-to-Implant Ratio and Its Relationship to Implant Survival and Crestal Bone Levels

Excessive crown-to-implant (C/I) ratios have been cited in the literature as a risk factor that may result in implant failure. However, no parameters exist that provide guidelines for making a clinical decision concerning C/I ratios. Natural teeth, which have reduced periodontal support resulting in a crown-to-root (C/R) ratio of 1:1, are considered to have a guarded prognosis. Teeth that have C/R ratios of 1.5:1 or larger are considered to have a poor long-term prognosis. A common practice is to apply the guidelines used for natural teeth to an implant-supported restoration or potential implant site.

A retrospective case series study was conducted to determine if there was a relationship between C/I ratios and implant survival. Additionally, the C/I ratios would be compared to the guidelines established for the C/R ratios of natural teeth (Schulte et al. 2007). This study included implants placed between May 1992 and April 2004. Measurements of standardized radiographs were made to calculate the C/I ratios. The time in function was defined by the date of abutment placement and last visit. Eight hundred and ninety-nine implants were included in the study. Sixteen failures were recorded, giving a 98.2% survival rate. The length of time the implants were in function was 4.2 ± 3.6 years. The mean C/I ratio of those implants in function was 1.3:1 (Fig. 18.7).

The mean C/I ratio of the 16 failures was 1.4:1. There were no significant differences between those that failed and those that continued to function. The distribution of the C/I ratios is illustrated in Figure 18.8.

The average length of the implants in this study was 8.6 mm.

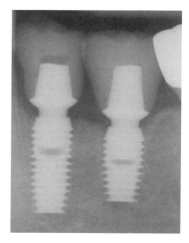

Figure 18.7. Example of a C/I ratio of 1.3:1.

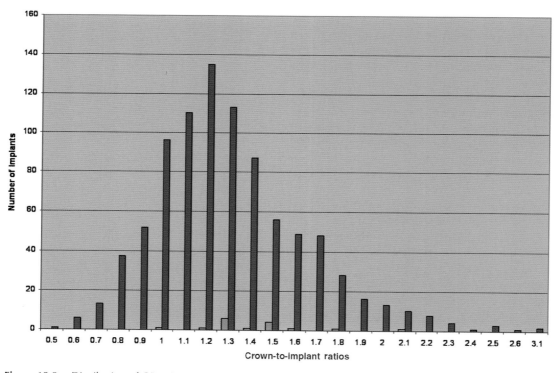

Figure 18.8. Distribution of C/I ratios.

Based on the findings of this study the guidelines associated with the C/R ratios of natural teeth should not be used to evaluate an implant-supported crown or potential implant site. There was no relationship established between C/I ratios and implant failure.

Crestal bone levels of the 5.7 and 6 mm length Bicon implants have been presented previously in this chapter. In addition to evaluating crestal bone levels, that study also calculated C/I ratios of the 5.7 and 6 mm length implants. The mean C/I ratio of the 534 single tooth-supported implants was 2:1 (Fig. 18.9).

The distribution of C/I ratios is illustrated in Figure 18.10.

The mean crestal bone levels were −0.2 ± 0.7 mm on the mesial surface and −0.2 ± 0.9 mm on the distal surface from the top of the implant.

In a similar study Rokni et al. (2005) reported a mean C/I ratio of 1.5:1. Their study included 198 sintered porous-surface implants of 5, 7, 9, and 10 mm lengths. Mean mesial and distal crestal bone levels were −0.3 ± 0.5 mm and −0.4 ± 0.5 mm, respectively. Crestal bone levels in the Bicon study were determined by measurement from the top of the implant. Bone levels were measured in Rokni et al.'s study from the junction of the smooth collar and porous surface, making comparison to the Bicon study impossible.

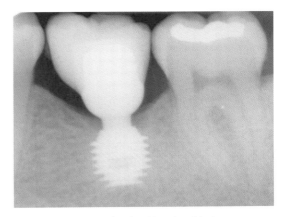

Figure 18.9. Example of a C/I ratio of 2:1.

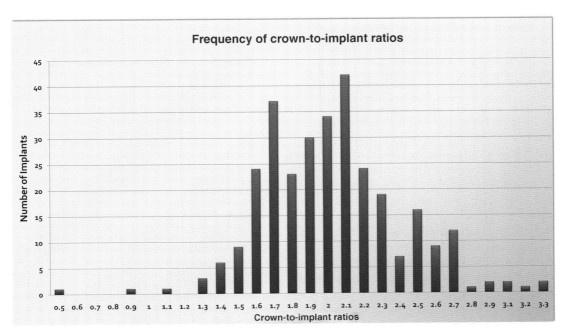

Figure 18.10. Distribution of C/I ratios.

Bone loss recorded for the shorter implants in the Rokni study was less than that of the longer implants. This trend is similar to the observations related to the Bicon implant.

THE INTERNAL CONNECTION: A CONTRIBUTING FACTOR TO ACHIEVING AN AESTHETIC RESULT

Antonio Sanz Ruiz

Restoring form, function, and aesthetics has always been the goal of oral rehabilitation (Adell et al. 1981; Brånemark et al. 1977; Laney et al. 1994).

A complex and challenging area of modern implant dentistry has been, and remains, the "Aesthetic Zone." An aesthetic zone may be defined as any area to be restored that is visible in the patient's full smile. An aesthetic restoration is one that duplicates every aspect of a natural tooth (Higginbottom et al. 1996; Laney 2001). Placing implants in the aesthetic zone is a technically sensitive procedure in which there is no room for error.

Considerations for Aesthetic Sites

Achieving favorable results in the aesthetic zone is dependent on many factors. Adequate bone volume (height and width), soft-tissue volume, the patient's biotype, and the spatial relationship of implant to tooth and implant to implant are important factors that require consideration. Implant design features, including shape, roughness, type of abutment connection, and microgap location, are fundamental in determining the final result (Higginbottom et al. 2004; Kazor et al. 2004; Sanz et al. 1998, 2001).

Among all these factors, marginal bone level is the key to aesthetic soft-tissue contours (Spear 1999). Alterations in the bone contours compromise the soft-tissue level, altering the aesthetic result. Therefore, preserving the marginal bone level must be one of the most important aims of our treatment plan.

Immediate implant placement and loading preserves the bone volume and optimizes the emergence profile of the tooth to achieve better aesthetic results (Kazor et al. 2004). Improvements in the design of implants have increased the success rate in immediate loading. Tapered implants have improved primary stability (Martinez et al. 2001; O'Sullivan et al. 2004) and reduced stress concentration at the bone-to-implant interface (Li Shi et al. 2007). Success rates of 93–100% have been reported with follow-up periods of 1–5 years on immediate placement and loading (Attard and Zarb 2005).

Stability of the abutment-to-implant interface is an important design factor that influences load distribution at the marginal bone. Implants with internal connections are currently provided by many implant companies. An important goal in the design of the internal connection is stability of the abutment-to-implant interface, especially when subjected to non-axial loads. Morse tapered, internal hexagon, and internal lobe type connections are some examples (Figs. 18.11a–c).

Internal connections also provide for an improved load distribution toward the center of the implant and protection of the prosthetic abutment screw (Chun et al. 2006; Merz et al. 2000; Niznick 1991). Furthermore, internal connections reduce stress concentration at the marginal bone level, thereby reducing marginal bone loss (Astrand et al. 2004; Engquist et al. 2002; Norton 1998, 2001, 2006).

Internal connections also reduce microleakage of bacteria (Norton 1998) and facilitate prosthetic procedures by reducing the height of prosthetic components.

Marginal bone loss has been used to evaluate implant health and clinical performance. Bone loss of up to 1.5 mm the first year and then 0.2 mm for subsequent years has been accepted (Brånemark et al. 1977.)

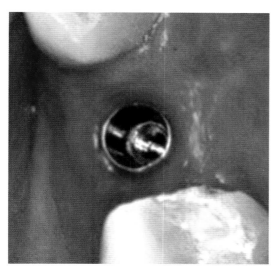

Figure 18.11a. Morse tapered connection.

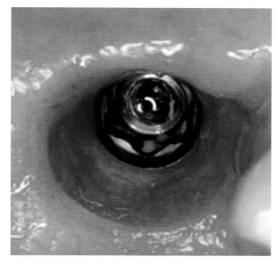

Figure 18.11c. PrimaConnex™ with TiLobe™ technology.

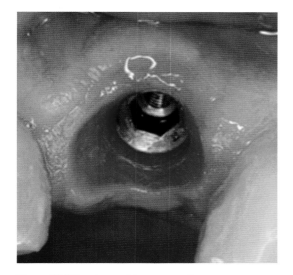

Figure 18.11b. Internal hex connection.

In the aesthetic zone marginal bone loss may compromise the result due to soft-tissue recession following bone loss. Unaesthetic changes could be even worse in soft-tissue contours associated with two adjacent implants where horizontal bone loss is followed by the formation of a bone crater between implants (Tarnow et al. 2002).

The etiologies of early marginal bone loss include surgical trauma, occlusal overload, the presence of microgap, reformation of biologic width, implant crest module, and others (Oh et al. 2002).

Marginal bone loss on single implants is related to load distribution. In flat-top interface implants the stress concentration is highest at the level of the bone crest, as has been demonstrated in finite element analysis (Chun et al. 2006; Hansson 2003; Merz et al. 2000). Studies comparing the performance of flat-top interface implants, such as the external hexagon, with internal conical connections have shown that in the latter, the peak bone-to-implant interfacial shear stresses generated by the conical implant-to-abutment interface were less than those produced in the flat-top interface (Hansson 2003).

Chun et al. (2006) studied the influence of the implant abutment type on stress distribution in bone under various loading conditions using finite element analysis. Three different types of implants were analyzed: one-piece, internal hexagon, and external hexagon implant systems. They concluded that the magnitude of maximum von Mises stresses increased as the inclination angle of applied load increased. Stresses were generated at the area of compact bone adjacent to the first implant micro-thread for all implant systems, and the difference in the level of maximum von Mises stress in peri-implant bone increased noticeably. The external hexagon implant generated the greatest von Mises stress, whereas the internal hexagon implant generated the lowest von Mises stress under all loading conditions. The maximum stress concentration at the cortical bone level observed in external hexagon implants could partially explain the marginal bone loss produced after loading during the first year. The internal hexagon implants presented a comparatively smaller stress concentration in the cortical bone, at the same loading conditions. In other words, there is a better redistribution of the load in these implants, which results in less marginal bone loss.

Norton (1998) evaluated bone loss in internal connection implants for 4 years and reported an average of 0.51 mm of marginal bone loss during the period. Palmer et al. (1997) published the results of a prospective study in single tooth replacement in 15 patients, using implants with an internal conical design. Their results show at the crown insertion a mean bone level of 0.46–0.48 mm apical to the top of the implant, and there were no statistically significant changes in the bone level over the 2-year study.

Another possible explanation of minimum marginal bone loss associated with internal connection implants may be minimal micro-leakage produced at the microgap level, in contrast with that observed in the flat-top interface of the Brånemark external hexagon design where the microleakage could be partially responsible for the bone loss (Persson et al. 1996; Quirynen and van Steenberghe 1993). Berglundh et al. (1992) also evaluated the microgap in second-stage Brånemark implants and found inflamed connective tissue 0.5 mm above and below the abutment-implant connection, which resulted in 0.5 mm bone loss within 2 weeks of the abutment being connected to the implant.

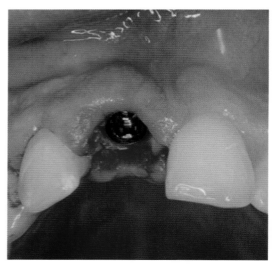

Figure 18.12a. Intrasurgical view of the immediate placement of the PrimaConnex™ implant RD 4.1 × 13 mm in the alveolar socket of tooth 11.

Beautiful aesthetic results are certainly difficult to attain with implants in the aesthetic zone. The alignment of the gingival margin and the presence of papilla are essential elements in the final result. These two soft-tissue entities, however, are closely related to the biotype and to the quality and quantity of underlying structural alveolar bone. The peri-implant mucosa, particularly if it is narrow, with a thin-scalloped biotype, inevitably retracts 6 months after abutment connection and restoration, due to the reformation of the biological space (Small and Tarnow 2000.)

Marginal bone loss reduction diminishes soft-tissue recession around the implants, which assures better aesthetic results by preserving the contour of soft tissue and interdental papilla (Figs. 18.12a–d).

Conclusions

Achieving aesthetic results in the aesthetic zone is always a challenge. Many variables must be considered: the remaining bone volume, the soft-tissue quality and quantity,

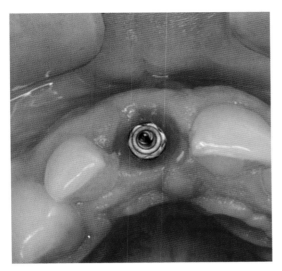

Figure 18.12b. The PrimaConnex™ implant 6 months after surgery.

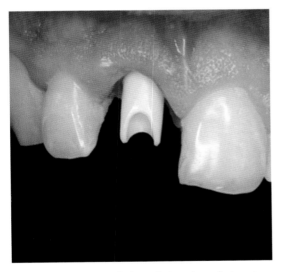

Figure 18.12c. Buccal view of zirconium abutment.

the patient's biotype, whether or not the placement is related to a tooth or to another implant, the height of the smile, and the occlusal contact relation. Among all these variables, bone tissue plays a fundamental role. Its presence assures more favorable results and its absence can cause failure.

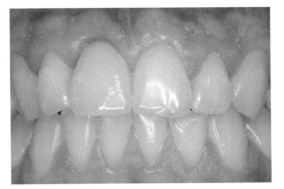

Figure 18.12d. Final rehabilitation of PrimaConnex™ implant in position 11.

The performance of internal connection implants has been evaluated and advantages have been attributed to them over the flat-top external hexagon connections. One of these advantages is the reduction of marginal bone loss, which has an important impact on the final aesthetic result. The reduction of marginal bone loss with internal connection implants may be attributed to better load distribution and transmission toward the bone, thereby reducing stress concentration at the marginal cortical bone level.

References

Adell R. 1983. Clinical results of osseointegrated implants supporting fixed prostheses in edentulous jaws. *J Prosthet Dent* 50:251–254.

Adell R, Ericksson B, Lekholm U, Brånemark PI, Jemt T. 1990. Long-term follow-up study of osseointegrated implants in the treatment of totally edentulous jaws. *Int J Oral Maxillofac Implants* 5:347–359.

Adell R, Lekholm U, Rockler B, Brånemark PI. 1981. A 15-year study of osseointegrated implants in the treatment of the edentulous jaw. *Int J Oral Surg* 10(6): 387–416.

Albrektsson T, Wennerberg A. 2004. Oral implant surfaces. Part 2: Review focusing on clinical knowledge of different surfaces. *Int J Prosthodont* 17(5):544–564.

Arlin ML. 2006. Short dental implants as a treatment option: Results from an observational study in a single private practice. *Int J Oral Maxillofac Implants* 21(5):769–776.

Astrand P, Engquist B, Dahlgren S, Gründahl K, Engquist E, Feldmann H. 2004. Astra Tech and Brånemark system implants: A 5-year prospective study of marginal bone reactions. *Clin Oral Implants Res* 15(4): 413–420.

Attard N, Zarb G. 2005. Inmediate and early Implant loading protocols: A literature review. *J Prosthet Dent* 94(3):242–257.

Bahat O. 1993. Treatment planning and placement of dental implants in the posterior maxillae: Report of 732 consecutive Nobelpharma implants. *Int J Oral Maxillofac Implants* 8:151–161.

Berglundh T, Lindhe J, Ericsson I, Liljenberg B. 1992. Soft tissue reaction to de novo plaque formation on implants and teeth. An experimental study in the dog. *Clin Oral Implants Res* 3:1–8.

Brånemark PI, Hansson BO, Adell R, Breine U, Lindström J, Hallen O, Ohman A. 1977. Osseointegrated implants in the treatment of the edentulous jaw. Experience from a 10-year period. *Scand J Plast Reconstr Surg* (Suppl) 16:1–132.

Chun HJ, Shin H, Han C, Lee S. 2006. Influence of implant abutment types on stress distribution in bone under various loading conditions using finite element analysis. *Int J Oral Maxillofac Implants* 21:195–202.

Elkhoury JS, McGlumphy EA, Tatakis DN, Beck FM. 2005. Clinical parameters associated with success and failure of single-tooth titanium plasma-sprayed cylindric implants under stricter criteria: A 5-year retrospective study. *Int J Oral Maxillofac Implants* 20:687–694.

Engquist B, Astrand P, Dahlgren S, Engquist E, Feldmann H, Gröndahl K. 2002. Marginal bone reaction to oral implant: A prospective comparative study of Astra Tech and Brånemark implant system implants. *Clin Oral Implants Res* 13:30–37.

Esposito M, Ekestubbe A, Grondahl K. 1993. Radiological evaluation of marginal bone loss at tooth surfaces facing single Brånemark implants. *Clin Oral Implants Res* 4:151–157.

Feldman S, Boitel N, Weng D, Kohles SS, Stach RM. 2004. Five-year survival distributions of short-length (10 mm or less) machined-surfaced and Osseotite™ implants. *Clin Implant Dent Relat Res* 6:16–23.

Friberg B, Grondahl K, Lekholm U, Brånemark PI. 2000. Long-term follow-up of severely atrophic edentulous mandibles reconstructed with short Brånemark implants. *Clin Implant Dent Relat Res* 2:184–189.

Gastaldo JF, Cury PF, Sendyk WR. 2004. Effect of the vertical and horizontal distances between adjacent implants and between a tooth and an implant on the incidence of interproximal papilla. *J Periodontol* 75(9):1242–1246.

Gentile MA, Chuang SK, Dodson TB. 2005. Survival estimates and risk factors for failure with 6×5.7-mm implants. *Int J Oral Maxillofac Implants* 20(6):930–937.

Goene R, Bianchesi C, Huerzeler M, Del Lupo R, Testori T, Davarpanah M, Jalbout Z. 2005. Performance of short implants in partial restorations: 3-year follow-up of Osseotite™ implants. *Implant Dent* 14(3): 274–280.

Goodacre CJ, Bernal G, Rungcharassaeng K, Kan JYK. 2003. Clinical complications with implants and implant prostheses. *J Prosthet Dent* 90(2):121–132.

Hagi D, Deporter DA, Pilliar RM, Arenovich T. 2004. A targeted review of study outcomes with short (<7 mm) endosseous dental implants placed in partially edentulous patients. *J Periodontol* 75:798–804.

Hansson SA. 2003. Conical implant-abutment interface at the level of marginal bone improves the distribution of stresses in the supporting bone. *Clin Oral Implants Res* 14:286–293.

Hatley CL, Cameron SM, Cuenin MF, Parker MH, Tompson SH, Harvey SB. 2001. The effect of dental implant spacing on peri-implant bone using the rabbit (*Oryctolagus cuniculus*) tibia model. *J Prosthodont* 10:154–159.

Herrmann I, Lekholm U, Holm S, Kultje C. 2005. Evaluation of patient and implant characteristics as potential prognostic factors for oral implant failures. *Int J Oral Maxillofac Implants* 20:220–230.

Higginbottom FL, Belser U, Jones J, Keith S. 2004. Prosthetic management of implants in the esthetic zone. *Int J Oral Maxillofac Implants* 19(Suppl):62–72.

Higginbottom FL, Wilson TG, Jr. 1996. Three-dimensional templates for placement of root-form dental implants: A technical note. *Int J Oral Maxillofac Implants* 6:787–795.

Jemt T. 1991. Failures and complications in 391 consecutively inserted fixed prostheses supported by Brånemark implant in edentulous jaws: A study of treatment from the time of prosthesis placement to the first annual checkup. *Int J Oral Maxillofac Implants* 6:270–276.

Jemt T, Lekholm U. 1995. Implant treatment in edentulous maxillae: A 5-year follow-up report on patients with different degrees of jaw resorption. *Int J Oral Maxillofac Implants* 10:303–311.

Kasemo B, Gold J. 1999. Implant surfaces and interface processes. *Adv Dent Res* 13:8–20.

Kazor CE, Al-Shamari K, Sarment DP, Misch CE, Wang HL. 2004. Implant plastic surgery: A review and rationale. *J Oral Implantology* 30:240–254.

Kemppanien P, Eskola S, Ylipaavalniemi P. 1997. A comparative prospective clinical study of two single-tooth implants: A preliminary report of 102 implants. *J Prosthet Dent* 77:382–387.

Krennmair G, Piehslinger E, Wagner H. 2003. Status of teeth adjacent to single-tooth implants. *Int J Prosthodont* 16:524–528.

Laney WR. 2001. The emphasis on esthetics. *Int J Oral Maxillofac Implants* 16:625.

Laney WR, Jemt T, Harris, D. 1994. Osseointegrated implants for single-tooth replacement: Progress report from a multicenter prospective study after 3 years. *Int J Oral Maxillofac Implants* 9:49–54.

Lee JH, Frias V, Lee KW, Wright RF. 2005. Effect of implant size and shape on implant success rates: A literature review. *J Prosthet Dent* 94:377–381.

Li Shi B, Haiyan B, Alex SL, Fok B, Cemal U, Devlin H, Horner K. 2007. Shape optimization of dental implants. *Int J Oral Maxillofac Implants* 22:911–920.

Malo P, de Araujo Nobre M, Rangert B. 2007. Short implants placed one-stage in maxillae and mandibles: A retrospective clinical study with 1 to 9 years of follow-up. *Clin Implant Dent Relat Res* 9(1):15–21.

Martinez H, Davarpanah M, Missika P, Celleti R, Lazzara R. 2001. Optimal implant stabilization in low density bone. *Clin Oral Implants Res* 12:423–432.

Merz BR, Hunenbart S, Belzer UC. 2000. Mechanics of the implant-abutment connection: An 8-degree taper compared to a butt joint connection. *Int J Oral Maxillofac Implants* 15:519–526.

Misch CE, Steignga J, Barboza E, Misch-Dietsh FM, Cianciola LJ, Kazor C. 2006. Short dental implants in posterior partial edentulism: A multicenter retrospective 6-year case series study. *J Periodontol* 77(8):1340–1347.

Misch CE, Suzuki JB, Misch-Dietsh FM, Bidez MW. 2005. A positive correlation between occlusal trauma and peri-implant bone loss: Literature support. *Implant Dent* 14(2):108–116.

Naert I, Koutsikakis G, Quirynen M, Jacobs R, Van Steenberghe D. 2002. Biologic outcome of implant-supported restorations in the treatment of partial edentulism. Part I: A longitudinal clinical evaluation. *Clin Oral Implants Res* 13:381–389.

Nedir R, Bischof M, Briaux JM, Beyer S, Szmukler-Moncler S, Bernard JP. 2004. A 7-year life table analysis from a prospective study on ITI implants with special emphasis on the use of short implants. Results from a private practice. *Clin Oral Implants Res* 15(2):150–157.

Niznick GA. 1991. The implant abutment connection: The key to prosthetic success. *Compendium* 12:932–937.

Norton MR. 1998. Marginal bone levels at single tooth implants with a conical fixture design. The influence of surface macro- and microstructure. *Clin Oral Implants Res* 9:91–99.

———. 2001. A 4–7 year follow-up on the biological and mechanical stability of single tooth implants. *Clin Implant Dent Relat Res* 3:214–220.

———. 2006. Multiple single-tooth implant restorations in the posterior jaws: Maintenance of marginal bone levels with reference to implant-abutment microgap. *Int J Oral Maxillofac Implants* 21:777–784.

Oh TJ, Yoon J, Mish CE, Wang L. 2002. The causes of early implant bone loss: Myth or science? *J Periodontol* 73:322–333.

O'Sullivan D, Senerby L, Meredith N. 2004. Influence of implant taper on the primary and secondary stability of osseointegrated titanium implants. *Clin Oral Implants Res* 15:474–480.

Palmer RM, Smith BJ, Palmer PJ, Floyd PD. 1997. A prospective study of Astra single tooth implants. *Clin Oral Implants Res* 8:173–179.

Persson LG, Lekholm U, Leonhardt A, Dahlen G, Lindhe J. 1996. Bacterial colonization on internal surfaces of Brånemark system implant components. *Clin Oral Implants Res* 7:90–95.

Quirynen M, Van Steenberghe D. 1993. Bacterial colonization of the internal part of two-stage implants. An in vivo study. *Clin Oral Implants Res* 4:158–161.

Renouard F, Nisand D. 2005. Short implants in the severely resorbed maxilla: A 2-year retrospective clinical study. *Clin Implant Dent Relat Res* 7(Suppl 1):104–110.

Renouard F, Nisand D. 2006. Impact of implant length and diameter on survival rates. *Clin Oral Implants Res* 17(Suppl 2):35–51.

Rokni S, Todescan R, Watson P, Pharoah M, Adegbembo AO, Deporter D. 2005. An assessment of crown-to-root ratios with short sintered porous-surfaced implants supporting prostheses in partially edentulous patients. *Int J Oral Maxillofac Implants* 20(1):69–76.

Romeo E, Ghisolfi M, Rozza R, Chiapasco M, Lops D. 2006. Short (8-mm) dental implants in the rehabilitation of partial and complete edentulism: A 3- to 14-year longitudinal study. *Int J Prosthodont* 19:586–592.

Saadoun AP, Landsberg TC. 1997. Treatment classifications and sequencing for post extraction implant therapy: A review. *Pract Periodont Restor Dent* 9:993–941.

Saadoun AP, Le Gall MG, Touati B. 2004. Current trends in implantology. Part II: Treatment planning, aesthetic considerations, and tissue regeneration. *Pract Proced Aesthet Dent* 16(10):707–714.

Salama H, Salama MA, Garber D, Adar P. 1998. The interproximal height of bone: A guidepost to predictable aesthetic strategies and soft tissue contours in anterior tooth replacement. *Pract Periodont Aesthet Dent* 10:1131–1141.

Sanz A, Farias D, Díaz I, Oyarzún A. 1998. Estudio experimental de la respuesta ósea sobre tres diferentes superficies de implantes titanio Cp, Ha, Tps. *Revista del Consejo de Odontólogos y Estomatólogos* 3:221–226.

Sanz A, Oyarzún A, Farias D, Díaz I. 2001. Experimental study of bone response to a new surface treatment of endosseous titanium implants. *Implant Dent* 10:127–129.

Schulte J, Flores AM, Weed M. 2007. Crown-to-implant ratios of single tooth implant-supported restorations. *J Prosthet Dent* 98(1):1–5.

Small P, Tarnow D. 2000. Gingival recession around implants: A 1-year longitudinal prospective study. *Int J Oral Maxillofac Implants* 15:527–532.

Spear FM. 1999. Maintenance of the interdental papilla following anterior tooth removal. *Pract Periodont Aesthet Dent* 11:21–28.

Tarnow DP, Cho SC, Wallace SS. 2002. The effect of inter-implant distance on the height of inter-implant bone crest. *J Periodontol* 71:546–549.

Tawil G, Younan R. 2003. Clinical evaluation of short, machined-surface implants followed for 12 to 92 months. *Int J Oral Maxillofac Implants* 18(6):894–901.

Ten Bruggenkate CM, Asikainen P, Foitzik C, Krekeler G, Sutter F. 1998. Short (6-mm) nonsubmerged dental implants: Results of a multicenter clinical trial of 1 to 7 years. *Int J Oral Maxillofac Implants* 13:791–798.

Van Staden RC, Guan H, Loo YC. 2006. Application of the finite element method in dental implant research. *Comp Methods Biomech Biomed Engr* 9(4):257–270.

Wagner WC. 1992. A brief introduction to advanced surface modification technologies. *J Oral Implantology* 18(3):231–235.

Weng D, Jacobson Z, Tarnow D, Hurzeler M, Faehn O, Sanavi F, Barkvoll P, Stach R. 2003. A prospective multicenter clinical trial of 3i machined-surfaced implants: Results after 6 years of follow-up. *Int J Oral Maxillofac Implants* 18:417–423.

Winkler S, Morris HF, Ochi S. 2000. Implant survival to 36 months as related to length and diameter. *Ann Periodontol* 5:22–31.

Wyatt CCL, Zarb GA. 1998. Treatment outcomes of patients with implant-supported fixed partial prostheses. *Int J Oral Maxillofac Implants* 13:204–211.

Zarb GA, Symington JM. 1983. Osseointegrated dental implants: Preliminary report on a replication study. *J Prosthet Dent* 50:271–276.

Loading Protocols and Clinical Outcomes

WHAT HAVE WE LEARNED ABOUT THE INFLUENCE OF LOADING ON THE QUALITY AND MAINTENANCE OF OSSEOINTEGRATION?

Ignace Naert, Katleen Vandamme, and Joke Duyck

Introduction

Brånemark et al. (1977) introduced the principles of osseointegration 30 years ago. Primary stability and lack of micromotion were considered to be two of the main factors necessary for achieving predictable high successes of 92–98% for osseointegrated oral implants after 10 years in the maxilla and mandibula, respectively (Adell et al. 1990). To minimize the risk of implant failure, a two-stage surgical technique was used and oral implants were kept load-protected during the healing period of 3–6 months for the mandible and maxilla, respectively (Brånemark et al. 1977). A longitudinal clinical trial suggested that implants could be loaded immediately or early in the mandibles of selected patients (Schnitman et al. 1990). Nowadays immediate and early loaded implants are frequently used in mandibles with sufficient jaw geometry and good bone quality. Nevertheless, prospective controlled studies are scarce that evidence the implant outcome in immediately or early loaded implants compared to delayed loaded ones and to understand the rationale behind early and immediate loading better. Apart from implant-related factors (material, design, topography, and surface chemistry), surgical technique, and patient variables (bone quantity and quality, health condition, smoking habit, bruxism), mechanical loading of the peri-implant bone is considered to be an important biomechanical factor in the implant outcome. During healing, excessive micromotion between the implant and the peri-implant bone is mentioned as a compromising factor, but the exact tolerance to micromotion is not known. After initial healing, mechanical overload is mentioned as one of the main reasons for late implant failure, because of component fractures or excessive marginal bone loss or implant mobility (Sennerby and Roos 1998). This contribution will deal with the influence of loading on healing and healed bone.

Bone Biology

Peri-implant endosseous healing is governed by three phases.

First, the inflammatory phase, where inflammatory cells are recruited for phagocytosis of wound debris and the diminishing oxygen gradient is chemotactic for endothelial and mesenchymal cells.

Second, a regeneration phase divided into (1) *angiogenesis* occurring in the first 48–72 hours, where the granulation tissue starts at day 4 until week 3, followed by (2) *osteogenesis*, where bone morphogenetic proteins, naturally released in response to trauma or at bone remodelling sites, are the only known inductive agents (Lind 1996). However, mechanical loading is known to be a particularly potent stimulus for bone cells if it does not exceed certain values (Frost 1987; Robling et al. 2006). Woven bone formation predominates within the first 4–6 weeks after implant placement.

Third is the remodelling phase, where in the second month after implant placement, woven bone is gradually replaced by lamellar bone. The packaging of the collagen fibrils gives lamellar bone the high strength necessary to resist implant loading. The maximum bone deposition is achieved only at 3–4 months.

While during bone modelling the bone architecture adapts under mechanical loading, during bone remodelling, the bone architecture remains the same, but the bone tissue is renewed. The main difference between delayed versus immediate loading is that in the former one waits to load until "secondary stability" is reached (after 3–4 months), while in the latter one relies on "primary stability" to load the implants (pure mechanical interlocking).

Frost (1987) pointed to the relationship between strain and modelling, described in the so-called "mechanostat." Although the parameters involved in mechanically mediated (mature) bone modelling have been well investigated experimentally (magnitude, distribution, frequency, duration, static vs. dynamic strain stimulus), the question of how they manifest around implants still remains.

In addition, biomechanical parameters involved in the initial healing process at the tissue-implant interface are not well understood, such as the effect of micromotion (Szmukler-Moncler et al. 1998). What is the critical threshold for implant integration? What is the effect of biomechanical coupling, such as the effects of macro- and micro-design? Does >150 μm displacement really lead to fibrous encapsulation (Duyck et al. 2006; Søballe et al. 1992). Biomechanical tissue-implant coupling exists when a force transfer takes place between both media. The implant surface must therefore establish a mechanical continuum with the surrounding tissues. For this to occur, intimate tissue adaptation is essential and dependent on the implant macro- and micro-design. We have searched for evidence at three levels: using the rabbit bone chamber model "gap interface," the tibial guinea pig model "direct contact," and the human mandible "direct contact."

Healing Bone

Rabbit Bone Chamber Model "Gap Interface"

Using the repeated sampling bone chamber methodology (Duyck et al. 2004) for the evaluation of tissue differentiation and bone adaptation around titanium implants under controlled mechanical conditions, Vandamme et al. (2007a) investigated the histodynamics of interfacial bone formation during immediate loading.

Controlled loading up to 50 μm displacement for a drawn cp Ti implant (Ra = 0.45 μm) increased bone formation after 12 weeks. In the clinic, *controlled* implant loading might be a key factor in stimulating bone formation.

The influence of controlled immediate loading on the implant macro-topography was also investigated (Vandamme et al. 2007b). Mean values of the bone area fraction were significantly larger for the loaded cylindrical and screw-shaped versus the unloaded screw-type implants. The bone-to-implant contact was only significantly higher for the loaded screw-type implants. Thus, the screw-shaped implant promoted osseointegration through a favorable local mechanical environment for bone formation compared to the cylindrical implant. In the clinic, screw-shaped implants not only favor the primary stability but might improve the so-called "secondary" stability achieved through physiological loading.

In another paper, Vandamme et al. (2008) investigated the effect of implant surface roughness and loading on peri-implant bone formation. They concluded that bone forms at a higher incidence adjacent to a roughened surface compared to a turned one in the unloaded mode. This is in agreement with clinical observations (Lazzara et al. 1999). However, in the loaded mode implant macrodesign (screw) was more significant than the micro-design (roughness). This is in agreement with clinical data (Al-Nawas et al. 2007).

Lastly, Vandamme et al. (2007c) investigated the effect of the magnitude of micromotion on the tissue response around an immediately loaded roughened screw-type titanium implant in the rabbit. They concluded that micromotion of up to 30 μm of a turned cylindrical and turned screw-shaped implant did not hamper the osseointegration. Moreover, micromotion of up to 90 μm of a roughened screw-shaped implant did not hamper the osseointegration either. Leucht et al. (2007) came to the same conclusions based on a 150 μm displacement of a Teflon screw-type implant.

Tibial Guinea Pig Model "Direct Contact"

De Smet (2006) installed 194 TiO$_2$-blasted (Ra: 1.74 μm) screw-type Ti-6Al-4V implants in 11 series of guinea pig tibial bones. The implants were left to heal for 1 week and then loaded with changing load parameters (frequency, magnitude, or number of cycles) for 4 weeks. One test implant (n = 97) and one control implant (n = 97) were lost over the course of the experiment. Differences in bone mass (bone mass test–bone mass control side) for the distal medullar 500 ROI in function of strain rate (strain × freq.) are shown in Figure 19.1.

Early controlled loading did not lead to a higher implant failure. An optimum stimulation was found combining a low frequency (3 Hz) with a force amplitude of 1 N, resulting in a calculated strain of 540 μɛ at the interface.

To the present the experimental literature on the loading of teeth and implants suggests that for teeth physiological loading + inflammation provokes bone loss; excessive loading without inflammation leads to tooth mobility; excessive loading + inflammation results in rapid bone loss. For implants, physiological loading + inflammation provokes bone loss; excessive loading without inflammation leads to bone/implant loss; not fully proven is that excessive loading + inflammation results in rapid bone/implant loss.

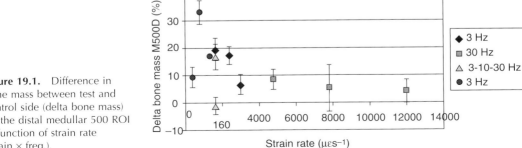

Figure 19.1. Difference in bone mass between test and control side (delta bone mass) for the distal medullar 500 ROI in function of strain rate (strain × freq.).

Human Mandible "Direct Contact"

Thirty edentulous patients were divided into three groups (De Smet 2006). In group I, two implants were loaded after 16 weeks (delayed) with a two-implant overdenture; in group II, the implants were loaded after 1 week (early); in group III, three implants were loaded the same day (immediate) with a fixed hybrid prosthesis (Brånemark et al. 1999). Patients in groups II and III were given verbal explanations and written soft diet instructions and asked to follow that diet for 8 weeks after prosthesis handover. Radiographic assessment, bite fork, and strain gauge measurements (groups I and II) were recorded. After 2 years implant outcomes for groups I, II, and III were 2/20, 2/20, and 6/30, respectively. The mean marginal bone loss (mean transversal and sagittal plane) between 1 week (baseline) and 20 months after loading for groups I, II, and III were 0.56, 0.75, and 0.85 mm respectively ($p > 0.05$).

The patients in groups II and III were instructed to follow a soft diet for the first 8 weeks, which resulted in lower maximum bite forces; however, mean peak axial and bending moments did not significantly differ between the loaded implants. From these data the following conclusions were formulated: Differences in implant outcome do not depend on the time of loading in the edentulous mandible. However, occlusal loading, and more particularly the magnitudes of bending moments, do seem to play an important role.

Mature Bone

Marginal bone loss is estimated to be the result of excessive loading for that particular local bone (Quirynen et al. 1992; Van Steenberghe et al. 1999). Implant overloading is associated with clinical complications such as screw loosening and fractures, veneering and prosthesis fractures, implant fractures, marginal bone loss, and ultimately implant loss. Risk factors seem to be short versus long

extensions in combination with bruxism or soft type IV bone, and excessive load during grinding; how does one control these loads? Clinical guidelines with biomechanical rationale were elegantly reported by Kim et al. 2005. Factors to consider in implant occlusion are increased support area and improved force direction; which occlusal design is best? The rationale for using a particular occlusal design in tooth and implant-borne reconstructions and complete dentures has recently been described by Klineberg et al. 2007. To summarize the latter: There is no research evidence from long-term outcome studies to suggest specifying a particular occlusal design for optimizing clinical outcomes for implant suprastructures. Best practice guidelines for implant suprastructure design have been developed by extrapolation from biomechanical studies on implant cantilevers and design features used for tooth-supported restorations. The latter lack evidence but are based on desirable patient outcomes. Another issue is dealing with the aging patient. The bone turn-over (δ = rho fraction) in humans is a minimum of 16 weeks (Frost 1994). In the initial phase of bone resorption, osteoid deposition and primary mineral formation lasts 4–5 weeks (or 30% (δ)). Gradual secondary mineralization takes another 11–12 weeks (70% (δ) (Parfitt 1990)). Thus maximal strength only gradually returns to the bone (Garetto et al. 1995; Parfitt 1990). Over time, by aging (hormonal, vascularity changes, etc.), this remodelling process may decline even though the occlusal environment has not changed, leading the implants to be at risk. More evidence needs to be collected. Indeed after 15 years an increased number of implants with more than a third thread bone loss in the maxilla was found (Jemt and Johansson 2006). Is the occlusion a determining factor for implant success? The type of occlusion that is used is of minor importance as long as occlusal loads are controlled, that is, they are within the physiological capacity of the local bone (healing or healed) to resist that loading. Measures to control these loads rest in good empirical prosthodontic handling, as has long been practiced in making restorations on teeth. These theories may open the way for the adoption of "smart" prostheses that warn the patient when the implant gets overloaded (http://imload.mech.kuleuven.ac.be).

Conclusions

Controlled implant loading leads to a positive effect on the initial bone formation. The importance of primary implant stability, implant geometry (screw vs. cylinder, implant surface texture (turned vs. roughened), bone bed status, and health status must all be considered as well. There is still a lack of randomized controlled clinical trials that may provide the risk factors for immediate loading in all areas and application in the human jaw. When it comes to healed bone, factors to consider in implant occlusion are increased support area and improved force direction. Measures to control these loads rest in good empirical prosthodontic handling.

Acknowledgements

The following sources for this research are acknowledged: the European community; the Research Council K.U.Leuven; the Fund for Scientic Research–Flanders; Astra Tech, Mölndal, Sweden; and Dentsply-Friadent®, Mannheim, Germany.

THE CONCEPT OF EARLY LOADING

Hans-Peter Weber

Dental implants have become an integral part of modern comprehensive dentistry. This development was possible through the discovery of osseointegration. This ankylotic anchorage of a cp titanium implant in the surrounding bone was first observed in animal experiments and verified in human studies in the late 1960s to early 1980s, and has since been accepted as the desirable interface between bone as a living tissue and a metal implant (Albrektsson et al. 1981; Brånemark et al. 1969, 1977; Schroeder et al. 1976, 1981). Osseointegration has rendered the needed short- and long-term predictability to implant-supported prostheses of all types after other modes of integration such as the fibrous-osseous interface postulated by Linkow et al. (1973) proved not to result in a clinically stable long-term treatment (Smithloff and Fritz 1976, 1987).

Biological and biomechanical principles and techniques to predictably achieve osseointegration in the clinical application were proposed in the early osseointegration literature (Albrektsson et al. 1981; Brånemark et al. 1969, 1977; Schroeder et al. 1976, 1981). Some of these principles were accepted as critically important by both Brånemark and Schroeder: commercially pure titanium as biomaterial of choice, importance of a low-trauma, high-precision implant site preparation without overheating the local bone, and a sufficiently long healing period without the application of load or stress to the implants. Differences existed in that Brånemark's approach included a submucosal implant placement and healing for 3–6 months, while Schroeder postulated transmucosal healing and a somewhat shorter healing period of 3–4 months. Notably, these healing times, which are defined as conventional healing times today (Aparicio et al. 2003; Cochran et al. 2004), were more empirical in nature than based on scientific evidence. The reasons for proposing such long healing times have to be seen in context with the level of understanding in the field at that time. Existing implant concepts such as subperiosteal implants or endosteal blades had proven clinically unsuccessful if not harmful (Smithloff and Fritz 1976, 1987). Since scientific evidence for minimal bone-healing times for dental implants could not easily be created in a short period of time, recommendations for clinical practice had to be conservative to minimize any risk for failure of the concept (Szmukler-Moncler et al. 2000). Additionally, the largest body of work on osseointegration was based on implants with turned surfaces (minimally rough in today's terms). This also impacted the recommendation for longer healing times prior to implant loading, primarily for jaw locations with bone of lesser quality.

While the above-described conventional loading protocol remains, of course, valid as the proven predictable approach, more aggressive implant treatment modalities like early and immediate loading have moved into the mainstream of implant dentistry. In this section of the chapter, the concept of early loading will be assessed for its clinical validity and predictability.

Although the number of publications on early and immediate loading has dramatically increased in recent years, the overall quality of evidence is still surprisingly low. Attard and Zarb (2005) found in their literature review on clinical studies involving early and immediate loading that there is a need for thorough investigation of clinical outcomes to measure the benefit of these protocols for a patient's quality of life as well as economically. They also strongly indicated that more accurate long-term studies are required to allow meaningful comparisons of such treatment protocols for different clinical situations. A recent systematic review on the effect of time to loading on implants and prosthetic outcomes (Jokstad and Carr 2007) demonstrated that while the average outcome was in favor of conventional loading protocols, there were no indications that immediate or early loading could not be safe procedures. This was confirmed and somewhat more specified in another recent systematic review by Esposito et al., who came to the following conclusion (Esposito et al. 2007a): "It is possible to successfully load dental implants immediately or early after their placement in selected patients, though not all clinicians may achieve optimal results when loading the

implant immediately. A high degree of primary implant stability (high value of insertion torque) seems to be one of the prerequisites for a successful immediate/early loading procedure. More well designed RCTs [Randomized Clinical Trials] are needed. Priority should be given to trials comparing immediately versus early loaded implants to improve patient satisfaction and decrease treatment time."

To complicate matters, there are differing opinions on what is considered immediate or early loading, and similarly, disagreements exist on what the term "loading" entails. For the purpose of this chapter, the definitions established by the 2003 ITI Consensus Conference are used (Cochran et al. 2004). Early loading is hereby defined as the placement of an implant-supported prosthesis into occlusal contact between 48 hours and 3 months following implant placement. It is apparent that the evolution of the early loading concept is closely tied to the advances in implant surface technology. According to numerous experimental studies, surface enhancements, that is, optimized roughness, morphology, and surface chemistry, will enhance the early wound-healing events and, thus, lead to improved peri-implant bone healing in time, quantity, and quality (Ellingsen 1998).

The application of surface coatings to create rough surfaces such as titanium plasma spraying (TPS) or hydroxyapatite (HA) represented early approaches to enhance dental implant surfaces for improved healing and stability. Schroeder and co-workers used TPS-coated implants and could demonstrate in numerous non-decalcified histological sections their excellent interaction with healing bone (Schroeder et al. 1976, 1981). In a canine study, Listgarten and co-workers (1992) assessed the intact tissue/implant interface of non-submerged dental implants with a rough titanium surface in the electron microscope and could show that the peri-implant bone was intimately adapted to the titanium surface without any intervening space. The improved bone anchorage of these rough surfaces made it clinically feasible to use shorter implants than commonly recommended for minimally rough screws, as well as to restore implants after shorter healing times (≤4 months) without reducing long-term predictability independent of jaw location (Buser et al. 1997, 1999a; Kim et al. 2008; Ten Bruggenkate et al. 1998; Weber et al. 2000). A true head-to-head comparison between rough and smooth-surfaced implants in the form of randomized controlled clinical trials was never conducted. This fact motivated Cochran to perform a meta-analysis to find out if an advantage in the clinical performance of rough versus turned surfaces was extractable from data in the literature (Cochran 1999). The results led him to conclude that the analyzed data from human clinical experiences support the documented advantage of implants with a roughened surface in animal and in vitro experimentation and indicate that the magnitude of the advantage is significant. In contrast, as a result of a more recent systematic review, Esposito et al. (2007b) found no evidence for any particular type of dental implant having superior long-term success. The authors caution, though, that these findings are based on a few RCTs, are often at high risk of bias, and also have few participants with relatively short follow-up periods.

Meanwhile, implant surface research and development continued to evolve. While some obvious advantages for the mentioned rough TPS and HA surfaces had been demonstrated in various studies, disadvantages were recognized as well. They included the greater potential for fracture of the implant-coating interface or coating dissolution in case of HA (Ong and Chan 2000), the risk for particle detachment and displacement for HA or TPS (Weingart et al. 1994), as well as the potential greater risk for peri-implantitis due to the porosity of these surfaces in addition to their roughness (Ong and Chan 2000). Therefore, the continued search for surfaces that would maintain or even enhance the positive effects on bone healing while eliminating or reducing the negative ones was important.

In 1991, Buser and co-workers could demonstrate the excellent osteoconductive potential of a moderately rough cp titanium surface, which was produced by blasting the endosseous portion of a cp titanium implant with a large grit powder followed by acid attacking (SLA), in a histometric study comparing six different surfaces in miniature pigs (Buser et al. 1991). Subsequent histological and biomechanical studies confirmed the superior stability of implants at earlier times in the healing process compared to rough (TPS) or minimally rough (turned) metallic implant surfaces (Buser et al. 1999b; Cochran et al. 1998). Similar experimental results showing improved osteoconductivity and peri-implant bone healing were reported for etched implant surfaces (Davies 1998; Trisi et al. 2003). Subsequently, clinical studies, in which shorter healing times of 6–8 weeks prior to loading were used, revealed success or survival rates of greater than 97% for implants with moderately rough surfaces after observation periods of up to 5 years (Bornstein et al. 2005; Cochran et al. 2002; Roccuzzo and Wilson 2002; Roccuzzo et al. 2001; Salvi et al. 2004; Sullivan et al. 2001; Testori et al. 2002). Although these published long-term documentations with moderately rough surfaces and a defined early loading approach do not yet reach the length of follow-up of those studies with minimally rough or rough surfaced implants and conventional loading, they have assured that the concept of early loading after 6–8 weeks leads to highly predictable treatment outcomes. In contrast to immediate loading or early loading with less than 6 weeks of healing, for which a successful outcome is fully dependent on excellent primary implant stability, the 6–8 weeks of bone healing on implants with optimized surfaces means that implants are not loaded until secondary stability through osseointegration has been achieved. This approach still allows for a substantial reduction of healing and overall treatment time compared to conventional loading, while maintaining the required high predictability. Figures 19.2a–h represent a clinical example of this treatment approach

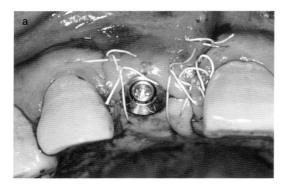
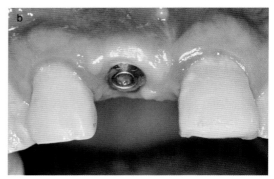
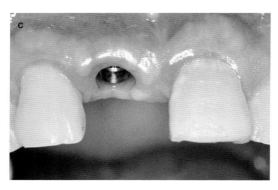
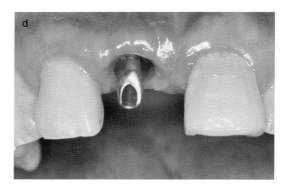

Figures 19.2a–d. The replacement of the missing right central incisor with an implant-supported single crown. The patient had been wearing a removable partial denture in an otherwise complete dentition for over 10 years after losing the tooth. a. A one-stage implant placement (semi-submerged technique using a 2 mm beveled extension healing cap). b. The completed tissue healing after 6 weeks. The healing cap was removed after 6 weeks and impression obtained for provisional crown (c) and the laboratory modified abutment inserted 7 weeks after surgery (d).

in a 72-year-old male patient, who was eager to have his treatment completed as soon as possible.

As the acceptance of this "safe" early loading concept continues to grow, further surface enhancements are already being proposed, enhancements that positively influence early bone-healing events. They include nanotechnology and changes in surface chemistry. One of these chemical modifications has succeeded in enhancing surface-free energy and hydrophilicity (Rupp et al. 2004, 2006). Subsequently, it could be demonstrated in vivo that this hydrophilic, that is, hydroxylated, chemically active SLA surface led to even earlier bone formation than observed with a conventional SLA surface (Buser et al.

2004). Similarly, implants with a fluoride-modified, moderately rough TiO_2-blasted surface demonstrated better retention in bone and greater bone integration than unmodified titanium implants after a shorter healing time in the rabbit tibia (Ellingsen et al. 2004). In a subsequent dog study, this fluoride-modified implant surface appeared to promote osseointegration in the early phase of healing following implant installation compared to a not-fluoride-modified control (Berglundh et al. 2007). While both these surfaces are already in clinical use, randomized controlled clinical trials will have to show if the observed stimulation of initial bone healing will indeed allow even earlier loading of dental implants without reducing predictability.

Table 19.6.   Levels of evidence as basis for advice about clinical treatment recommendations. Adapted from the Oxford Centre for Evidence-based Medicine (http://www.cebm.net).

The Evidence-Based View	The Experience-Based View
1. Science and scientific methods are relevant to practitioners 2. Benefits and usefulness of science have been demonstrated 3. Testimonies, case studies, non-objective experience not adequate to make relevant judgments 4. Refereed research journals are not biased 5. Clinical research is adequately performed and published	1. Only clinical experience, and years of it, is relevant to the practitioner 2. Denies the usefulness of science 3. Anecdotal evidence is adequate to make clinical judgments and better than science 4. Research journals are biased against the experience-based view 5. There are no good clinical studies or clinical researchers

described by another philosopher, Thomas Kuhn (1962). Kuhn maintained that the choice of paradigm, in this case immediate loading versus conventional loading, was sustained, but not ultimately determined, by logical processes. In the case of a general acceptance of one paradigm or another, Kuhn believed that it represented the consensus of the community of clinicians/scientists and that the acceptance or rejection of some paradigm is more a social than a logical process. The last group of clinicians practice critical rationalism as a basis for clinical practice, as they have been training in academic institutions (Brunette 2007; Popper 1934). Within this theoretical framework, it is essential to understand that scientific studies cannot prove anything beyond doubt, but claims or hypotheses can be disproved by a properly designed experiment or clinical trial.

Conclusion

So what do we do after we weigh all the evidence about immediate loading and realize that uncertainty reigns? Many would say that the ability to make a clinical judgment in the face of uncertainty defines the art of medicine and sets it apart from reductionist science.

Thus the bottom line is that the literature has not shown that a shortened loading protocol in itself is harmful. Considerations beyond this must be based on individual patient needs and expectations, and the tacit understanding that the clinician works in the best interest of the patient.

References

Adell R, Eriksson B, Lekholm U, Brånemark PI, Jemt T. 1990. Long-term follow-up study of osseointegrated implants in the treatment of totally edentulous jaws. *Int J Oral Maxillofac Implants* 5:347–359.

Albrektsson T, Brånemark PI, Hansson HA, Lindström J. 1981. Osseointegrated titanium implants. Requirements for ensuring a long-lasting, direct bone-to-implant anchorage in man. *Acta Orthopedica Scandinavica* 52:155–170.

Albrektsson T, Wennerberg A. 2004. Oral implant surfaces. Part 1: Review focusing on topographic and chemical properties of different surfaces and in vivo responses to them. *Int J Prosthodont* 17:536–543.

Al-Nawas B, Hangen U, Duschner H, Krummenauer F, Wagner W. 2007. Turned, machined versus double-etched dental implants in vivo. *Clin Implant Dent Relat Res* 2:71–78.

Aparicio C, Rangert B, Sennerby L. 2003. Immediate/early loading of dental implants: A report from the Sociedad Española de Implantes World Congress consensus meeting in Barcelona, Spain, 2002. *Clin Implant Dent Relat Res* 5:57–60.

Attard NJ, Zarb GA. 2005. Immediate and early implant loading protocols: A literature review of clinical studies. *J Prosthet Dent* 94:242–258.

Berglundh T, Abrahamsson I, Albouy JP, Lindhe J. 2007. Bone healing at implants with a fluoride-modified surface: An experimental study in dogs. *Clin Oral Implants Res* 18:147–152.

Bornstein MM, Schmid B, Belser UC, Lussi A, Buser D. 2005. Early loading of nonsubmerged titanium implants with a sandblasted and acid-etched surface. 5-year results of a prospective study in partially edentulous patients. *Clin Oral Implants Res* 16:631–638.

Brånemark PI, Adell R, Breine U, Hansson BO, Lindström J, Ohlsson A. 1969. Intraosseous anchorage of dental prostheses. I: Experimental studies. *Scand J Plast Reconstr Surg* 3:81–100.

Brånemark PI, Engstrand P, Öhrnell LO, Gröndhal K, Nilsson P, Hagberg K, Darle C, Lekholm U. 1999. Brånemark Novum: A new treatment concept for rehabilitation of the edentulous mandible. Preliminary results from a prospective clinical follow-up study. *Clin Implant Dent Relat Res* 1:2–16.

Brånemark PI, Hansson BO, Adell R, Breine U, Lindström J, Hallen O, Ohman A. 1977. Osseointegrated implants in the treatment of the edentulous jaw. Experience from a 10-year period. *Scand J Plast Reconstr Surg* (Suppl) 16:1–132.

Brunette DM. 2007. *Critical Thinking: Understanding and Evaluating Dental Research*, 2nd ed. Chicago: Quintessence.

Buser D, Broggini N, Wieland M, Schenk RK, Denzer AJ, Cochran DL, Hoffmann B, Lussi A, Steinemann SG. 2004. Enhanced bone apposition to a chemically modified SLA titanium surface. *J Dent Res* 83:529–533.

Buser D, Mericske-Stern R, Bernard JP, Behneke A, Behneke N, Hirt HP, Belser UC, Lang NP. 1997. Long term evaluation of nonsubmerged ITI implants. Part 1: 8 year life table analysis of a prospective multi-center study with 2359 implants. *Clin Oral Implants Res* 8:161–172.

Buser D, Mericske-Stern R, Dula K, Lang NP. 1999a. Clinical experience with one-stage, non-submerged dental implants. *Adv Dent Res* 13:153–161.

Buser D, Nydegger T, Oxland T, Schenk RK, Hirt HP, Cochran DE, Snétivy D, Nolte LP. 1999b. The interface shear strength of titanium implants with a sandblasted and acid-etched surface. A biomechanical study in the maxilla of miniature pigs. *J Biomed Mater Res* 45:75–83.

Buser D, Schenk RK, Steinmann S, Fiorellini JP, Fox CH, Stich H. 1991. Influence of surface characteristics on bone integration of titanium implants. A histometric study in miniature pigs. *J Biomed Mater Res* 25:889–902.

Cochran DL. 1999. A comparison of endosseous dental implant surfaces. *J Periodontol* 70:1523–1539.

Cochran DL, Buser D, Ten Bruggenkate CM, Weingart D, Taylor TM, Bernard JP, Peters F, Simpson JP. 2002. The use of reduced healing times on ITI® implants with a sandblasted and acid-etched (SLA) surface: Early results from clinical trials on ITI® SLA implants. *Clin Oral Implants Res* 13:144–153.

Cochran DL, et al. 2004. Loading protocols for endosseous dental implants. ITI Workshop. Presented material for review and consensus guidelines. *Int J Oral Maxillofac Implants* 19(Suppl): 75–113.

Cochran DL, Schenk RK, Lussi A, Higginbottom FL, Buser D. 1998. Bone response to unloaded and loaded titanium implants with a sandblasted and acid-etched surface: A histometric study in the canine mandible. *J Biomed Mater Res* 40:1–11.

Davies JE. 1998. Mechanisms of endosseous integration. *Int J Prosthodont* 11:391–401.

De Smet E. 2006. Mechanical determinants of bone (re)modelling around implants. K.U.Leuven. PhD thesis.

Del Fabbro M, Testori T, Francetti L, Taschieri S, Weinstein R. 2006. Systematic review of survival rates for immediately loaded dental implants. *Int J Periodontics Restorative Dent* 26(3):249–263

Duyck J, Cooman MD, Puers R, Van Oosterwyck H, Sloten JV, Naert I. 2004. A repeated sampling bone chamber methodology for the evaluation of tissue differentiation and bone adaptation around titanium implants under controlled mechanical conditions. *J Biomechanics* 37:1819–1822.

Duyck J, Vandamme K, Geris L, Van Oosterwyck H, De Cooman M, Vandersloten J, Puers R, Naert I. 2006. The influence of micro-motion on the tissue differentiation around immediately loaded cylindrical turned titanium implants. *Archives Oral Biology* 51:1–9.

Ellingsen JE. 1998. Surface configurations of dental implants. *Periodontology 2000* 17:36–46.

Ellingsen JE, Johansson CB, Wennerberg A, Holmén A. 2004. Improved retention and bone-to-implant contact with fluoride-modified titanium implants. *Int J Oral Maxillofac Implants* 19:659–666.

Esposito M, Grusovin MG, Willings M, Coulthard P, Worthington HV. 2007a. Interventions for replacing missing teeth: Different times for loading dental implants. (Update of *Cochrane Database of Systematic Reviews* 2004 (3):CD003878.) *Cochrane Database of Systematic Reviews* (1):CD003878.

Esposito M, Murray-Curtis L, Grusovin MG, Coulthard P, Worthington HV. 2007b. Interventions for replacing missing teeth: Different types of dental implants. *Cochrane Database of Systematic Reviews* 17(4): CD003815.

Feyerabend P. 1975. *Against Method: Outline of an Anarchistic Theory of Knowledge*. London: Humanities Press.

Fischer K, Stenberg T. 2004. Early loading of ITI implants supporting a maxillary full-arch prosthesis: 1-year data of a prospective, randomized study. *Int J Oral Maxillofac Implants* 19:374–381.

Fischer K, Stenberg T. 2006. Three-year data from a randomized, controlled study of early loading of single-stage dental implants supporting maxillary full-arch prostheses. *Int J Oral Maxillofac Implants* 21:245–252.

Frost HM. 1987. Bone "mass" and the "mechanostat": A proposal. *Anatomical Record* 219:1–9.

———. 1994. Wolff's Law and bones' structural adaptations to mechanical usage: An overview for clinicians. *Angle Orthodontist* 64(3):175–188.

Garetto LP, Chen J, Parr JA, Roberts WE. 1995. Remodelling dynamics of bone supporting rigidly fixed titanium implants: A histomorphometric comparison in four species including humans. *Implant Dentistry* 4:235–243.

IMLOAD EU-project. http://imload.mech.kuleuven.ac.be.

Jemt T, Johansson J. 2006. Implant treatment in the edentulous maxillae: A 15-year follow-up study on 76 consecutive patients provided with fixed prostheses. *Clin Implant Dent Relat Res* 8:61–69.

Jokstad A, Carr A. 2007. What is the effect on outcomes of time-to-loading of a fixed or removable prosthesis placed on implant(s)? *Int J Oral Maxillofac Implants* 22(Suppl):19–48.

Kim DM, Badovinac RM, Lorenz RL, Fiorellini JP, Weber HP. 2008. A 10-year prospective clinical and radiographic study of one-stage dental implants. *Clin Oral Implants Res* 19:254–258.

Kim Y, Oh TJ, Misch C, Wang HL. 2005. Occlusal considerations in implant therapy: Clinical guidelines with biomechanical rationale. *Clin Oral Implants Res* 16:26–35.

Klineberg I, Kingston D, Murray G. 2007. The bases for using a particular occlusal design in tooth and implant-borne reconstructions and complete dentures. *Clin Oral Implants Res* 18 (Suppl 3):151–167.

Kuhn TS. 1962. *The Structure of Scientific Revolutions*. Chicago: University of Chicago Press.

Lambrecht JT, Hodel Y. 2007. Long-term results of immediately loaded interforaminal implants. *Quintessence International* 38:111–119.

Lazzara RJ, Testori T, Trisi P, Porter SS, Weinstein RL. 1999. A human histologic analysis of Osseotite™ and machined surfaces using implants with 2 opposing surfaces. *Int J Periodontics Restorative Dent* 19:117–129.

Leucht P, Kim J-B, Wazen R, Currey JA, Nanci A, Brunski J, Helms JA. 2007. Effect of mechanical stimuli on skeletal regeneration around implants. *Bone* 40:919–930.

Lind M. 1996. Growth factors: Possible new clinical tools. A review. *Acta Orthopaedica Scand* 67:4074–4117.

Linkow LI, Glassman PE, Asnis ST. 1973. Macroscopic and microscopic studies of endosteal bladevent implants (six-month dog study). *Oral Implantology* 3:281–309.

Listgarten MA, Buser D, Steinemann SG, Donath K, Lang NP, Weber HP. 1992. Light and transmission electron microscopy of the intact interfaces between non-submerged titanium-coated epoxy resin implants and bone or gingiva. *J Dent Res* 71:364–371.

Moradi DR, Moy PK, Chiappelli F. 2006. Evidence-based research in alternative protocols to dental implantology: A closer look at publication bias. *J Calif Dent Assoc* 34(11):877–886.

Nkenke E, Fenner M. 2006. Indications for immediate loading of implants and implant success. *Clin Oral Implants Res* 17(Suppl 2):19–34.

Ong JL, Chan DC. 2000. Hydroxyapatite and their use as coatings in dental implants: A review. *Crit Rev Biomed Engr* 28:667–707.

Parfitt AM. 1990. Calcitriol for postmenopausal osteoporosis. *Ann Internal Med* 15:112–147.

Popper KR. 1934. *Logik der Forschung*. Vienna: Springer. (Also as: *The Logic of Scientific Discovery*. London: Routledge, 2002.)

Quirynen M, Naert I, Van Steenberghe D. 1992. Fixture design and overload influence marginal bone loss and fixture success in the Brånemark system. *Clin Oral Implants Res* 3:104–111.

Rinchuse DJ, Rinchuse DJ, Kandasamy S. 2005. Evidence-based versus experience-based views on occlusion and TMD. *Am J Orthod Dentofacial Orthop* 127(2):249–254.

Robling AG, Castillo AB, Turner CH. 2006. Biomechanical and molecular regulation of bone remodelling. *Ann Rev Biomed Engr* 8:455–498.

Roccuzzo M, Aglietta M, Bunino M, Bonino L. 2008. Early loading of sandblasted and acid-etched (SLA) implants: A randomized-controlled double-blind split-mouth study. Five-year results. *Clin Oral Implants Res* 19:148–152.

Roccuzzo M, Bunino M, Prioglio F, Bianchi SD. 2001. Early loading of sandblasted and acid-etched (SLA) implants: A prospective split-mouth comparative study. *Clin Oral Implants Res* 12:572–578.

Roccuzzo M, Wilson T. 2002. A prospective study evaluating a protocol for 6 weeks loading of SLA implants in the posterior maxilla: One year results. *Clin Oral Implants Res* 13:502–507.

Rupp F, Scheideler L, Olshanska N, de Wild M, Wieland M, Geis-Gerstorfer J. 2006. Enhancing surface free energy and hydrophilicity through chemical modification of microstructured titanium implant surfaces. *J Biomater Res* 76:323–334.

Rupp L, Scheideler D, Rehbein D, Axmann D, Geis-Gerstörfer J. 2004. Roughness induced dynamic changes of wettability of acid-etched titanium implant modifications. *Biomaterials* 25:1429–1438.

Salvi GE, Gallini G, Lang NP. 2004. Early loading (2 or 6 weeks) of sandblasted and acid-etched (SLA) ITI® implants in the posterior mandible. A 1-year randomized clinical trial. *Clin Oral Implants Res* 15:142–149.

Schnitman PA, Wöhrle PS, Rubenstein JE. 1990. Immediate fixed interim prostheses supported by two-stage threaded implants: Methodology and results. *J Oral Implantology* 16:96–105.

Schroeder A, Pohler O, Sutter F. 1976. Tissue reaction to an implant of a titanium hollow cylinder with a titanium surface spray layer. *Schweiz Monatsschrift Zahnheilkunde* 86:713–727.

Schroeder A, Van der Zypen E, Stich H, Sutter F. 1981. The reactions of bone, connective tissue, and epithelium to endosteal implants with titanium-sprayed surfaces. *J Maxillofac Surg* 9:15–25.

Sennerby L, Roos J. 1998. Surgical determinants of clinical success of osseointegrated oral implants: A review of the literature. *Int J Prosthodont* 11:408–420.

Smithloff M, Fritz ME. 1976. The use of blade implants in a selected population of partially edentulous adults: A five-year report. *J Periodontol* 47:19–24.

Smithloff M, Fritz ME. 1987. The use of blade implants in a selected population of partially edentulous adults: A 15-year report. *J Periodontol* 58:589–593.

Søballe K, Brockstedt-Rasmussen H, Hansen ES, Bünger C. 1992. Hydroxyapatite coating modifies implant membrane formation. Controlled micromotion studied in dogs. *Acta Orthopaedica Scand* 63:128–140.

Sullivan, DY, Sherwood, RL, Porter, SS. 2001. Long-term performance of Osseotite™ implants: A 6-year clinical follow-up. *Compendium* 22:326–328.

Szmukler-Moncler S, Piattelli A, Favero GA, Dubruille JH. 2000. Considerations preliminary to the application of early and immediate loading protocols in dental implantology. *Clin Oral Implants Res* 11:12–25.

Szmukler-Moncler S, Salama H, Reingewirtz Y, Dubruille JH. 1998. Timing of loading and effect of micromotion on bone-dental implant interface: Review of experimental literature. *J Biomed Mater Res* 43:192–203.

Ten Bruggenkate CM, Asikainen P, Foitzik C, Krekeler G, Sutter F. 1998. Short (6mm) non-submerged dental implants: Results of a multicenter clinical trial of 1–7 years. *Int J Oral Maxillofac Implants* 13:791–798.

Testori T, Del Fabbro M, Feldman S, Vincenzi G, Sullivan D, Rossi R, Jr., Anitua E, Bianchi F, Francetti L, Weinstein RL. 2002. A multicenter prospective evaluation of 2-month loaded Osseotite® implants in the posterior jaws: 3-year follow-up results. *Clin Oral Implants Res* 13:154–161.

Testori T, Galli F, Capelli M, Zuffetti F, Esposito M. 2007. Immediate nonocclusal versus early loading of dental implants in partially edentulous patients: 1-year results from a multicenter, randomized controlled clinical trial. *Int J Oral Maxillofac Implants* 22(5):815–822.

Trisi P, Lazzara R, Rebaudi A, Rao W, Testori T, Porter SS. 2003. Bone-implant contact on machined and dual acid-etched surfaces after 2 months of healing in the human maxilla. *J Periodontol* 74:945–956.

Van Steenberghe D, Naert I, Jacobs R, Quirynen M. 1999. Influence of inflammatory reactions vs. occlusal loading on peri-implant marginal bone level. *Adv Dent Res* 13:130–135.

Vandamme K, Naert I, Geris L, Vander Sloten J, Puers R, Duyck J. 2007a. Histodynamics of bone tissue formation around immediately loaded cylindrical implants in the rabbit. *Clin Oral Implants Res* 18:471–480.

Vandamme K, Naert I, Geris L, Vander Sloten J, Puers R, Duyck J. 2007b. Influence of controlled immediate loading and implant design on peri-implant bone formation. *J Clin Periodontol* 34:172–181.

Vandamme K, Naert I, Geris L, Vander Sloten J, Puers R, Duyck J. 2007c. The effect of micro-motion on the tissue response around immediately loaded roughened titanium implants in the rabbit. *Eur J Oral Sci* 115:21–29.

Vandamme K, Naert I, Vander Sloten J, Puers R, Duyck J. 2008. Effect of implant surface roughness and loading on peri-implant bone formation. *J Periodontol* 79:150–157.

Weber HP, Crohin CC, Fiorellini JP. 2000. A 5-year prospective clinical and radiographic study of non-submerged dental implants. *Clin Oral Implants Res* 11:144–153.

Weingart D, Steinemann S, Schilli W, Strub JR, Hellerich U, Assenmacher J, Simpson J. 1994. Titanium deposition in regional lymph nodes after insertion of titanium screw implants in the maxillofacial region. *Int J Oral Maxillofac Surg* 23:450–452.

Patient Focus on Neurophysiology

20

A NEUROPHYSIOLOGIC PERSPECTIVE ON REHABILITATION WITH ORAL IMPLANTS AND THEIR POTENTIAL SIDE EFFECTS

Barry J. Sessle, Iven Klineberg, and Peter Svensson

Introduction

Numerous studies reviewed in this book have addressed the biomechanics, tissue reactions, and the benefits of oral implants to restore function impaired by the loss of teeth. Some neurophysiologic studies have provided an initial understanding of the potential neural substrate contributing to this restoration of function, for example, by documenting that stimulation of oral implants evokes neural activity in the sensorimotor cortex as well as jaw reflexes in humans. Nevertheless, the exact site(s) of the sense organs ("receptors") activated by such stimulation (e.g., bone, other peri-implant tissues) and their func-tional properties are still unclear (for review, see Abarca et al. 2006; Feine et al. 2006; Sessle 2006). Also lacking are detailed inves-tigations of the learning and adaptive proc-esses in the brain that may be associated with the loss of teeth in the first place, or with their replacement. How do we adapt (or not) to such an altered oral environment and learn to function with the modified occlusion? How do clinical approaches aimed at restoring orofacial function (e.g., bridges, dentures, implants) produce their rehabilitative effect? There is emerging evidence that alterations to the occlusion or other intraoral tissues produce neuroplastic changes in areas of the central nervous system (CNS) such as the sen-sorimotor cerebral cortex that are crucial for our ability to learn and adapt our sensorimo-tor system to the new intraoral environment. There is also evidence that dysfunctional neuro-plastic changes in the CNS may occur in response to installation of oral implants and in some patients lead to serious side effects such as pain and dysesthesia. This evidence will be reviewed, but first a brief overview of the sensorimotor cortex is provided.

Overview of the Sensorimotor Cortex

The sensorimotor cortex includes a precentral gyrus containing the primary motor cortex (MI) and the postcentral gyrus that includes the primary somatosensory cortical area (SI). Studies employing cortical surface electrical stimulation, intracortical microstimulation (ICMS), or cortical neural recordings in animals, or electrical stimulation, transcranial magnetic stimulation (TMS), or brain imaging techniques in humans have documented the topographic representation of muscles or movements in MI and shown that the major role of MI is in the initiation, control, and execution of limb and orofacial movements; it also contributes to the learning of new motor skills (for review, see Sanes and Donoghue 2000; Sessle et al. 1999, 2005). In addition, studies of the so-called face MI have revealed its involvement in the control not only of elemental and learned movements of the face, jaw, and tongue (e.g., jaw-opening, tongue protrusion) but also of semi-automatic movements such as mastication and swallowing.

MI and also SI receive afferent inputs from different regions of the body. In SI in particular they are represented in a topographical arrangement. In processing the somatosensory information generated by these sensory inputs, SI plays a critical role in somatosensory acuity, detection, and documentation of stimuli applied to the body. It also contributes to motor control through its interconnections with MI and its descending connections to lower parts of the CNS by which it can exert corticofugal modulation of CNS regions transmitting sensory information that is generated during movements and transmitted to the cortex (for review, see Buonomano and Merzenich 1998; Ebner 2005).

Sensorimotor Cortex Neuroplasticity

Learning a new motor skill is associated with, and indeed may be dependent upon, functional and structural changes in MI, with the size of a motor representation in MI related to the motor skill, for example, expansion of the digits' neural representation in limb MI when a subject is trained in a novel task involving the fingers. Such a change reflects so-called neuroplasticity and may also occur when there are alterations in the somatosensory inputs to the sensorimotor cortex, for example, as a consequence of peripheral sensory or motor nerve lesions or manipulations (for review, see Buonomano and Merzenich 1998; Chen et al. 2002; Ebner 2005; Sanes and Donoghue 2000). SI may also undergo neuroplastic changes in association with motor skill acquisition, sensory manipulations, or loss of sensory inputs ("deafferentation" by traumatic injury of a sensory nerve; see section below), for example, expansion within SI of body representations adjacent to a deafferented peripheral site. These neuroplastic changes in MI and SI may last months or longer, and comparable alterations in auditory and visual cortices underscore what appears to be a general principle of neuroplasticity of sensory and motor cortices in relation to motor learning or changes in the sensory environment. Neuroplastic changes in subcortical regions (as well as other cortical areas) may also contribute, as noted below.

Recent studies indicate that neuroplasticity occurs in the face sensorimotor cortex in association with orofacial motor skill acquisition or following manipulations of orofacial sensory inputs. After a 1–2 month period of training awake monkeys in a novel tongue-protrusion task, a significant increase occurs in the proportion of discrete ICMS-defined efferent zones for tongue protrusion in the monkey's face MI and a significant decrease in MI zones for lateral tongue movement. This is associated with a significant increase in the proportion of MI (and SI neurones) showing tongue protrusion-related activity and the proportion of neurones receiving tactile sensory inputs from the tongue (see Sessle et al. 2005, 2007). Comparable neuroplastic changes may also occur in humans since after only 1 hour or less of successful training in a tongue-protrusion task analogous to that used in the monkey studies, human subjects show a significant increase in the MI tongue representation, a significant decrease in the TMS-evoked thresholds for tongue activation, and an increase in the amplitude of TMS-evoked tongue motor potentials (Boudreau et al. 2007; Svensson et al. 2003, 2006).

Also of interest in these human studies was the finding that pain induced by intraoral application of the irritant capsaicin interfered with both the face MI neuroplasticity and the acquisition of the tongue motor skill (Boudreau et al. 2007). This novel finding is consistent with other studies reporting that manipulating facial sensory inputs or motor function is associated with neuroplastic changes in face MI (for review, see Sessle et al. 2005, 2007). The Sessle laboratory has also documented face MI neuroplasticity following changes in the oral environment (Adachi et al. 2008; Sessle et al. 2007). Trimming of the rat mandibular incisors (to take them out of occlusion with the maxillary incisors) or loss of one incisor (through extraction) or transection of the lingual nerve produces neuroplastic changes within days in the ICMS-defined parameters of face MI. Whereas altering the occlusion of the teeth by incisor trimming induces a significant reduction (compared to sham treatment) in the anterior digastric representation in face MI, incisor extraction induces a significantly increased digastric representation of this jaw muscle. Lingual nerve trauma initially produces a decreased digastric and genioglossus representation followed later by an increased genioglossus representation. Neuroplasticity of face SI has also been reported after incisor extraction and other orofacial manipulations (see Henry et al. 2005; Sessle et al. 2007).

Other Examples of Central Neuroplasticity

In addition to the cortical changes noted above, neuroplastic changes may also occur in subcortical regions following orofacial stimulation, trauma, or other alterations in the orofacial region. Especially notable is the cascade of intracellular events in the second-order nociceptive neurons of the trigeminal brainstem sensory nuclear complex (VBSNC) that can occur after peripheral tissue injury or inflammation, and can lead to spontaneous discharges, reduced thresholds, and increased responses to peripheral stimuli, as well as expansion of receptive fields of the neurons. This "central sensitization" is important in spontaneous pain, pain referral, and hyperalgesia and allodynia (see below), features that are typical of many neuropathic pain conditions; peripheral sensitization reflecting an increased excitability of nociceptive afferents may also contribute to some of these features (see Hansson et al. 2001; Sessle 2006). Let's now consider further the clinical significance of such neuroplastic changes.

Clinical Implications of Central Neuroplasticity

Biological adaptability of the stomatognathic system to restorations and prostheses is an expectation, but also includes the key paradigm of psychosocial factors for aesthetic acceptance and well-being, and neurophysiological factors of central neuroplasticity that provide mechanisms for task-dependent adaptation to changes in dental status as described previously (see also Sessle 2005; Sessle et al. 2007). These mechanisms allow patients to develop confidence and competence with their oral rehabilitation (fixed and removable appliances) (Feine and Lund 2006; Feine et al. 2006; Klineberg et al. 2007; Miyaura et al. 2000; Sessle 2005; Sessle et al. 2005).

Although the masticatory system has a remarkable capacity to adapt, this capacity may be compromised by many factors including parafunction, psychosocial, and neurological influences. As a result, maladaption may occur and lead to physiological developments including chronic pain and temporomandibular disorders. For example, tissue injury with trauma to peripheral nerve branches and possible aberrant nerve repair are recognized as a trigger for chronic symptoms, since injury may provoke neurological change with alteration of neural sodium channels and development of peripheral and central sensitization associated with neuropathic pain (see below). Longstanding dental symptoms may arise from a cusp or crown fracture (so called "split-tooth") and require progressively complex dental treatment including restorations, endodontic treatment, post-core, and crown as a not-infrequent approach to the management of persistent dental pain. It is also acknowledged that extraction of such teeth does not necessarily result in pain relief. Continuing symptoms under such circumstances are recognized as chronic pain of neuropathic origin. Neuropathic pain in medical and dental practice presents a management challenge, as it may be a manifestation of altered endogenous pain control affecting the balance of inhibitory and facilitatory influences leading to pain persistence. These aspects will be considered in more detail in the following section.

Neuropathic Orofacial Pain

Traumatic events such as mechanical, thermal, or chemical stimuli to trigeminal nerve branches can lead to primary lesions that may be, but are not always, associated with neuropathic orofacial pain (NOP). In fact, the trigeminal system seems to be less vulnerable compared to the spinal system in the risk of developing neuropathic pain following a nerve injury (Bennett 2004). Operationalized criteria for the diagnosis of NOP have only very recently been proposed (Treede et al. 2007) together with a suggestion for a new definition of neuropathic pain as "pain arising as a direct consequence of a lesion or disease affecting the somatosensory system." Similar criteria need to be developed and tested for NOP (Drangsholt et al. 2007). Many diseases can cause

lesions to the somatosensory system, for example, autoimmune diseases, metabolic diseases, infections, vascular diseases, and cancer, but here we will only consider dental procedures and trauma that may potentially induce NOP of a peripheral origin.

Epidemiology

Extraction of a tooth is a deafferentation (see Klineberg and Murray 1999) of the nerve supply to the tooth pulp. Fortunately, these procedures, which still are very common in dental practice due to advanced caries and periodontitis, only appear to carry a very small risk for development of NOP. It has been proposed that chronic infections and inflammatory reactions in the tooth pulp or periapical region may in some cases increase the risk, but there are no systematic data available on this topic (Woda and Pionchon 2000). The increasing use of oral implants and the associated surgical procedures may also contribute to risk for trigeminal nerve injuries (Jaaskelainen et al. 2005). The literature is, however, scarce on this topic, most likely as a reflection of the problems with an operationalized classification of NOP. There is some information on the prevalence of somatosensory dysfunction following rehabilitation with oral implants. Ellies (1992) found in a retrospective study (n = 266) that about one-third of the patients had short-term somatosensory changes and 13% had long-term changes. Walton (2000) reported in a prospective study that 24% of patients (n = 75) had short-term changes and only 1% long-term (1 year) changes in somatosensory function. In general, the prevalence of somatosensory disturbances following insertion of oral implants appears to vary between zero and 44%, but the numbers are dependent on how somatosensory function is assessed, for example, patient-based reports or psychophysical tests. Dao and Mellor (1998) pointed out that the site of implant placement, the type of surgical procedure, the design of the study, the sensitivity of the testing methods, the choice of outcome parameters, and the terminology used could have a significant impact on the prevalence of somatosensory disturbances and NOP. There is clearly a need for a standardization of questionnaires and psychophysical testings (Abarca et al. 2006; Svensson et al. 2004).

Symptomatology of Neuropathic Orofacial Pain

Patients with NOP often complain of a constant burning pain starting with a clear traumatic onset; there may, however, be a delay between trauma and development of pain. Burning is frequently used to describe the pain, but other descriptors such as dull, aching, sharp, and shooting are also commonly reported. In addition to the spontaneous pain, there is frequently stimulus-evoked pain triggered mainly by mechanical stimuli (allodynia and hyperalgesia), for example, touching the skin or oral mucosa, or intensified by normal oral functions such as chewing, talking, and jaw opening.

Clinical findings are normally rare. There are no visible signs of inflammation and only in very rare cases may there be swelling and reddening of the facial skin or oral mucosa, possibly mimicking complex regional pain syndromes (Lewis et al. 2007). One of the hallmark findings in neuropathic pain is change in somatosensory function (Treede et al. 2007). The use of quantitative sensory tests (QSTs) has revealed a number of somatosensory disturbances with both hypo- and hyperesthesia. According to the new criteria suggested by Treede et al. (2007), there may be either gain or loss in somatosensory function within the painful area, possibly because deafferentation of small areas can potentially be masked by hyperphenomona from the surrounding areas (Finnerup and Jensen 2006). It should be noted that although a number of QST techniques are available for intraoral use (Jacobs et al. 2002; Svensson et al. 2004), there are no widely accepted guidelines for the standardized assessment of intraoral sen-

sitivity, which varies substantially from region to region and with type, thickness, and vascularisation of the tissues. However, in the painful facial areas of patients with NOP, increased temperature and tactile thresholds have been demonstrated in addition to abnormal temporal summation of painful stimuli (e.g., Eide and Rabben 1998). Relatively few QST studies are available and there appear to be modality-specific differences, which suggests that a comprehensive battery of QST techniques should be used (Rolke et al. 2006).

A number of electrophysiological tests may be of help in the diagnosis of neuropathic pain (Cruccu et al. 2004). For example, the blink reflex and recording of sensory nerve action potentials can provide important diagnostic information about the integrity of trigeminal nerve fibers (Jaaskelainen et al. 2005). In addition, laser-evoked potentials and brain stem reflexes can be used (Cruccu et al. 2004).

Pathophysiology of Neuropathic Orofacial Pain

The underlying pathophysiology of NOP involves the same basic mechanisms linked with lesions of spinal nerves and an illustration of dysfunctional neuroplasticity (Baron 2006; Campbell and Meyer 2006). In brief, the mechanisms involved in an injury to a peripheral nerve can be summarized as sensitization of the primary afferent due to up-regulation of sodium channels and ectopic activity. One of the many consequences is an increased release of glutamate and activation of ionotropic NMDA receptors and metabotropic glutamate receptors on second-order neurons in the CNS, for example, in the VBSNC, where it can lead to the central sensitization mentioned above. In addition, loss of inhibitory control and involvement of glia in the CNS, as well as the interaction between somatic afferent fibers and sympathetic activity, may contribute (see Hansson et al. 2001; Marchand et al. 2005; Sessle 2006).

Management

There are relatively few controlled clinical trials on the specific management of NOP, but generally the same principles and guidelines for other neuropathic pain conditions should be followed. Thus, low doses of tricyclic antidepressants and selective serotonin and norepinephrine reuptake inhibitors would be the first choice (Dworkin et al. 2007). Antiepileptics with calcium channel alpha2-delta ligands such as gabapentin and pregabalin would be second choices, followed by opioids and tramadol. Capsaicin and other topical formulations such as lidocaine patches have been reported to be effective in some NOP conditions but mainly in open trials. The advantage of topical medication is the potential to reduce the side effects, but so far there is only limited evidence for their efficacy (Lewis et al. 2007). An important point is to avoid further trauma to the area by avoiding further explorative oral surgery (e.g., tooth extraction, endodontics).

Knowledge about the sensory manifestations and the neuroplasticity in peripheral tissues as well as CNS is essential for correct diagnosis and management of NOP associated with insertion of oral implants. Interestingly, recent studies have suggested the usefulness of sensory retraining to combat the unwarranted somatosensory side effects ("a sensory rehabilitation strategy"), and this appears to be a promising avenue (Phillips et al. 2007). In the following section, the effects of implants on oral sensorimotor function will be considered.

Sensorimotor Function and Its Control

The complex regulation of chewing and swallowing is dependent on a learned pattern of jaw movements through progressive peripheral feedback, which develops from sucking during oro-facial maturation; it is encoded in the brain stem and sensorimotor cortex, through peripheral afferent input from mechanoreceptors including periodontium, jaw muscles, temporomandibular joints, and skin. Of special importance in dentate situations are periodontal mechanoreceptors around tooth roots, which provide an exquisitely sensitive feedback system to monitor tooth loading and the directional specifics of occlusal forces.

The following briefly summarizes the key differences in proprioceptive feedback between teeth and dental implants in the control of jaw function with restorative and prosthodontic restorations. Data has been derived from clinical studies in humans, supported by correlated studies in animals.

Proprioception Associated with Teeth as Indications for Occlusal Scheme Design

Details of periodontal mechanoreceptor function have been progressively acquired through microneurographic recordings in human subjects (see Trulsson 2005, 2006; Trulsson and Essick 2004). Periodontal afferents signal the effects of vertical and horizontal forces on teeth to the brain through "population" effects, where many mechanoreceptors are evoked, but feedback from individual teeth dominate at a particular time depending on bite force location. The "population" effect allows encoding of load magnitude and direction.

Afferents from periodontal mechanoreceptors are especially sensitive to low forces, and there are specific differences between load thresholds for anterior and posterior teeth: Anterior teeth have a dynamic sensitivity to low forces $<1.0 \, N$ and posterior teeth to higher forces of $4.0 \, N$ or greater. Anterior teeth are able to detect varying loads in all directions (presumably arising from the relatively greater number of mechanoreceptor afferents associated with anterior teeth; Trulsson 2006); posterior tooth afferents appear to detect loads only in distal and lingual directions. By contrast, static sensitivity increases progressively from anterior to posterior teeth, which is of particular importance in the control of increases in bite force on posterior teeth to generate the power stroke required for crushing food.

These features differentiate neurophysiological roles of anterior and posterior teeth, where static responses are similar yet dynamic responses are different: Anterior teeth have higher sensitivity to low forces but reach their force limit early, while posterior teeth have higher sensitivity at higher force levels and for longer periods. The data also define the role of periodontal mechanoreceptors in providing fine control of jaw movements required for food manipulation during chewing, and in providing dynamic and static influences on muscle spindle activity.

The clinical implications of these data are significant, as they provide evidence for occlusal scheme design. In particular, (1) anterior guidance on teeth is desirable based on the dynamic sensitivity data (above), as a specific requirement for anterior tooth form (aesthetics) and function providing the delicate control for anterior bite force; and (2) the lower periodontal innervation of posterior teeth (see Trulsson 2006) is associated with the generation of larger posterior chewing forces, while the reduced directionally specific feedback appears to be appropriate for the control of vertically and laterally directed forces. The provision of narrow posterior occlusal width and reduced cuspal inclines may be justified to reduce vertical and lateral forces.

Proprioception Associated with Implants: Osseoperception

The peripheral feedback system is different for implants, as a result of the absence in peri-implant tissues of similar mechanoreceptors to those located in periodontal tissues. However, given the successful functional rehabilitation outcomes in short- and long-term studies of implants supporting tooth crowns and larger prostheses, other peripheral mech-

anisms appear to play a role (Jacobs and van Steenberghe 2006; Klineberg and Murray 1999; Van Steenberghe and Jacobs 2006). In addition, central neuroplasticity (see above) is likely to be a feature of restoration of jaw function with implants, as noted below.

Functional loading is in general transient, unless the food bolus is dense and difficult to break down. In the latter situation, crown load points or areas are important with implants, and high loads in posterior quadrants are best dissipated (in a mechanical context) along the long axis of the implant or tooth. However desirable, vertical loads are not consistent and heavy loads generate bending moments that are transferred to the supporting bone. Gotfredsen et al. (2001) reported evidence that static continuous loads on implants resulted in increased bone density, which is supported by data of Heitz-Mayfield et al. (2004) data indicating that transient functional loads are acceptable physiologically as a trigger for bone remodeling.

Modulation of function where implant crowns and bridges are located between natural teeth requires minimal adaptation due to the established control mechanisms associated with surrounding teeth, but is likely to involve central neuroplasticity in response to the changed intraoral situation.

More extensive segmental and full-arch implant restorations involve a major change in mechanotransduction and feedback associated with progressive osseointegration of the implant-bone interface supporting fixed implant or implant-supported superstructures, as osseointegration-linked "osseoperception." Osseointegration was initially described as a "direct anchorage to the bone tissue" (Brånemark et al. 1977), recognizing the unique properties of commercially pure titanium (CPTi) when atraumatically placed into bone. Research on interface biology over the last two decades has included implant surface modification of the CPTi to develop a polycrystalline surface with surface irregularities of prescribed size and periodicity. The resulting increase in surface crystalinity enhances the bone response (Buser et al. 2004;

Hall and Lausmaa 2000; Larsson 2000; Sul et al. 2005, 2006), which is complex and involves stem cell recruitment, cell proliferation, and extracellular matrix production with progressive mineralization. The latter specifically includes the release of extracellular matrix proteins osteocalcin and osteopontin during bone matrix expression (for review, see Klineberg and Calford 2005). The continuity of osseointegration linked to a more broadly based view of osseoperception as the functional requirement is now recognized (Feine et al. 2006; Jacobs and van Steenberghe 2006; Klineberg and Calford 2005; Van Steenberghe 2000).

It is evident that the face sensorimotor cortex also has a crucial role in the neuroplasticity associated with rapid adaptation to dental-specific changes. Data on neuroplastic changes in face MI and SI, derived primarily from animal studies (see above and Sessle et al. 2007), have shown that changes occur in association with changes in tooth form and tooth loss. It is a reasonable expectation that neuroplasticity also has a crucial role with the restoration of function with implant replacement of lost teeth and occlusal form in implant rehabilitation. The human data from Svensson et al. (2006) of rapid neuroplastic changes in MI, as a task-specific response, by implication supports the concept of similar adaptive mechanisms with implant replacement of lost teeth and tissues.

The contemporary data on central neuroplasticity and its role in adaptation to changed intraoral conditions is compelling, as is the recognition of the continuous and changing peripheral mechanoreceptor feedback required for function with teeth and with changes in their form with intracoronal restorations, crowns, and bridgework, as well as with implant rehabilitation of lost teeth and tissues. These data for the first time provide the clinician with an evidence-based explanation for the remarkable adaptive capacity of the jaw sensorimotor system, with dental restorative and oral rehabilitation treatment, to ensure that function is maintained and possibly enhanced.

Conclusions, and a New Paradigm for Integrating Form and Function

Clinical outcomes are related to psychosocial factors and are dependent primarily on clinician-patient interaction, but not dependent on the number of natural teeth remaining, nor necessarily on their condition (pain is an exception, as described above), nor bite force or chewing efficiency. This is clearly indicated with complete dentures for totally edentulous patients, as well as with maxillofacial prostheses, where the "prosthetic condition" (defined by De Baat et al. 1997) has no correlation with the patient's subjective judgment of his or her prostheses (De Baat et al. 1997; Schoen et al. 2007; Takata et al. 2006). The recognition by clinicians of the need for a patient-centered focus ensures that each patient's psychological needs are addressed through informed consent to optimize patient satisfaction including a sense of well-being, while background neurophysiological adaptation ensures optimization of function.

Clinical treatment is in general provided in the wishful expectation that the system will continue to function or that function will be enhanced, and also is often designed with emphasis on specific occlusal form and tooth contact relationships, without any validated clinical evidence to justify these specific requirements apart from personal preference and that it "works in my hands."

The emerging data on cortical neuroplasticity following intraoral changes provides an explanation for adaptation to variations in occlusal form and clinical treatment success, which is independent of occlusal form or tooth contact specifics. This prompts a new paradigm for understanding clinical outcomes since the data available from animal and clinical studies outlined earlier has indicated that subtle and gross changes to tooth form (or other changes in the oral cavity) lead rapidly to changes in somatosensory or motor representations in the face sensorimotor cortex. These data, by implication, confirm that plasticity of the face sensorimotor cortex, provoked to accommodate changes to tooth form and occlusal relationships, is crucially important for maintaining and enhancing masticatory function. The novel findings of face MI and SI neuroplasticity suggest that it reflects dynamic, adaptive constructs that underlie our ability to learn new motor skills but is also responsive to changes in the oral sensory environment to the extent that face MI and SI neuroplasticity is crucial for the adaptation and learning of new motor skills and behavior appropriate to the altered sensory environment. It is clear from the dental literature that adaptive behaviors occur when the occlusion is modified or lingual or dental nerve damaged, and in some cases maladaptive behaviors and development of somatosensory disturbances and neuropathic pain may result that compromises even the best-intentioned rehabilitative approaches. Building upon its recent findings in rat and monkey models, the Sessle laboratory is currently examining whether oral implants and their loading also are associated with neuroplastic changes in face MI and SI that may account for our ability to adapt to the altered oral environment and acquire the necessary motor skill to function within the new dental framework. Such studies to clarify the cortical, and also subcortical, mechanisms associated with changes in the oral sensory environment and the adaptive mechanisms associated with these changes are crucial for understanding how humans learn, or re-learn, oral motor behaviors or adapt or not to an altered oral environment. Advances in brain imaging techniques as well as other non-invasive neurophysiological measures in humans will facilitate such research avenues. The findings will also be important for developing even better rehabilitative strategies to exploit these mechanisms in humans suffering from orofacial sensorimotor deficits.

References

Abarca M, Van Steenberghe D, Malevez C, De Ridder J, Jacobs R. 2006. Neurosensory disturbances after immediate loading of implants in the anterior mandible: An initial questionnaire approach followed by a psychophysical assessment. *Clin Oral Investig* 10:269–277.

Abarca M, Van Steenberghe D, Malevez C, Jacobs R. 2006. The neurophysiology of osseointegrated oral implants. A clinically underestimated aspect. *J Oral Rehabil* 33:161–169.

Adachi K, Lee J, Hu J, Yao D, Sessle BJ. 2007. Motor cortex neuroplasticity associated with lingual nerve injury in rats. *Somatosens Motor Res* 24:1–13.

Baron R. 2006. Mechanisms of disease: Neuropathic pain—a clinical perspective. *Nature Clin Practice Neurology* 2:95–106.

Bennett GJ. 2004. Neuropathic pain in the orofacial region: Clinical and research challenges. *J Orofac Pain* 18:281–286.

Boudreau S, Romaniello A, Wang K, Svensson P, Sessle BJ, Arendt-Nielsen L. 2007. The effects of intra-oral pain on motor cortex neuroplasticity associated with short-term novel tongue-protrusion training in humans. *Pain* 132:169–178.

Brånemark PI, Hansson BO, Adell R, Breine U, Lindström J, Hallen O, Ohman A. 1977. Osseointegrated implants in the treatment of the edentulous jaw. Experience from a 10-year period. *Scand J Plast Reconstr Surg* (Suppl) 16:1–132.

Buonomano DV, Merzenich MM. 1998. Cortical plasticity: From synapses to maps. *Ann Rev Neurosci* 21:149–186.

Buser D, Broggini N, Wieland M, Schenk RK, Denzer AJ, Cochran DL, Hoffmann B, Lussi A, Steinemann SG. 2004. Enhanced bone apposition to a chemically modified SLA titanium surface. *J Dent Res* 83:529–533.

Campbell JN, Meyer RA. 2006. Mechanisms of neuropathic pain. *Neuron* 52:77–92.

Chen R, Cohen LG, Hallett M. 2002. Nervous system reorganization following injury. *Neuroscience* 111:761–773.

Cruccu G, Anand P, Attal N, Garcia-Larrea L, Haanpää M, Jørum E, Serra J, Jensen

TS. 2004. EFNS guidelines on neuropathic pain assessment. *Eur J Neurol* 11:153–162.

Dao TT, Mellor A. 1998. Sensory disturbances associated with implant surgery. *Int J Prosthodont* 11:462–469.

De Baat C, Van Aken AA, Mulder J, Kalk W. 1997. "Prosthetic condition" and patients' judgment of complete dentures. *J Prosthet Dent* 78:472–478.

Drangsholt M, Nguyen K, Svensson P. 2007. Systematic review of orofacial pain mechanisms: Which conditions are neuropathic? *J Dent Res* abstract #261.

Dworkin RH, O'Connor AB, Backonja M, Farrar JT, Finnerup NB, Jensen TS, Kalso EA, Loeser JD, Miaskowski C, Nurmikko TJ, Portenoy RK, Rice AS, Stacey BR, Treede RD, Turk DC, Wallace MS. 2007. Pharmacologic management of neuropathic pain: Evidence-based recommendations. *Pain* 132:237–251.

Ebner FF (ed.). 2005. *Neural Plasticity in Adult Somatic Sensory-Motor Systems.* Boca Raton, FL: CRC Press.

Eide PK, Rabben T. 1998. Trigeminal neuropathic pain: Pathophysiological mechanisms examined by quantitative assessment of abnormal pain and sensory perception. *Neurosurgery* 43:1103–1110.

Ellies LG. 1992. Altered sensation following mandibular implant surgery: A retrospective study. *J Prosthet Dent* 68:664–671.

Feine JS, Jacobs R, Lobbezoo F, Sessle BJ, Van Steenberghe D, Trulsson M, Fejerskov O, Svensson P. 2006. A functional perspective on oral implants—state-of-the-science and future recommendations. *J Oral Rehabil* 33:309–331.

Feine JS, Lund JP. 2006. Measuring chewing ability in randomized controlled trials with edentulous populations wearing implant prostheses. *J Oral Rehabil* 33:301–308.

Finnerup NB, Jensen TS. 2006. Mechanisms of disease: Mechanism-based classification of neuropathic pain—a critical analysis. *Nat Clin Pract Neurol* 2(2):107–115.

Gotfredsen K, Berglundh T, Lindhe J. 2001. Bone reactions adjacent to titanium implants subjected to static load. A study in the dog (I). *Clin Oral Implants Res* 12:1–8.

Hall J, Lausmaa J. 2000. Properties of a new porous oxide surface on titanium implants. *Appl Osseointeg Res* 1:5–8.

Hansson P, Lacerenza M, Marchettini P. 2001. Aspects of clinical and experimental neuropathic pain: The clinical perspective. In: *Neuropathic Pain: Pathophysiology and Treatment.* PT Hansson, HL Fields, RG Hiel, and P Marchettini (eds.). Progress in Pain Research and Management, Vol 21. Seattle: IASP Press. 1–18.

Heitz-Mayfield LJ, Schmid B, Weigel C, Gerber S, Bosshardt DD, Jonsson J, Lang NP. 2004. Does excessive occlusal load affect osseointegration? An experimental study in the dog. *Clin Oral Implants Res* 15:259–268.

Henry EC, Marasco PD, Catania KC. 2005. Plasticity of the cortical dentition representation after tooth extraction in naked mole-rats. *J Comp Neurol* 485:64–74.

Jaaskelainen SK, Teerijoki-Oksa T, Forssell H. 2005. Neurophysiologic and quantitative sensory testing in the diagnosis of trigeminal neuropathy and neuropathic pain. *Pain* 117:349–357.

Jacobs R, Van Steenberghe D. 2006. From osseoperception to implant-mediated sensory-motor interactions and related clinical implication. *J Oral Rehabil* 33:282–292.

Jacobs R, Wu CH, Van Loven K, Desnyder M, Kolenaar B, Van Steenberghe D. 2002. Methodology of oral sensory tests. *J Oral Rehabil* 29:720–730.

Klineberg I, Calford M. 2005. Introduction: From osseointegration to osseoperception. The functional translation. *Clin Exp Pharmacol Physiol* 32:97–99.

Klineberg I, Kingston D, Murray G. 2007. The bases for using a particular occlusal design in tooth and implant-borne reconstructions and complete dentures. *Clin Oral Implants Res* 18:151–167.

Klineberg I, Murray G. 1999. Osseoperception: Sensory function and proprioception. *Adv Dent Res* 13:120–129.

Larsson C. 2000. The interface between bone and implants with different surface properties. *Appl Osseointeg Res* 1:9–14.

Lewis MA, Sankar V, De Laat A, Benoliel R. 2007. Management of neuropathic orofacial pain. *Oral Surg Oral Med Oral Pathol Oral Radiol Endod* 103 Suppl:S32.e1–24.

Marchand F, Perretti M, McMahon SB. 2005. Role of the immune system in chronic pain. *Nature Rev Neuroscience* 6:521–532.

Miyaura K, Morita M, Matsuka Y, Yamashita A, Watanabe T. 2000. Rehabilitation of biting abilities in patients with different types of dental prostheses. *J Oral Rehabil* 27:1073–1076.

Phillips C, Essick G, Preisser JS, Turvey TA, Tucker M, Lin D. 2007. Sensory retraining after orthognathic surgery: Effect on patients' perception of altered sensation. *J Oral Maxillofac Surg* 65:1162–1173.

Rolke R, Baron R, Maier C, Tölle TR, Treede RD, Beyer A, Binder A, Birbaumer N, Birklein F, Bötefür IC, Braune S, Flor H, Huge V, Klug R, Landwehrmeyer GB, Magerl W, Maihöfner C, Rolko C, Schaub C, Scherens A, Sprenger T, Valet M, Wasserka B. 2006. Quantitative sensory testing in the German Research Network on Neuropathic Pain (DFNS): Standardized protocol and reference values. *Pain* 123:231–243.

Sanes N, Donoghue JP. 2000. Plasticity and primary motor cortex. *Ann Rev Neurosci* 23:393–415.

Schoen PJ, Reintsema H, Bourma J, Roodenburg JLN, Vissink A, Raghoebar GM. 2007. Quality of life related to oral function in edentulous head and neck cancer patients posttreatment. *Int J Prosthodont* 20:469–477

Sessle BJ. 2005. Biological adaptation and normative values. *Int J Prosthodont* 18:280–282.

———. 2006. Mechanisms of oral somatosensory and motor functions and their clinical correlates. *J Oral Rehabil* 33:243–261.

Sessle BJ, Adachi K, Avivi-Arber L, Lee J, Nishiura H, Yao D, Yoshino K. 2007. Neuroplasticity of face primary motor cortex control of orofacial movements. *Arch Oral Biol* 52:334–337.

Sessle BJ, Yao D, Nishiura H, Yoshino K, Lee JC, Martin RE, Murray GM. 2005. Properties and plasticity of the primate somatosensory and motor cortex related to orofacial sensorimotor function. *Clin Exp Pharmacol Physiol* 32:109–114.

Sessle B, Yao D, Yamamura K. 1999. Face primary motor cortex and somatosensory cortex: Input and output properties and functional interrelationships in the awake monkey. In: *Neurobiology of Mastication—From Molecular to Systems Approach*. Y Nakamura and BJ Sessle (eds.). Amsterdam: Elsevier. 482–493.

Sul YT, Johansson C, Albrektsson T. 2006. Which surface properties enhance bone response to implants? Comparison of oxidized magnesium, TiUnite®, and Osseotite™ implant surfaces. *Int J Prosthodont* 19:319–328.

Sul YT, Johansson C, Wennerberg A, Cho LR, Chang BS, Albrektsson T. 2005. Optimizing surface oxide properties of oxidized implants for reinforcement of osseointegration: Surface chemistry, oxide thickness, porosity, roughness, crystal structure. *Int J Oral Maxillofac Implants* 20:349–359.

Svensson P, Baad-Hansen L, Thygesen T, Juhl GI, Jensen TS. 2004. Overview on tools and methods to assess neuropathic trigeminal pain. *J Orofac Pain* 18:332–338.

Svensson P, Romaniello A, Arendt-Nielsen L, Sessle BJ. 2003. Plasticity in corticomotor control of the human tongue musculature induced by tongue-task training. *Exp Brain Res* 152:42–51.

Svensson P, Romaniello A, Wang K, Arendt-Nielsen L, Sessle BJ. 2006. One hour of tongue-task training is associated with plasticity in corticomotor control of the human tongue musculature. *Exp Brain Res* 173:165–173.

Takata Y, Ansai T, Awano S, Fukuhara M, Sonoki K, Wakisaka M, Fujisawa K, Akifusa S, Takehara T. 2006. Chewing ability and quality of life in an 80-year-old population. *J Oral Rehabil* 33:330–334.

Treede RD, Jensen TS, Campbell JN, Cruccu G, Dostrovsky JO, Griffin JW, Hansson P, Hughes R, Nurmikko T, Serra J. 2007. Neuropathic pain. Redefinition and a grading system for clinical and research purposes. *Neurology* [Epub ahead of print].

Trulsson M. 2005. Sensory and motor function of teeth and dental implants: A basis for osseoperception. *Clin Exp Pharmacol Physiol* 32:119–122.

———. 2006. Sensory-motor function of human periodontal mechanoreceptors. *J Oral Rehabil* 33:262–273.

Trulsson M, Essick GK. 2004. Mechanosensation. In: *Clinical Oral Physiology*. T Miles, B Nauntofte, and P Svensson (eds.). Copenhagen: Quintessence. 165–198.

Van Steenberghe D. 2000. From osseointegration to osseoperception. *J Dent Res* 11:1833–1837.

Van Steenberghe D, Jacobs R. 2006. Jaw motor inputs originating from osseointegrated oral implants. *J Oral Rehabil* 33:274–281.

Walton JN. 2000. Altered sensation associated with implants in the anterior mandible: A prospective study. *J Prosthet Dent* 83:443–449.

Woda A, Pionchon P. 2000. A unified concept of idiopathic orofacial pain: Pathophysiologic features. *J Orofac Pain* 14:196–212.

21

Patient Focus on Expected and Unexpected Outcomes

DENTAL IMPLANT INNOVATIONS—GROWING EVIDENCE FOR BEST DECISIONS

Kent Knoernschild

Introduction

Use of dental implants to address disabilities for partially and completely edentulous patients continues to revolutionize patient care. With advances in medicine and technology has come recognition that tooth replacement using dental implants is not only predictable but also the best solution for many. Implant-supported overdentures are first-choice options for completely edentulous patients (Feine et al. 2002). Implant-supported single- or multi-unit fixed partial dentures may be at least as predictable or more predictable than natural tooth prostheses depending upon the patient situation and time of follow-up (Iqbal and Kim 2007; Pjetursson et al. 2004; Salinas and Eckert 2007; Torabinejad et al. 2007). Such statements were not made with confidence in 1982, because osseointegrated implant and

prosthesis longevity was less well documented, and because documentation of tooth-borne prosthesis longevity was limited. Psychosocial impact of therapy on patient quality of life and satisfaction with therapy was also lacking. The current volume of evidence, although heterogeneous in study design, reported outcomes, and clinical interpretations, has allowed us to begin developing systematic reviews that investigate patient care predictability at implant, restoration, and patient levels for the completely and partially edentulous. Such analyses further assist in identifying areas for future research with the vision of effectively mitigating patient oral disability.

Comprehensive therapy is the goal, and the clinical focus must be to best fulfill needs from the patient perspective. Breadth of knowledge and skills required for predictable, patient-centered, comprehensive, prosthetically driven therapy continue to increase, and lines that have historically separated the restoring from the surgical clinician have become increasingly transparent. Categories for describing patient outcomes (Guckes et al. 1996) are presented in Table 21.1. Each outcome directly influences patient

Table 21.1.   Patient outcome categories for therapy with dental implants (adapted from Guckes et al. 1996).

Longevity/Survival	Physiologic	Psychological	Economic
Implant survival	Bone response	Patient satisfaction	Direct cost
Implant success	Bite force	Quality of life	Indirect cost
Prosthesis survival	Masticatory efficiency	Body image	Cost-benefit
Prosthesis success	Diet	Self-concept	Maintenance
Morbidity	Nutrition		Complications
Mortality			

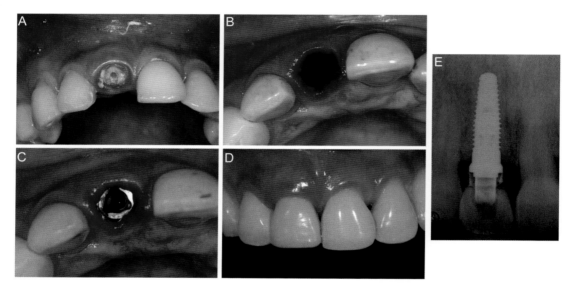

Figure 21.1.   Maxillary right central incisor single-tooth implant therapy: (a) pre-extraction, (b) atraumatic tooth extraction, (c) immediate implant placement, (d) provisional restoration on day of surgery, (e) radiographic result 3 months post-surgery. (Photos courtesy of Dr. M. Hallas, UIC Advanced Prosthodontics.)

perceptions. For example, implant or prosthesis survival or success would affect patient maintenance needs while improving masticatory efficiency and patient satisfaction. Patients neither desire nor expect implant or prosthesis complications, the incidence of which has been well summarized (Berglundh et al. 2002; Goodacre et al. 2003). Patients expect satisfaction with therapy provided in a timely manner with predictable comfort, function, and aesthetic results that ultimately improve their quality of life (Fig. 21.1). These

goals will be reached only with credible assessment of therapy innovations and analysis of published clinical evidence from those assessments.

Clinical Evidence Growth and Focus

Ongoing clinical research provides substantive resources for evidence-based decision making. In 1982 fewer than 1,000 citations

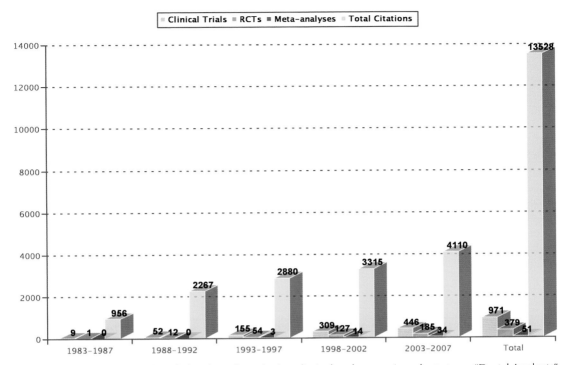

Figure 21.2. Number of PubMed dental implant citations limited to humans (search strategy: "Dental Implants" [Mesh] OR "Dental Implants, Single-Tooth"[Mesh] OR "Dental Prosthesis, Implant-Supported"[Mesh] OR "Osseointegration"[Mesh] OR "Dental Implantation"[Mesh]).

existed that supported decisions for implant patients. Figure 21.2 identifies the number of publications reported on MEDLINE as one measure of evidence production from January 1, 1983, through December 31, 2007. The MEDLINE PubMed search strategy performed on March 11, 2008, identified 16,396 citations, which represented 85% of all citations indexed with the specified dental implant terms. When citations were limited to humans, 13,528 remained. The number of human publications increased for each 5-year period beginning in 1983, and 55% of identified citations were published from 1998 to 2007. Since the 1982 Toronto Consensus Conference a more than ten-fold increase in dental implant publications has occurred. The magnitude of increase in publications is likely greater because the search strategy did not necessarily represent all research areas related

to implants, and because other electronic and manual searching methods were not completed.

Expansion in dental implant use led to increased numbers of published studies with greater rigor in research design including clinical trials, randomized controlled trials (RCTs), and meta-analyses. Figure 21.2 identifies the number of citations of each study type by 5-year period using PubMed search limits. From the search described above, a total of 1,401 citations were indexed as human clinical trials (69%), RCTs (27%), or meta-analyses (4%), and the incidence of each publication type increased over each 5-year period. The number of publications from 1998 to 2007 represented 80% of the total clinical trials, RCTs, and meta-analyses. Many publications including Cochrane Collaboration systematic reviews were recognized with this search strategy. As previously stated, additional publications could be identified with other search methods.

Evidence quality was also categorized by reported outcome. The distribution of publications identified by clinical outcome category (Fig. 21.3) shows that most studies have had a focus on bone response and maintenance and complications. Although most publications report implant survival, only those explicitly categorized as such through PubMed are reported. Table 21.2 shows the distribution of citations further identified by the proportion of clinical trials, RCTs, or meta-analyses. By comparison, fewer studies addressed psychological and economic cate-

gories, and those studies generally focused on completely edentulous patients.

More research for in-depth understanding of the impact of implants is particularly necessary for partially edentulous patients who, as a diagnostic group, present complex therapy decision-making issues. Data is necessary to support decision making with indications for endodontic therapy, single- or multi-unit implant restoration, selection of restoration design, timing of implant placement after extraction, and timing of loading after surgical placement. Systematic reviews (Esposito et al. 2006a, 2007a; Jokstad and Carr 2007; Quirynen et al. 2007; Torabinejad et al. 2007; Weber and Sukotjo

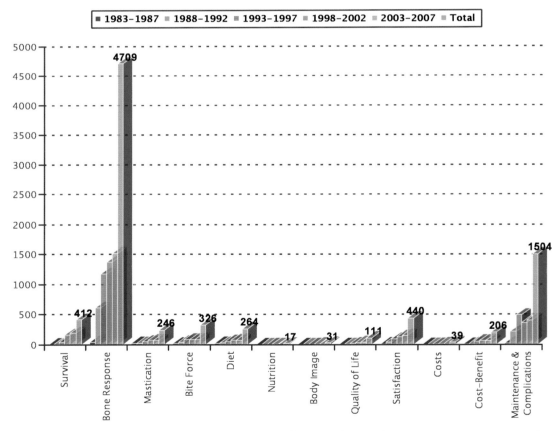

Figure 21.3. Number of PubMed dental implant citations limited to humans by patient outcome category. Values over each category represent total number of identified citations from 1983 to 2007.

Table 21.2. Number of PubMed Citations by Outcome Category (Total/[clinical trial + RCT + meta-analyses]; search strategy: ("Dental Implants"[Mesh] OR "Dental Implants, Single-Tooth"[Mesh] OR "Dental Prosthesis, Implant-Supported"[Mesh] OR "Osseointegration"[Mesh] OR "Dental Implantation"[Mesh]) AND (search terms for each outcome category in the table).

Category	Search Terms	1983–1987	1988–1992	1993–1997	1998–2002	2003–2007	Total
Survival	"Survival"[Mesh] OR "Survival Rate"[Mesh] OR "Survival Analysis"[Mesh] OR "Kaplan-Meiers Estimate"[Mesh]	0/0	8/0	44/9	164/53	196/48	412/110
Physiologic	"Bone Resorption"[Mesh] OR "Bone Remodeling"[Mesh] OR "Alveolar Bone Loss"[Mesh]	44/0	611/31	1,172/103	1,367/197	1,515/258	4,709/589
	"Mastication"[Mesh]	23/0	27/2	52/11	72/15	72/19	246/47
	"Bite Force"[Mesh]	20/0	45/0	86/4	84/4	91/8	326/16
	"Nutrition Disorders"[Mesh] OR "Nutritional Status"[Mesh] OR "Nutrition Physiology"[Mesh] OR "Nutritional Sciences"[Mesh] OR "Nutrition Assessment"[Mesh] OR "Nutrition Therapy"[Mesh] OR "Nutrition Surveys"[Mesh] OR "Nutrition Processes"[Mesh]	25/0	29/2	58/11	75/15	77/21	264/49
	"Diet"[Mesh] OR "Diet Surveys"[Mesh] OR "Food Habits"[Mesh]	2/0	0/0	3/0	9/2	2/2	16/4
Psychological	"Body Image"[Mesh] OR "Self-Concept"[Mesh] OR "Personal Autonomy"[Mesh]	3/0	3/0	5/1	13/1	7/3	31/5
	"Quality of Life"[Mesh] OR "Life Style"[Mesh] OR "Health Behavior"[Mesh] OR "Karnofsky Performance Status"[Mesh] OR "Activities of Daily Living"[Mesh]	0/0	6/0	21/3	35/6	49/13	111/22
	"Personal Satisfaction"[Mesh] OR "Patient Satisfaction"[Mesh] OR "Consumer Satisfaction"[Mesh]	14/1	40/3	96/22	135/32	155/50	440/108
Economic	Cost-Benefit Analysis[Mesh]	0/0	4/0	8/0	11/3	16/3	39/6
	"Costs and Cost Analysis"[Mesh] OR "Economics"[Mesh] OR "Cost Allocation"[Mesh] OR "Health Care Costs"[Mesh] OR "Direct Service Costs"[Mesh]	6/0	16/0	56/0	64/3	64/7	206/10
	"Maintenance"[Mesh] OR "Complications" [Subheading] OR "Intraoperative Complications"[Mesh] OR "Postoperative Complications"[Mesh] OR "complications" [Subheading]	24/1	216/11	491/47	395/29	408/46	1,534/134

2007) in these areas have produced encouraging but inconclusive prognostic results due to study heterogeneity. Further, carefully designed studies with long-term follow-up must be completed to give deeper insight for implant and prosthesis survival and success, soft and osseous tissue response, patient satisfaction, and the benefits and risks of those therapy approaches.

Prognostic Factors, Outcomes, and Patient Benefit

Outlining the growth in understanding of benefits for all types of patients is unrealistic in a short chapter, because partially and completely edentulous patients differ in disabilities, treatment needs, and therapy expectations as diagnostic groups and as individual patients. Associations have been made with patient, implant, and prosthesis prognostic factors and implant or restoration survival and success. Bone quantity, bone quality, implant site, and implant length are widely documented factors for implant survival. Fewer prognostic factors have been associated with physiologic, psychological, and economic impact due to the plethora of confounding variables. A challenge has been that standardized inclusion criteria and assessment mechanisms pre- and post-therapy were not developed until CONSORT guidelines were established. Data reporting methods have been highly variable, and the inclusion and assessment of reported data in meta-analyses and systematic reviews has been difficult.

Factors affecting healing and ongoing adaptive remodeling with function affect osseointegration, yet linking specific systemic or local prognostic factors to patient prognoses has been challenging. Although subjectively determined poorer bone quality from radiological and clinical assessments has been associated with implant failure, definitive parameters that objectively define bone quality and link quality to implant survival

and rehabilitation success are lacking. Attempts to link suspected systemic conditions to osseointegration have not been conclusive. Smoking may be associated with a greater incidence of implant failure, but studies have often analyzed data at the implant rather than the patient level, thereby biasing conclusions. Diabetic patients may have greater risk of implant failure, but evidence is not strongly supportive due to liberal study inclusion criteria. Compelling evidence does not exist to link osteoporosis or use of oral bisphosphonates to implant failure, yet concern does exist with possible postsurgical side effect of osteonecrosis with bisphosphonates. Grafting for adequate bone volume has been achieved successfully using many site-specific procedures (Aghaloo and Moy 2007; Esposito et al. 2006b; Wallace and Froum 2003), yet implant survival may be more a function of residual bone supporting the dental implant than the means used to obtain viable grafted bone (Aghaloo and Moy 2007). Implant designs vary widely, yet evidence is currently lacking to support selection of one implant design over another among well-documented systems (Esposito et al. 2007c; Jokstad et al. 2003). One- and two-stage surgical procedures may have similar results in achieving osseointegration (Esposito et al. 2007b). Although various prosthesis designs have had documented success, the best prosthesis design for optimum load distribution and adaptive remodeling for partially edentulous or completely edentulous patients is uncertain (Weber and Sukotjo 2007). Future research is necessary in all areas to improve predictability and meet patient expectations.

The following sections briefly summarize evidence that supports clinical decisions for patient benefit. Systematic reviews and meta-analyses were included for reference, but they are based upon a wide array of studies that are retrospective and prospective with differences in patient inclusion and treatment. Cochrane Collaboration Systematic Reviews that answer more explicit clinical research questions are also included.

Completely Edentulous
Patient Benefits

Implant and Prosthesis Predictability

Overdenture and fixed complete denture patient studies reported an implant survival weighted mean greater than 91% at 5 years for both treatment groups (Berglundh et al. 2002). Studies continue to confirm these trends for both prosthesis groups. Clinical results are not yet available to recommend design for long-term prosthesis survival for either arch due to widely varying designs and their application. A possible recognized difference in implant survival by prosthesis type was found at 60 months between maxillary fixed designs (CI: 82.7–92.7%) compared to maxillary removable designs (CI: 70.9–82.3%) (Bryant et al. 2007). Observed weighted mean prosthesis 5-year survival rate in studies was often 90% and often approached 100%.

Increased Bite Force; Improved Diet and Nutrition

Although bite force can be greater for edentulous patients with implant prostheses, the degree of improvement is not predictable by patient. Bite force may be a surrogate for functional stability, but evidence does not exist that bite force directly and consistently correlates to patient adaptation. Tooth loss can lead to dietary change and compromised nutrition (Allen and McMillan 2002; Fontijn-Tekamp et al. 1996; Hutton et al. 2002; Sheiham et al. 2001), and implant-supported prostheses, both fixed and removable, have the potential to improve patient-perceived ability to masticate and swallow foods that are more difficult to chew (Allen and McMillan 2002).

Positive Psychosocial Impact

Smith and Sheiham (1979) first documented a relationship between compromised oral health in edentulous patients, unsatisfactory prostheses, and daily activities. Survey instruments have been developed for assessment of patient perspectives, and the Oral Health Impact Profile (OHIP) (Slade and Spencer 1994) is the most widely used to assess oral health-related quality of life (OHRQoL). Impact of implant-supported prostheses on the completely edentulous patient's self-esteem, quality of life, and satisfaction has been documented. A recent analysis (Strassburger et al. 2006) of 114 studies suggested patient ratings for satisfaction, aesthetics, chewing ability, cleaning ability, stability, and speech can be improved with removable or fixed prostheses in either arch, but the degree of satisfaction may be dependent upon prognostic factors that were not assessed. The number of implants needed for a specific patient may be based upon the prosthesis design, which is driven by the patient's expectations of the comprehensive rehabilitation. Two implants may be adequate to achieve patient satisfaction with mandibular overdentures (Feine et al. 2002; Geertman et al. 1996; Naert et al. 2004; Stoker et al. 2007), but patients differ in their preference for fixed or removable prostheses (Feine et al. 1994). Little information is available regarding pre-therapy patient expectations based upon comprehensive prosthodontic diagnosis. Linking of comprehensive diagnoses and patient expectations with therapy outcomes has not occurred. This is important because patients' desire for a fixed or removable prosthesis design and their ability to accommodate to their prosthesis varies. Focus in these clinical research areas is necessary.

Economic Impact

Understanding of costs for therapy is in the early stages, and trials have assessed costs and cost-benefit with implant-supported fixed or removable prostheses (Attard et al. 2005; Heydecke et al. 2005; MacEntee and Walton 1998; Palmqvist et al. 2004; Stoker et al. 2007). With advances in implant therapy has come documentation of complications. Incidence of these complications was frequently reported as indicated in Figure 21.3, and a summary of complication has been published (Goodacre et al. 2003). These complications must be considered in the context of alternative therapies, benefits, and risks. A standardized method for documentation of complications with linking to potential prognostic factors does not exist.

Partially Edentulous Patient Benefits

Implant and Prosthesis Predictability

One systematic review suggested implant survival for single- and multi-unit prostheses may be similar at 5 years, at 94% (Weber and Sukotjo 2007), whereas another meta-analysis (Lindh et al. 1998) showed greater implant survival at 5 years with single-unit (97.5%) restorations compared to multi-unit (94.0%). Timing of loading is important, and early or immediate restoration after placement can be successful in selected patients (Esposito et al. 2007c; Jokstad and Carr 2007). Survival of prostheses in both reviews was greater than 90%. Greater risk of failure may occur in the maxillary posterior, and implants in grafted sinus have increased risk (Graziani et al. 2004). To maintain a specific tooth compared to its extraction and placement of a tooth or implant-supported restoration must be focused on patient factors often not recorded in studies. However, endodontic therapy for periodontally sound teeth with pulpal or periapical pathosis compared to a single-tooth implant-supported prosthesis have substantial and similar long-term prognoses (Torabinejad et al. 2007). Implant pooled success and survival rates were 95% (CI: 93–96%) and 97% (CI: 95–99%), respectively. Tooth-borne FPDs exhibited success and survival rates of appro-

ximately 80% at 6 or more years, which was consistent with the results of several previous meta-analyses. The Pjetursson et al. (2004) meta-analysis indicated an estimated survival of implants in implant-supported FPDs of 95.4% (CI 93.9–96.5%) after 5 years and 92.8% (CI: 90–94.8%) after 10 years. The survival rate of FPDs supported by implants was 95% (CI: 92.2–96.8%) after 5 years and 86.7% (CI: 82.8–89.8%) after 10 years.

Bite Force, Diet, and Nutrition

Evidence linking comprehensive restoration to physiologic assessments is largely inferred from completely edentulous or completely tooth-borne situations. Patients may find masticatory efficiency acceptable with a shortened dental arch (Sarita et al. 2003; Witter et al. 2001; Wolfart et al. 2005). Further research is necessary.

Psychosocial Impact

Few studies are available. Research study analyses (Strassburger et al. 2006; Torabinejad et al. 2007) report overall satisfaction with therapy, mastication, phonetics, and aesthetics with single-tooth or fixed partial denture restorations. Aesthetic results may be less predictable due to soft-tissue considerations (Levine et al. 2005). As for completely edentulous patients, potential associations with prosthodontic diagnoses, patient expectations, and patient-reported outcomes must be assessed.

Economic Impact

Little information regarding the costs of therapy is available. Prosthesis designs, complications, and maintenance costs vary and a standardized means to assess these issues has not been developed. Incidence of complications has been reported (Berglundh et al. 2002; Goodacre et al. 2003), but the long-term economic impact of ameliorating these complications must be addressed in future research.

Growth in Evidence Over the Next 25 Years

Several factors have led to evidence growth since 1982: (1) dentistry's embrace of evidence-based decision making, which reinforced the need for identification and use of best available information in decisions for individual patients; (2) establishment of the Cochrane Collaboration Research Group protocols that led to a population of systematic reviews with well-defined inclusion criteria; and (3) establishment of the CONSORT guidelines to standardize approaches for prospective clinical research. Although clinical decisions have been based largely on case series studies and retrospective data analysis, the above factors facilitated identification of evidence with strength, fostered development of new, well-designed clinical trials, and reinforced the need for standardized RCTs for patient care applicability and future meaningful systematic reviews.

Future clinical care and research will be driven by patients' expectations of predictable care, aesthetic outcomes, and effective function. Such research will be based on the available foundational information, which will only be best applied by specific patient diagnosis. Clinical research to support therapy has made enormous progress, yet the published results applicable to any individual patient situation are still limited for the practicing clinician. Evidence growth has led to clinician confidence in patient care using implants. In the next 25 years confidence will increase because careful analysis of the evidence will provide clinician reassurance for decisions as they apply to new patient situations. Emerging technology and clinical techniques guided by practitioner focus on patient expectations will continue to reinforce the need for evidence-based analytical principles in practice.

Future research efforts in all areas described in Table 21.1 will continue with recognition that each outcome fundamentally contributes to patient satisfaction and quality of life. Many questions must be more fully addressed: (1) Do patients realize the extent of their functional disabilities? (2) How can patient-recognized disabilities be well documented? (3) What expectations do patients have? (4) How well do implant interventions meet expectations? Furthermore, the greater proportion of future implant patients will be partially edentulous (Naert et al. 2002a, 2002b), and further research for that diagnostic group is particularly necessary.

To facilitate growth of best evidence to substantiate patient benefits, the following will occur in the next 25 years:

1. *Validation and adoption of a standardized comprehensive diagnostic system for data collection:* Elements from the American College of Prosthodontists Prosthodontic Diagnostic Index (McGarry et al. 1999, 2002) could serve as a framework for a standardized comprehensive diagnostic and research instrument.
2. *Embracing of advancing technology to optimize therapy outcomes:* Beyond 2030 patients will most commonly receive predictable, definitive implant-supported prostheses at the time of implant placement, which could often be immediately after extraction. Ability to better predict implant/prosthesis survival and therapy success through appropriate application of advanced technology is therefore necessary to achieve this scenario, along with innovative approaches for diagnosis and therapy using existing technology (e.g., computerized tomography, radiofrequency analysis, 3-D imaging for treatment planning, 3-D imaging for restoration fabrication) and new technology known or not yet discovered (e.g., identification host genomic characteristics, systemic and cellular metabolic characteristics, use of local or systematic bioactive substances for osseointegration).

3. *Development of a worldwide multicenter research database:* Multicenter study design and data collection with centralized data analysis will occur to increase the power of research conclusions and applicability.
4. *Validation and adoption of standardized instruments* for prospective assessment of objective clinical outcomes, patient expectations, and outcomes from psychological and economic perspectives.
5. *Ongoing application of a standardized instrument (e.g., OHIP)* to objectively assess effects of implant therapy on OHQOL issues.
6. *Correlation of prosthodontic diagnosis with patient expectations and patient-perceived benefit:* Clear evaluation of patient expectations and patient-perceived benefit based on comprehensive diagnosis will lead to better prediction of treatment outcomes.
7. *Widespread use of a single-care provider model for implant placement and restoration:* For thoughtfully selected situations this will effectively meet expectations for many patients.
8. *Widespread application of a clinician-friendly evidence-based decision-making model* that facilitates identification and use of the best evidence for patient benefit. Clinician expectations from published research, quality of published clinical studies, and accuracy in clinician prognostic abilities will increase. The best plans will be developed to meet patient expectations based on best evidence.

SUBJECTIVE AND OBJECTIVE EVALUATION OF IMPLANT-SUPPORTED RECONSTRUCTIONS FOR PARTIALLY EDENTULOUS PATIENTS

Klaus Gotfredsen

Subjective evaluation is of great importance when the indication for, and the outcome of, implant-supported reconstructions are evaluated and compared. Patient subjective assessments were once regarded as a secondary outcome occasionally useful to complement biologic and technical evaluation of implant-supported reconstructions, but currently the subjective evaluation is at the forefront. The indication for treatment is normally based on insufficient masticatory, aesthetics, phonetics, and/or psychosocial function (Gotfredsen and Walls 2007). Subjective evaluation is especially important for decision making as patients may have the same objective need for improving an oral function, but subjective need may be the contributing factor in the decision for starting a treatment. When patient-generated aspects are incorporated into the decision-making process, decisions initiate treatment and the evaluation of the outcome of the treatment becomes easier.

A number of publications have demonstrated that implant-supported reconstructions may also increase masticatory efficiency as well as masticatory ability and psychosocial factors, and thereby patient satisfaction (Gotfredsen and Walls 2007). To obtain information regarding these parameters the dentist normally talks to the patient in a relatively unstructured manner. More information may, however, be collected if structured interview methods are used, for example, schedule for the evaluation of individual quality of life—direct weighting (SEIQoL-DW), or standardized oral health-related quality of life (OHRQoL) questionnaires (Slade 2002). Implant-supported reconstructions increase the number of prosthetic treatment approaches, and incorporation of perspectives gained from instruments such as these is critical.

An appealing method to assess OHRQoL is to create global questions about a patient's self-rated oral health before and after treatment. The responses may be rated on an ordinal scale ranging from "excellent" to "very poor" or on a numerical scale, such as a visual analog scale (VAS). Numerous specific questions are sometimes used to evaluate multiple dimensions of OHRQoL. This approach attempts to delineate the specific experiences that encompass the researcher's definition of OHRQoL.

One of the most widely used and validated multi-item questionnaires is the Oral Health Impact Profile (OHIP). The questionnaire is based on a theoretical framework derived from the World Health Organization's International Classification of Impairments, Disabilities, and Handicaps. The OHIP-49 has been used in a number of studies comparing conventional prosthesis with implant-supported prosthesis and has consistently demonstrated improvements in OHRQoL (Allen et al. 2001; Awad et al. 2000).

A number of cohort studies have evaluated the subjective as well as the objective outcome of implant treatment. For subjective evaluation, global self-ratings have been used with a VAS, and the OHIP-49 was used before and after implant treatment. The following describes these studies.

In a 5-year prospective study of implant-supported single-tooth replacements 20 patients were asked to evaluate the functional and aesthetic outcome of the treatment using a VAS (Gotfredsen 2004). Patient inclusion criteria included (1) healthy patients without periodontal disease; (2) single-tooth loss in the anterior maxilla; and (3) mesio-distal bone width >6.5 mm in the region planned for implant therapy. A dentist not involved in the study but working with implant-supported reconstructions evaluated the aesthetic outcome of the same treatments using a VAS. The objective evaluation criteria evaluated yearly were plaque index score, bleeding score, probing pocket depth, papilla height, crown length, marginal bone level, and technical complications. A force discrimination test was performed at the implant crown as well as at the contralateral natural tooth. All the implant-supported crowns were followed for >10 years with few complications. Only one implant lost more than 1.5 mm of marginal bone during a 10-year follow-up. One crown was remade due to abutment screw loosening and another due to ceramic fracture (Fig. 21.4). The result of greatest importance was that demands for prosthetic treatment were very different among patients and between patient and dentist.

Another study entitled "Oral Function and Quality of Life for Patients with Tooth Agenesis after Oral Rehabilitation" (Dueled et al. 2008) evaluated implant-supported reconstructions subjectively and objectively. The test group consisted of 129 patients prosthetically treated for tooth agenesis. Nineteen patients were treated with tooth-supported fixed dental prostheses (FDP), and 116 were

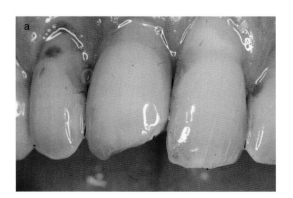
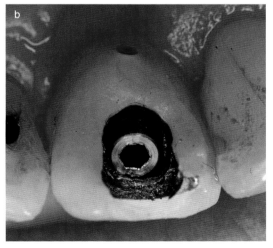

Figure 21.4.   A PFM crown with a ceramic fracture six and a half years after the baseline examination (a). The crown could easily be removed by a drilling access to the abutment screw (b).

treated with implant-supported reconstructions. Six patients were treated with both types of reconstruction. A control group of 58 patients without agenesis and matched in age and sex were included in the subjective part of the study. Before and after implant treatment all patients filled out an OHIP-49 questionnaire for an evaluation of the oral health-related quality of life. Generally, the total OHIP scores were low for both test and control group and the dimensions concerning functional limitation and physical pain were the items with highest impact (Table 21.3). The mean of the total OHIP score was higher for the patients with tooth agenesis treated with prosthetic reconstructions compared to the control group without tooth agenesis. When specific OHIP questions were analyzed, the major concerns for the patients treated with prosthetic reconstructions related to the aesthetic result. A subjective aesthetic evaluation was performed based on OHIP questions 3, 4, 20, 22, 31, and 38. The prevalence of patients reporting aesthetic problems occa-

sionally, fairly often, or very often was higher for patients treated with tooth-supported fixed partial dentures compared to patients treated with implant-supported reconstructions (Table 21.4). There was no difference in the number of tooth agenesis between the two groups. When the total test group, prosthetically treated patients with tooth agenesis, was compared with the control group the frequency of patients with aesthetic concerns was highest in the test group. In the same study an objective index score was calculated based on modified USPHS criteria for buccal, mucosal discoloration, crown morphology, crown color match score, occlusal harmony score, and papilla level score. There was no significant correlation between the objective aesthetic score and the subjective aesthetic score.

In a parallel prospective study (Dueled et al. 2008) of patients with tooth agenesis of the maxillary lateral incisor, 40 patients treated with 58 implant-supported single crowns were divided into two groups. Thirty zirconium oxide crowns were retained with ceramic abutment and compared with 28 metal-ceramic crowns retained with metallic abutments. Differences were observed between the two groups (ceramic abutment with all-ceramic crowns vs. metallic abutment with metal-ceramic crowns) following objective evaluation of the buccal, mucosal discoloration, and the crown color match score measured at the baseline examination. The subjective evaluation was also done with the OHIP-49 questionnaire before treatment and at the baseline examination. No significant differences at these two examination times were seen for the aesthetic-related questions in the OHIP-49 (i.e., OHIP-3, OHIP-4, OHIP-20, OHIP-22, OHIP-31, and OHIP-38).

In summary, the following can be concluded:

1. The demands for implant-supported reconstructions are very different among patients and between patient and dentist.
2. Whereas a great number of studies have evaluated objective variables for implant-

Table 21.3.   Oral health impact profile for patients with (test) and without (control) maxillary anterior tooth agenesis (Dueled et al. 2008).

	OHIP Score	
	Test	Control
1. Functional limitations (OHIP 1–9)	3.9	2.5
2. Physical pain (OHIP 10–18)	3.8	3.4
3. Psychological discomfort (OHIP 19–23)	2.1	1.1
4. Physical disability (OHIP 24–32)	1.2	0.5
5. Psychological disability (OHIP 33–38)	1.1	0.5
6. Social disability (OHIP 39–43)	0.4	0.1
7. Handicap (OHIP 44–49)	0.7	0.1
Total mean OHIP score	13.2	8.2

Table 21.4. Subjective aesthetic evaluations by patients with maxillary anterior tooth agenesis who have implant-supported single crowns or tooth-supported fixed partial dentures compared to untreated control patients without agenesis—prevalence (%) of patients reporting item occasionally, fairly often, or very often (Dueled et al. 2008).

	Test		Control
	ISSC* n = 116	FPD* n = 19	n = 58
OHIP 3: Have you noticed a tooth which doesn't look right?	20	28	2
OHIP 4: Have you felt that your appearance has been affected because of problems with your teeth, mouth, or dentures?	9	16	2
OHIP 20: Have you been self-conscious because of your teeth, mouth, or dentures?	9	11	9
OHIP 22: Have you felt uncomfortable about the appearance of your teeth, mouth, or dentures?	8	11	7
OHIP 31: Have you avoided smiling because of problems with your teeth, mouth, or dentures?	10	11	3
OHIP 38: Have you been a bit embarrassed because of problems with your teeth, mouth, or dentures?	5	5	5

*6 patients had implant-supported and tooth-supported reconstructions.

supported reconstructions, only a few studies have used subjective variables.

3. Whereas a great number of objective variables have been used to evaluate the outcome of implant-supported reconstructions, only a few subjective variables have been reported.

4. There is a need for more studies evaluating the subjective indication for treatment and the treatment result.

References

Aghaloo T, Moy P. 2007. Which hard tissue augmentation techniques are the most successful in furnishing bone support for implant placement? *Int J Oral Maxillofac Implants* 22(Suppl):49–77.

Allen F, McMillan A. 2002. Food selection and perceptions of chewing ability following provision of implant and conventional prostheses in complete denture wearers. *Clin Oral Implants Res* 13:320–326.

Allen PF, McMillan AS, Walshaw D. 2001. A patient-based assessment of implant-stabilized and conventional complete dentures. *J Prosthet Dent* 85:141–147.

Attard NJ, Zarb GA, Laporte A. 2005. Long-term treatment costs associated with implant-supported mandibular prostheses in edentulous patients. *Int J Prosthodont* 18:117–123.

Awad MA, Locker D, Korner-Bitensky N, Feine JS. 2000. Measuring the effect of intra-oral implant rehabilitation on health-related quality of life in a randomized controlled clinical trial. *J Dent Res* 79:1659–1663.

Berglundh T, Persson L, Klinge B. 2002. A systematic review of the incidence of biological and technical complications in implant dentistry reported in prospective longitudinal studies of at least 5 years. *J Clin Periodontol* 29(Suppl)3: 197–212.

Bryant SR, MacDonald-Jankowski D, Kim K. 2007. Does the type of implant prosthesis affect outcomes for the completely edentulous arch? *Int J Oral Maxillofac Implants* 22(Suppl):117–139.

Dueled E, Gotfredsen K, Damsgaard M, Hede B, Özhayat E. 2008. Oral function and quality of life for patients with tooth agenesis after oral rehabilitation. Abstract. Scandinavian Society of Prosthetic Dentistry Annual Meeting, Copenhagen, Denmark.

Esposito M, Grusovin MG, Martinis E, Coulthard P, Worthington HV. 2007b. Interventions for replacing missing teeth: 1- versus 2-stage implant placement. *Cochrane Database of Systematic Reviews* 18(3):CD006698.

Esposito M, Grusovin MG, Willings M, Coulthard P, Worthington HV. 2007a. The effectiveness of immediate, early, and conventional loading of dental implants: A Cochrane systematic review of randomized controlled clinical trials. *Int J Oral Maxillofac Implants* 22(6):893–904.

Esposito M, Grusovin MG, Worthington HV, Coulthard P. 2006b. The efficacy of various bone augmentation procedures for dental implants: A Cochrane Systematic Review of randomized controlled clinical trials. *Int J Oral Maxillofac Implants* 21:696–710.

Esposito M, Kokoulopoulou A, Couthard P, Worthington HV. 2006a. Interventions for replacing missing teeth: Dental implants in fresh extraction sockets (immediate, immediate-delayed and delayed implants). *Cochrane Database of Systematic Reviews* Oct 18(4):CD005968.

Esposito M, Murray-Curtis L, Grusovin MG, Coulthard P, Worthington HV. 2007c. Interventions for replacing missing teeth: Different types of dental implants. *Cochrane Database of Systematic Reviews* 17(4):CD003815.

Feine JS, Carlsson GE, Awad MA, Chehade A, Duncan WJ, Gizani S, Head T, Lund JP, MacEntee M, Mericske-Stern R, Mojon P, Morais J, Naert I, Payne AG, Penrod J, Stoker GT, Jr., Tawse-Smith A, Taylor TD, Thomason JM, Thomson WM, Wismeijer D. 2002. The McGill Consensus Statement on Overdentures. Montreal, Quebec,

Canada. May 24–25, 2002. *Int J Prosthodont* 5(4):413–414.

Feine JS, De Grandmont P, Boudrias P, Brien N, LaMarche C, Tache R, Lund JP. 1994. Within-subject comparisons of implant-supported mandibular prostheses: Choice of prosthesis. *J Dent Res* 73:1105–1111.

Fontijn-Tekamp FA, Van't Hof MA, Slater AP, Van Waas MA. 1996. The state of dentition in relation to nutrition in elderly Europeans in the SENECA study of 1993. *Eur J Clin Nutrition* 50(Suppl 2):S117–122.

Geertman M, Van Waas M, Van't Hof M, Kalk W. 1996. Denture satisfaction in a comparative study of implant-retained mandibular overdentures: A randomized clinical trial. *Int J Oral Maxillofac Implants* 11:194–200.

Goodacre CJ, Bernal G, Rungcharassaeng K, Kan JY. 2003. Clinical complications with implants and implant prostheses. *J Prosthet Dent* 90(2):121–132.

Gotfredsen K. 2004. A 5-year prospective study of single-tooth replacements supported by the Astra Tech implant. *Clin Implant Dent Relat Res* 6(1):1–8.

Gotfredsen K, Walls AWG. 2007. What dentition assures oral function. *Clin Oral Implants Res* 18(Suppl 3):34–45.

Graziani F, Donos N, Needleman I, Gabriele M, Tonetti M. 2004. Comparison of implant survival following sinus floor augmentation procedures with implants placed in pristine posterior maxillary bone: A systematic review. *Clin Oral Implants Res* 15(6):677–682.

Guckes AD, Scurria MS, Shugars DA. 1996. A conceptual framework for understanding outcomes of oral implant therapy. *J Prosthet Dent* 75(6):633–639.

Heydecke G, Penrod JR, Takanashi Y, Lund JP, Feine JS, Thomason JM. 2005. Cost-effectiveness of mandibular two-implant overdentures and conventional dentures in the edentulous elderly. *J Dent Res* 84:794–799.

Hutton B, Feine J, Morais J. 2002. Is there an association between edentulism and nutritional state? *J Can Dent Assoc* 68:182–187.

Iqbal M, Kim S. 2007. For teeth requiring endodontic treatment, what are the differences in outcomes of restored endodontically treated teeth compared to implant-supported restorations? *Int J Oral Maxillofac Implants* 22(Suppl):96–116.

Jokstad A, Braegger U, Brunski JB, Carr A, Naert I, Wennerberg A. 2003. Quality of dental implants. *Int Dent J* 53(6 Suppl 2): 409–443.

Jokstad A, Carr A. 2007. What is the effect on outcomes of time-to-loading of a fixed or removable prosthesis placed on implant(s)? *Int J Oral Maxillofac Implants* 22(Suppl):19–48.

Levine RA, Clem DS, 3rd, Wilson TG, Jr., Higginbottom F, Solnit G. 2005. Multicenter retrospective analysis of the ITI implant system used for single-tooth replacements: Results of loading for 2 or more years. *Int J Oral Maxillofac Implants* 14:516–520.

Lindh T, Gunne J, Tillberg A, Molin M. 1998. A meta-analysis of implants in partial edentulism. *Clin Oral Implants Res* 9(2):80–90.

MacEntee MI, Walton JN. 1998. The economics of complete dentures and implant-related services: A framework for analysis and preliminary outcomes. *J Prosthet Dent* 79:24–29.

McGarry TJ, Nimmo A, Skiba JF, Ahlstrom RH, Smith CR, Koumajian JH. 1999. Classification system for complete edentulism. The American College of Prosthodontists. *J Prosthodont* 8:27–39.

McGarry TJ, Nimmo, A, Skiba JF, Ahlstrom RH, Smith CR, Koumajian JH, Arbree NS. 2002. Classification system for partial edentulism. *J Prosthodont* 11:181–193.

Naert I, Alsadi G, Van Steenberghe D, Quirynen M. 2004. A 10-year randomized clinical trial on the influence of splinted and unsplinted oral implants retaining mandibular overdentures. *Int J Prosthodont* 19:695–702.

Naert I, Koutsikakis G, Duyck J, Quirynen M, Jacobs R, Van Steenberghe D. 2002a. Biologic outcome of implant-supported restoration in treatment of partial edentulism. Part 1: A longitudinal clinical evaluation. *Clin Oral Implants Res* 13:381–389.

Naert I, Koutsikakis G, Quirynen M, Duyck J, Van Steenberghe D, Jacobs R. 2002b. Biologic outcome of implant-supported restoration in the treatment of partial edentulism. Part 2: A longitudinal radiographic evaluation. *Clin Oral Implants Res* 13:390–395.

Palmqvist S, Owall B, Schou S. 2004. A prospective randomized clinical study comparing implant-supported fixed prostheses and overdentures in the edentulous mandible: Prosthodontic production time and costs. *Int J Prosthodont* 17:231–235.

Pjetursson BE, Tan K, Lang NP, Bragger U, Egger M, Zwahlen M. 2004. A systematic review of the survival and complication rates of fixed partial dentures (FPDs) after an observation period of at least 5 years. I: Implant-supported FPDs. *Clin Oral Implants Res* 15:625–642.

Quirynen M, Van Assche N, Botticelli D, Berglundh T. 2007. How does the timing of placement to extraction affect outcome? *Int J Oral Maxillofac Implants* 22(Suppl): 203–223.

Salinas T, Eckert S. 2007. In patients requiring single-tooth replacement, what are the outcomes of implant—as compared to tooth-supported restorations? *Int J Oral Maxillofac Implants* 22(Suppl):71–95.

Sarita PT, Witter DJ, Kreulen CM, Van't Hof MA, Creugers NH. 2003. Chewing ability of subjects with shortened dental arches. *Comm Dentistry Oral Epidemiol* 31:328–334.

Sheiham A, Steele JG, Marcenes W, Lowe C, Finch S, Bates CJ, Prentice A, Walls AW. 2001. The relationship among dental status, nutrient intake, and nutritional status in older people. *J Dent Res* 80(2):408–413.

Slade GD. 2002. Assessment of oral health-related quality of life. In: *Oral Health-Related Quality of Life*. MR Inglehart and

RA Bagramian (eds.). Chicago: Quintessence. 29–45.

Slade G, Spencer A. 1994. Development and evaluation of the oral health impact profile. *Comm Dental Health* 11:3–11.

Smith J, Sheiham A. 1979. How dental conditions handicap the elderly. *Comm Dentistry Oral Epidemiol* 7:305–310.

Stoker G, Wismeijer D, Van Waas MA. 2007. An eight-year follow-up to a randomized clinical trial of aftercare and cost-analysis with three types of mandibular implant-retained overdentures. *J Dent Res* 86: 276–280.

Strassburger C, Kirschbaum T, Heydecke G. 2006. Influence of implant and conventional prostheses on satisfaction and quality of life: A literature review. Part 2: Qualitative analysis and evaluation of the studies. *Int J Prosthodont* 19:339–348.

Torabinejad M, Anderson P, Bader J, Brown LJ, Chen LH, Goodacre CJ, Kattadiyil MT, Kutsenko D, Lozada J, Patel R, Petersen F, Puterman I, White SN. 2007. Outcomes of root canal treatment and restoration, implant-supported single crowns, fixed partial dentures, and extraction without replacement: A systematic review. *J Prosthet Dent* 98:285–311.

Wallace S, Froum S. 2003. Effect of maxillary sinus augmentation on the survival of endosseous dental implants. A systematic review. *Ann Periodontol* 8(1):328–343.

Weber HP, Sukotjo C. 2007. Does the type of implant prosthesis affect outcomes in the partially edentulous patient? *Int J Oral Maxillofac Implants* 22(Suppl):140–172.

Witter DJ, Creugers NH, Kreulen CM, De Haan AF. 2001. Occlusal stability in shortened dental arches. *J Dent Res* 80:432–436.

Wolfart S, Heydecke G, Luthardt RG, Marre B, Freesmeyer WB, Stark H, et al. 2005. Effects of prosthetic treatment for shortened dental arches on oral health-related quality of life, self-reports of pain and jaw disability: Results from the pilot-phase of a randomized multicentre trial. *J Oral Rehabil* 32:815–822.

Patient Focus on Function and Quality of Life and Future Implementation

J. Mark Thomason, Jocelyne S. Feine, and Daniel Wismeijer

Patient-Based Outcomes

The assessment of the quality and perform-ance of an oral prosthesis has traditionally focused on clinical assessment and laboratory testing. Until the end of the last century these outcomes were largely the standard, and it was rare to find studies in which patient-based assessments were measured. Carlsson and his colleagues appear to have been the first to use patient-based outcomes when investigating the performance of conventional dentures (Bergman and Carlsson 1972; Carlsson et al. 1967). Later, the same team included patient-based outcomes in their studies of implant prostheses (Haraldson et al. 1979). In addi-tion to measuring bite force and masticatory muscle activity, they asked participants to indicate their satisfaction with their chewing capacity (Haraldson et al. 1979). It was only in the early 1990s that other groups began to publish studies in which patient-based out-comes were included (De Grandmont et al. 1994; Wismeijer et al. 1992).

The increased interest in patient-based assessment coincided with changes in com-munication between health care providers

and their patients. Decision making began to move away from the provider being the prime decision maker, to shared decision making with informed patients with the explanation and information often based on discussions with their health care providers. Furthermore, there was increasing awareness in the profes-sion that edentulism is a chronic condition, for which treatment is by definition palliative and aimed at improving satisfaction with function and improving quality of life. No matter how efficient a prosthesis, it can not be considered successful unless the patient finds it easy to use and comfortable. There-fore laboratory assessments became less important than information from patients about how well they could chew and speak, how comfortable the prosthesis felt, and other prosthetic factors the patients consid-ered to be important to them (Feine and Lund 2006). A variety of methods has been used to gain information and to assist in understand-ing how implant support for various types of prostheses improve the lives of edentulous patients. These methods range from question-naires designed to measure satisfaction and quality of life to interviews and focus groups with edentulous individuals (De Grandmont et al. 1994; Heydecke et al. 2005a). Our profession now has a better understanding of how implant support for dentures improves patients' lives. The overwhelming majority of the studies based on patient satisfaction and quality of life outcomes published to date within the whole of restorative dentistry involved the assessment of treatment of edentulous patients, and most of these involved treatment of the edentulous mandible (Thomason et al. 2007).

The Edentulous Mandible

Most of the studies that compared conventional dentures with implant overdentures were from seven randomized controlled trials. Raghoebar and co-workers reported significantly better satisfaction scores for groups having implants or preprosthetic surgery compared with patients receiving conventional complete dentures with no surgical intervention by the end of year 1. At the end of year 5 it was the implant overdenture group that showed significantly better scores when compared to the other two groups (Raghoebar et al. 2000). These satisfaction findings were shown to impact on the patient's quality of life, certainly in terms of dental health-related quality of life (at 1 year), although they were not able to show an effect on general quality of life markers (Bouma et al. 1997).

Meijer and colleagues reported greater satisfaction with implant supported overdentures than conventional dentures at 1, 5, and 10 years. Within this study series subjects not initially allocated to the implant group were offered the opportunity to have implants. Despite the conventional denture group containing some patients converted to implants, the mean ratings of the conventional denture group were still lower than the designated implant overdenture group (Meijer et al. 1999, 2003).

Although Kapur and colleagues reported no significant differences in patient satisfaction between implant overdenture and conventional denture groups at 6 months post-treatment, the within-group changes were significantly better in the implant overdenture group (Kapur et al. 1998). In both groups, however, patients reported a decline in perceived taste and texture acceptability of almost all test foods (Roumanas et al. 2002). A similar situation has been reported by Allen and colleagues (Allen et al. 2006). Improvements in both oral health-related quality of life (OHRQoL) and satisfaction were reported for both conventional denture and implant overdenture groups; nevertheless, analysis showed no significant post-treatment differences between the groups. The authors suggested that the use of the "intention to treat" analysis may have masked the differences between groups and reported that the Oral Health Impact Profile (OHIP) change scores for those receiving implants were significantly greater than for those who refused them. Unfortunately the study was not able to show subgroup differences when analyzed "per-protocol."

The positive association between patient satisfaction and its impact on quality of life (QoL) has been reported in a series of studies based on a population of 102 middle-aged subjects (age 35–65 years) (Awad and Feine 1998; Awad et al. 2000a, 2000b, 2003a, 2003b; Heydecke et al. 2005a; Thomason et al. 2003). Satisfaction was measured using the McGill Satisfaction Questionnaire, which comprises a series of 100 mm visual analog scales (VAS) on which the patient can mark his or her level of satisfaction. The VAS are anchored by phrases indicating "completely satisfied with . . ." and "completely unsatisfied with . . ." At 2 months post-delivery general satisfaction was significantly higher in the overdenture group than in the conventional denture group, as it was for the three additional measures: comfort, stability, and ease of chewing (Awad et al. 2003a, 2003b). These general satisfaction scores can largely be explained by gender, patient's rating of comfort, stability, aesthetics, and the ability to chew (Awad and Feine 1998). At the same time point, the implant group reported significantly better QoL scores (OHIP) (Awad et al. 2000a). The implant group also reported less post-treatment looseness during eating, speaking, kissing, and yawning. They also associated less unease during kissing and during sexual activity than conventional denture subjects; a reduction in unease of around 34% (Heydecke et al. 2005b). At 6 months the implant group reported a significant difference in ability to speak, not present at 2 months, suggesting that some improvements take longer than others to establish. Overall the difference between the two groups at 6 months was greater than at 2 months (Thomason et al. 2003).

Similar results were reported by the McGill group for a senior population comparing conventional dentures with implant overdentures supported by ball attachments (Awad et al. 2003a, 2003b; Heydecke et al. 2003a). The reports that general satisfaction and ratings for comfort, stability, and ability to chew were also reflected in the observation that the implant overdenture subjects rated their OHRQoL greater than the conventional denture group (OHIP-EDENT) (Awad et al. 2003a, 2003b). These differences were not detected when using the SF36 (Heydecke et al. 2003a).

The Edentulous Maxilla

Although there are no available reports on the effect of implant rehabilitation in the maxilla with relation to OHRQoL, a number of studies report the effect on patient satisfaction of maxillary rehabilitation. In a series of case reports Naert and colleagues reported high satisfaction ratings with four splinted implants supporting a removable prosthesis (Naert et al. 1998). The Montreal group used a standard crossover trial design to compare maxillary long-bar implant overdentures with and without palatal coverage; these were opposed in the mandibular arch by a fixed implant-supported prosthesis (De Albuquerque Jr. et al. 2000). There were no significant differences between treatments, nor

significant differences compared with the new maxillary conventional denture. As a result, the authors suggested that maxillary implant prostheses should not be considered as a general treatment of choice in patients with good bony support for maxillary conventional prostheses (De Albuquerque Jr. et al. 2000).

By contrast, the same team demonstrated that long-bar overdentures were rated significantly higher than fixed prostheses in the maxilla for general satisfaction and also speaking (Heydecke et al. 2003a). In this study the majority of subjects chose to keep the removable prosthesis. The patient's reported speech ratings coincided with those of external speech assessors (Heydecke et al. 2004).

In a separate study, two groups of ten patients were treated with either a fixed prosthesis or a removable implant overdenture in a non-randomized parallel arm study. Greater within-group changes for aesthetics, taste, and speech were shown in the implant overdenture group, although there were no significant differences between groups for the major satisfaction outcomes (Zitzmann and Marinello 2000).

Attachment Systems

It is possible to draw out a little more information relating to patient satisfaction with implants from studies comparing different types of implant attachment systems where patient-centered outcomes have been used.

Naert and colleagues reported an RCT comparing three attachment types over a 10-year period (Naert et al. 1997a, 1999, 2004). Each type of attachment showed improved satisfaction compared with the old prosthesis; at 5 years there were no significant between-group differences (bar, ball, or magnet group). Findings were largely the same at 10 years for general satisfaction, although stability and chewing comfort were rated significantly lower for the magnet group compared to the ball and bar groups.

Similar findings have been reported by other authors (Karabuda et al. 2002; MacEntee et al. 2005; Stellingsma et al. 2003; Timmerman et al. 2004; Visser et al. 2005; Walton et al. 2002; Wismeijer et al. 1997). This raises the question of the design of these studies with regard to their statistical power to test differences in satisfaction; was there in fact no difference between attachments or were the studies lacking the ability to show such a difference? This is not clear from the current literature.

Although not stated in the paper, the cross-over study from the Montreal group examining long-bar overdenture and hybrid implant-supported mandibular overdentures (Tang et al. 1997) used the same design as a previous study (De Grandmont et al. 1994), which was powered to see a VAS difference of 10 mm or more. They demonstrated that factors apart from cleaning were rated better with the long-bar overdenture and that all subjects chose the long-bar overdenture (Tang et al. 1997).

Methodological Issues

The increasing use of validated questionnaires such as the Montreal Satisfaction VAS or the OHIP is encouraging, and allows a very real way of collecting patient-centered outcome and comparing effects between different studies. There is now an accumulating body of patient-centered data for implant treatment of the edentulous mandible, although still very little in other areas of implant-supported dentistry or restorative dentistry in general. Because of this it is not possible to compare different treatment modalities in terms of patient satisfaction or QoL in relationship to the economics of these different treatment modalities except to a limited degree. This is an important next step. Nevertheless, progress has been made in terms of determining the cost of treating edentulous patients either with conventional or implant-supported dentures. From this starting point we welcome further development and expansion into other treatment areas.

General Evaluation and Options for Future Research

Costs Involved with Treating Edentulous Patients with Dental Implants

Studies published in the last 25 years have shown the benefit of implant over dentures in terms of stability, function, speech, and patient satisfaction. The McGill Consensus suggested implant overdenture on two implants as the standard of care for edentulous patients (Feine et al. 2002). This raises the question as to whether the benefit of implant overdentures is large enough to be proposed as a standard of care with their inherently larger costs. The first studies analyzing the costs and cost-effectiveness of dental implants were published in the beginning of the nineties (Jacobson et al. 1990; Jonsson and Karlsson 1990). During the last 8 years more studies have been published on this subject looking further than the initial costs of the treatment and going into the costs of after-care as well.

When treating patients with any form of care, the costs generated are diverse but include the following: labor, practice, materials, patient, and environmental costs. The direct costs involved with dental care are of interest when informing patients about the proposed treatment; they can then relate this to a long-term prognosis and an idea of likely satisfaction levels, so allowing them to estimate their views of the value for money of the procedure. These costs are also vital when planning the targeting of resources by funding agencies or government.

Within the available literature there have been diverse ways of defining these costs. Some authors have calculated labor costs based on the tariff structure of the country they work in (Attard et al. 2003, 2005a,

2005b, 2006; Zitzmann et al. 2005, 2006), while others have based their calculations on the time spent treating patients (Heydecke et al. 2005a; Palmqvist et al. 2004; Stoker et al. 2007; Takanashi et al. 2004). Some authors then multiply the treatment time by the mean hourly wages of the dental professional (Heydecke et al. 2005a; Stoker et al. 2007; Takanashi et al. 2004).

The problem involved when calculating with standardized tariffs is that these fees include a lot of general costs that play a role at individual levels. Fees as such do not allow for a clean comparison of costs between centers or countries. Apart from treatment time, one could argue that any general practice costs should include materials, overhead, maintenance, and capital costs of the hospital or clinic (building and equipment) where the patient is treated. The overhead itself may also include cleaning, laundry, electricity, heating/cooling, and administration. It is not always clear in the literature if these factors have been included in the calculations.

Some articles also calculate the patient's costs involved with acquiring the treatment (Attard et al. 2003, 2005a, 2005b, 2006; Heydecke et al. 2005a; Takanashi et al. 2004). These were labeled as indirect costs. When considering which indirect costs could be considered the following come to mind: travel, loss of free time, loss of time at work (income) and the impact thereof at the place of work, costs involved with replacement, impact at home, medication, and impact on accompanying family and friends. As this is rather complex these costs are then often simplified to mean wages defined by gender and occupation. Some studies gave housewives the mean salary of a housekeeper and those patients who said they were retired were evaluated at the mean retirement income. A cost aspect that has not been explored in the cost analysis reported in the literature is environmental costs. The environmental impact of disposables, the heating/cooling of the building, building costs (building construction), or the environmental cost of travel and transportation have not been reported to date.

When analyzing the studies on costs of implant treatment we see that some studies divided the costs into direct and indirect costs. Direct costs include the costs of labor, materials, medication, laboratory costs, radiography fees, and so forth. Indirect costs include the patient's time costs and out-of-pocket costs (Anderson 1998; Heydecke et al. 2005a; Takanashi et al. 2004; Zitzmann et al. 2005, 2006).

Other studies performed a slightly different analysis. Total costs = (total clinical costs) + (time costs). Time costs = (salary per hr) × (clinical treatment time). Total clinical costs = (initial treatment costs) + (maintenance costs). Maintenance costs = (prosthetic costs for work other than the first implant-supported prosthesis) + (recall costs). These studies excluded the patient's travel expenses from their equation (Attard et al. 2003, 2005a, 2005b, 2006).

The study by Heydecke et al. (2005a) used the Delphi method and a panel of experts to estimate the costs of after-care in the long term. Their results are based on expert assumptions and not on actual costs, as these figures were not available in the literature for these procedures, so weakening the cost prognosis. As different groups use different strategies to define the costs of the treatment it is not easy to compare the results.

Attard and colleagues compared fixed mandibular prostheses (FDPs) with mandibular implant overdentures and concluded that after a period of 10 years the implant overdentures were a significantly cheaper treatment option (45–70% depending on the evaluation period) (Attard et al. 2003).

Palmqvist and colleagues compared the costs of an FDP with an implant overdenture. Both were placed on three implants, which makes a comparison with other studies rather difficult, as implant overdentures are generally made on two or four implants and FDPs on four or more. The authors stated that, due to future milling procedures, they expect the costs of dental technicians to fall (Palmqvist et al. 2004). Their dental technicians spent more time fabricating FDPs than they did implant overdentures. The clinicians on the other hand needed about 25% more time to provide patients with their implant overdentures. The authors stated that in their opinion an implant overdenture and an FDP on three implants had comparable costs and the FDP formed a lower biological risk (combination syndrome). The treatment groups were small (11 and 6 patients) and the conclusions are speculative. Their report does not differentiate between direct costs and costs concerning after-care.

Stoker et al. (2007) compared three different types of overdentures (two implants with ball attachments, two implants with a bar, and four interconnected implants). The initial costs after 8 years were about 75% of the total costs. He concluded that the costs of after-care did not differ for the three treatment groups. However, the number of unscheduled visits for patients in the two implant ball attachment groups was significantly higher than in the other groups and, based on the number of after-care visits, two interconnected implants would be the treatment of choice. More studies reported that implant-retained overdentures with ball attachments needed unscheduled checkups to reactivate the retentive system (Davis and Packer 1999; Stoker et al. 2007; Walton et al. 2002). Abutment design and choice of materials in time might lead to other conclusions.

Takanashi compared two implants with ball attachment implant overdenture to conventional denture treatment (Takanashi et al. 2004). The evaluation time was only 1 year, so conclusions on the long-term after-care of this treatment modality cannot be drawn. From the same Montreal group, however, Heydecke, using the Delphi method, asked 30 experts about their expectations concerning after-care for implant overdentures and conventional dentures (Heydecke et al. 2005a). They came up with estimated per-year costs for implant overdentures of C$395 and for the conventional dentures of C$273. This was based on Takanashi's 1-year costs, which included all indirect costs, and so seems high when compared to the other estimates in Table 22.1 (Takanashi et al. 2004). Neverthe-

Table 22.1　Treatment costs involved with implant treatment in the edentulous mandible. Patient's time and environmental cost have been excluded.

Author	Year	Denture	N	Initial Costs	Maintenance Costs	Evaluation Period Years	% per Year	Total Costs
Stoker	2007	2IOD ball	36	2413 euro	997 euro	8	5%	3410 euro
		2IOD	37	2602 euro	961 euro	8	4.6%	3563 euro
		4IOD	37	3564 euro	984 euro	8	3.5%	4548 euro
Takanashi	2004	2IOD ball	30	2332 Can$	85 Can$	1	3.6%	2417 Can$
		CD	30	814 Can$	64 Can$	1	7.8%	87 Can$
Zitzmann	2006	2IOD ball	20	6935 CH	271 CH	3	1.3%	7206 CH
		4IOD	20	15805 CH	364 CH	3	1%	16169 CH
		CD	20	2525 CH	126 CH	3	1.6%	2651 CH
Attard	2005	FDP	20	7621 Can$	1259 Can$	10	1.6%	8880 Can$
		IOD	20	4609 Can$	528 Can$	10	1%	5137 Can$
Attard	2003	FDP	25	7567 Can$	2527 Can$	9	3.7%	10094 Can$
		IOD	25	2505 Can$	830 Can$	9	3.7%	3343 Can$
Palmqvist	2004	FDP	11	3.1 hrs				1700 + 3.1 hrs
		IOD	6	4.1 hrs				1350 + 4.1 hrs

less, the point that is made by the group is that the cost difference between treatment modalities is still small.

Zitzmann et al. (2005) presented a paper where they plotted the costs of a conventional denture, an implant overdenture, and an FDP against the effects of the treatment options. The study showed that FPDs were six times more expensive, and implant overdenture treatment three times more expensive, than conventional denture treatment. The treatment effect was much higher for the implant treatment options. There was, however, no significant difference in treatment effects between the FDP and implant overdenture groups. This is in line with the study by Attard et al. (2003) where it was concluded that the implant overdenture was more cost-effective than the FDP.

The Montreal group presented a model to analyze lifetime cost-effectiveness following the cost per quality of life unit (Heydecke et al. 2005a). This is a method to measure the effectiveness of the treatment, and they calculated the cost per quality of life score for conventional denture and implant overdenture treatments. The additional cost of an implant overdenture over its expected lifetime was 226CAD per year for an average between-group difference of 15.7 OHIP-20 points, which equated to 14.41CAD per OHIP point per year. They suggested that "providing the implant overdenture instead of the conventional denture improved ORQoL by 33%, approximately one standard deviation and that compared to this the incremental cost of the implant overdenture of $226 per year seems relatively modest."

During the last few years several prospective studies have been published on immediate loading of implant-supported overdentures in the edentulous mandible, but they all relate to four or more implants (Chiapasco and Gatti 2003; Degidi and Piattelli 2003). Immediate loading is defined by the ITI Consensus group (Cochran et al. 2004) as a restoration placed in occlusion with the opposing dentition within 48 hours of implant placement. The conclusions of the ITI Consensus Confer-

ence based on a literature review on this subject were that the immediate loading of a minimum of four rigidly connected implants with a bar in the intraforaminal area showed results comparable to the treatment carried out with conventional loading procedures. Engelke et al. (2005) published a study in which they placed two implants in the edentulous mandible but added another two satellite implants for support during the healing period.

There are a few publications on the subject of early loading of implant-supported overdentures in the edentulous mandible using two implants. Roynesdal and co-workers published a study on 11 patients with ball attachments that were loaded after 14–21 days (Roynesdal et al. 2001). Studies by Payne and colleagues (2002) (12 patients, 10 mm implants) and Tawse-Smith et al. (2002) (24 patients) loaded implants that were either connected by a bar or on ball attachments after 2 weeks. (Admittedly, treatment groups with very small numbers.) Attard et al. (2005a, 2005b) reported on a group of 35 patients with a bar attachment in which the prosthodontic treatment was performed 10 days after surgery. They report on a study again in 2006 (Attard et al. 2006) but do not describe the prosthetic protocol in that paper. It seems that they are referring to the above-mentioned study published in 2005. It is in this study that they conclude that the immediate protocol is not cheaper than the conventional loading protocol. It seemed that the prosthetic phase of the treatment was associated with higher maintenance costs. Ormianer et al. (2006) describe what they call a modified loading protocol for the immediate loading of implant overdentures (n = 10), where they use an impression material as a buffer to reduce forces in the initial loading phase. This material was replaced every 2 weeks during the first 3 months after surgery. There was no direct attachment of the overdentures to the implants. Stricker et al. (2004) reported in a paper on immediate loading of two implants with a bar and a mandibular overdenture (n = 10), a relining procedure in which the overdenture is delivered 7 days after implant placement. The patients function without an overdenture for 7 days. No studies were found where two implants were loaded by a bar and an overdenture within 48 hours after implant insertion. This leads to the conclusion that this treatment strategy is at present not a predictable (evidence-based) treatment option for the edentulous mandible.

The studies outlined in this chapter show that there is compelling evidence that patients are more satisfied with implant overdentures than conventional dentures and that a similar picture is seen for OHRQoL. These improvements in satisfaction also apply to parameters such as aesthetics, chewing ability, stability, comfort, and speech as well as the impact on social and sexual activities. An emerging trend is for studies with simpler rather than involved treatment, which offers the opportunity to introduce these treatments to a wider group than previously considered. The impact of early implant loading and the overall real cost implications still need further work. Nevertheless, the evidence is strong that OHRQoL and patient satisfaction can be significantly improved by mandibular prostheses stabilized by two implants in edentulous patients compared with a conventional denture.

References

Allen PF, Thomason JM, Jepson NJ, Nohl F, Smith DG, Ellis J. 2006. A randomized controlled trial of implant-retained mandibular overdentures. *J Dent Res* 85(6): 547–551.

Anderson J. 1998. The need for criteria on reporting treatment outcomes. *J Prosthet Dent* 79(1):49–55.

Attard N, David LA, Zarb GA. 2005a. Immediate loading of implants with mandibular overdentures: One-year clinical results of a prospective study. *Int J Prosthodont* 18(6):463–470.

Attard N, Laporte A, Locker D, Zarb GA. 2006. A prospective study on immediate loading of implants with mandibular overdentures: Patient-mediated and economic outcomes. *Int J Prosthodont* 19(1): 67–73.

Attard N, Wei X, Laporte A, Zarb GA, Ungar WJ. 2003. A cost minimization analysis of implant treatment in mandibular edentulous patients. *Int J Prosthodont* 16(3): 271–276.

Attard N, Zarb GA, Laporte A. 2005b. Long-term treatment costs associated with implant-supported mandibular prostheses in edentulous patients. *Int J Prosthodont* 18(2):117–123.

Awad M, Feine J. 1998. Measuring patient satisfaction with mandibular prostheses. *Comm Dentistry Oral Epidemiol* 26:400–405.

Awad M, Locker D, Korner-Bitensky N, Feine J. 2000a. Measuring the effect of intra-oral implant rehabilitation on health-related quality of life in a randomized controlled clinical trial. *J Dent Res* 79(9):1659–1663.

Awad M, Lund JP, Dufresne E, Feine JS. 2003a. Comparing the efficacy of mandibular implant-retained overdentures and conventional dentures among middle-aged edentulous patients: Satisfaction and functional assessment. *Int J Prosthodont* 16(2): 117–122.

Awad M, Lund JP, Shapiro SH, Locker D, Klemetti E, Chehade A, Savard A, Feine JS. 2003b. Oral health status and treatment satisfaction with mandibular implant overdentures and conventional dentures: A randomized clinical trial in a senior population. *Int J Prosthodont* 16(4):390–396.

Awad M, Shapiro SH, Lund JP, Feine JS. 2000b. Determinants of patients' treatment preferences in a clinical trial. *Comm Dentistry Oral Epidemiol* 28(2):119–125.

Bergman B, Carlsson GE. 1972. Review of 54 complete denture wearers. Patients' opinions 1 year after treatment. *Acta Odontol Scand* 30(4):399–414.

Bouma J, Boerrigter L, Van Ooort RP, Van Sonderen E, Boering G. 1997. Psychosocial effects of implant-retained overdentures.

Int J Oral Maxillofac Implants 12(4):515–522.

Carlsson GE, Otterland A, Wennstrom A. 1967. Patient factors in appreciation of complete dentures. *J Prosthet Dent* 17(4): 322–328.

Chiapasco M, Gatti C. 2003. Implant-retained mandibular overdentures with immediate loading: A 3- to 8-year prospective study on 328 implants. *Clin Implant Dent Relat Res* 5(1):29–38.

Cochran DL, Morton D, Weber HP. 2004. Consensus statements and recommended clinical procedures regarding loading protocols for endosseous dental implants. *Int J Oral Maxillofac Implants* 19(Suppl): 109–113.

Davis D, Packer M. 1999. Mandibular overdentures stabilized by Astra Tech implants with either ball attachments or magnets: 5-year results. *Int J Prosthodont* 12(3): 222–229.

De Albuquerque R, Jr., Lund J, Tang L, Larivee J, De Grandmont P, Gauthier G, Feine J. 2000. Within-subject comparison of maxillary long-bar implant-retained prostheses with and without palatal coverage: Patient-based outcomes. *Clin Oral Implants Res* 11(6):555–565.

De Grandmont P, Feine J, Tache R, Boudrias P, Donohue W, Tanguay R, Lund J. 1994. Within-subject comparisons of implant-supported mandibular prostheses: Psychometric evaluation. *J Dent Res* 73(5): 1096–1104.

Degidi M, Piattelli A. 2003. Immediate functional and non-functional loading of dental implants: A 2- to 60-month follow-up study of 646 titanium implants. *J Periodontol* 74(2):225–241.

Engelke W, Decco OA, De las Mercedes Capobianco M, Schwarzwaller W, Villavicencio MM. 2005. Immediate occlusal loading of freestanding implants using cortical satellite implants: Preliminary report of a prospective study. *Implant Dent* 14(1):50–57.

Feine JS, Carlsson GE, Awad MA, Chehade A, Duncan WJ, Gizani S, Head T, Lund JP,

MacEntee M, Mericske-Stern R, Mojon P, Morais J, Naert I, Payne AG, Penrod J, Stoker GT, Tawse-Smith A, Taylor TD, Thomason JM, Thomson WM, Wismeijer D. 2002. The McGill consensus statement on overdentures. Mandibular two-implant overdentures as first choice standard of care for edentulous patients. Montreal, Quebec, May 24–25, 2002. *Int J Oral Maxillofac Implants* 17(4):601–602.

Feine JS, Lund JP. 2006. Measuring chewing ability in randomized controlled trials with edentulous populations wearing implant prostheses. *J Oral Rehabil* 33(4): 301–308.

Haraldson T, Carlsson GE, Ingervall B. 1979. Functional state, bite force and postural muscle activity in patients with osseointegrated oral implant bridges. *Acta Odontol Scand* 37(4):195–206.

Heydecke G, Boudrias P, Awad M, De Albuquerque R, Lund J, Feine J. 2003a. Within-subject comparisons of maxillary fixed and removable implant prostheses. *Clin Oral Implants Res* 14:125–130.

Heydecke G, Locker D, Awad MA, Lund JP, Feine JS. 2003b. Oral and general health-related quality of life with conventional and implant dentures. *Comm Dentistry Oral Epidemiol* 31(3):161–168.

Heydecke G, McFarland DH, Feine JS, Lund JP. 2004. Speech with maxillary implant prostheses: Ratings of articulation. *J Dent Res* 83(3):236–240.

Heydecke G, Penrod JR, Takanashi Y, Lund JP, Feine JS, Thomason JM. 2005a. Cost-effectiveness of mandibular two-implant overdentures and conventional dentures in the edentulous elderly. *J Dent Res* 84(9): 794–799.

Heydecke G, Thomason JM, Lund JP, Feine JS. 2005b. The impact of conventional and implant supported prostheses on social and sexual activities in edentulous adults—results from a randomized trial 2 months after treatment. *J Dent* 33(8): 649–657.

Jacobson J, Maxson B, Mays K, Peebles J, Kowalski C. 1990. Cost-effectiveness of dental implants: A utility analysis. *J Dent Educ* 54(11):688–689.

Jonsson B, Karlsson G. 1990. Cost-benefit evaluation of dental implants. *Int J Technol Assess Health Care* 6(4):545–557.

Kapur K, Garrett N, Hamada M, Roumanas E, Freymiller E, Han T, Diener R, Levin S, Ida R. 1998. A randomized clinical trial comparing the efficacy of mandibular implant-supported overdentures and conventional dentures in diabetic patients. Part I: Methodology and clinical outcomes. *J Prosthet Dent* 79(5):555–569.

Karabuda C, Tosun T, Ermis E, Ozdemir T. 2002. Comparison of 2 retentive systems for implant-supported overdentures: Soft tissue management and evaluation of patient satisfaction. *J Periodontol* 73(9): 1067–1070.

MacEntee MI, Walton JN, Glick N. 2005. A clinical trial of patient satisfaction and prosthodontic needs with ball and bar attachments for implant-retained complete overdentures: Three-year results. *J Prosthet Dent* 93(1):28–37.

Meijer HJ, Raghoebar GM, Van't Hof MA. 2003. Comparison of implant-retained mandibular overdentures and conventional complete dentures: A 10-year prospective study of clinical aspects and patient satisfaction. *Int J Oral Maxillofac Implants* 18(6):879–885.

Meijer H, Raghoebar G, Van't Hof M, Geertman M, Van Oort R. 1999. Implant-retained mandibular overdentures compared with complete dentures: A 5-years' follow-up study of clinical aspects and patient satisfaction. *Clin Oral Implants Res* 10(3): 238–244.

Naert I, Alsaadi G, Quirynen M. 2004. Prosthetic aspects and patient satisfaction with two-implant-retained mandibular overdentures: A 10-year randomized clinical study. *Int J Prosthodont* 17(4):401–410.

Naert I, Gizani S, Van Steenberghe D. 1998. Rigidly splinted implants in the resorbed maxilla to retain a hinging overdenture: A series of clinical reports for up to 4 years. *J Prosthet Dent* 79(2):156–164.

Naert I, Gizani S, Vuylsteke M, Van Steenberghe D. 1997a. A randomized clinical trial on the influence of splinted and unsplinted oral implants in mandibular overdenture therapy: A 3-year report. *Clin Oral Investig* 1:81–88.

Naert I, Gizani S, Vuylsteke M, Van Steenberghe D. 1999. A 5-year prospective randomized clinical trial on the influence of splinted and unsplinted oral implants retaining a mandibular overdenture: Prosthetic aspects and patient satisfaction. *J Oral Rehabil* 26(3):195–202.

Naert I, Hooghe M, Quirynen M, Van Steenberghe D. 1997b. The reliability of implant-retained hinging overdentures for the fully edentulous mandible. An up to 9-year longitudinal study. *Clin Oral Investig* 1(3):119–124.

Ormianer Z, Garg AK, Palti A. 2006. Immediate loading of implant overdentures using modified loading protocol. *Implant Dent* 15(1):35–40.

Palmqvist S, Owall B, Schou S. 2004. A prospective randomized clinical study comparing implant-supported fixed prostheses and overdentures in the edentulous mandible: Prosthodontic production time and costs. *Int J Prosthodont* 17(2):231–235.

Payne AG, Tawse-Smith A, Duncan WD, Kumara R. 2002. Conventional and early loading of unsplinted ITI implants supporting mandibular overdentures. *Clin Oral Implants Res* 13(6):603–609.

Raghoebar GM, Meijer HJ, Stegenga B, Van't Hof MA, Van Oort RP, Vissink A. 2000. Effectiveness of three treatment modalities for the edentulous mandible. A five-year randomized clinical trial. *Clin Oral Implants Res* 11(3):195–201.

Roumanas ED, Garrett NR, Hamada MO, Diener RM, Kapur KK. 2002. A randomized clinical trial comparing the efficacy of mandibular implant-supported overdentures and conventional dentures in diabetic patients. Part V: Food preference comparisons. *J Prosthet Dent* 87(1):62–73.

Roynesdal AK, Amundrud B, Hannaes HR. 2001. A comparative clinical investigation of 2 early loaded ITI dental implants supporting an overdenture in the mandible. *Int J Oral Maxillofac Implants* 16(2):246–251.

Stellingsma K, Bouma J, Stegenga B, Meijer HJ, Raghoebar GM. 2003. Satisfaction and psychosocial aspects of patients with an extremely resorbed mandible treated with implant-retained overdentures. A prospective, comparative study. *Clin Oral Implants Res* 14(2):166–172.

Stoker GT, Wismeijer D, Van Waas MA. 2007. An eight-year follow-up to a randomized clinical trial of aftercare and cost-analysis with three types of mandibular implant-retained overdentures. *J Dent Res* 86(3):276–280.

Stricker A, Gutwald R, Schmelzeisen R, Gellrich NG. 2004. Immediate loading of 2 interforaminal dental implants supporting an overdenture: Clinical and radiographic results after 24 months. *Int J Oral Maxillofac Implants* 19(6):868–872.

Takanashi Y, Penrod JR, Lund JP, Feine JS. 2004. A cost comparison of mandibular two-implant overdenture and conventional denture treatment. *Int J Prosthodont* 17(2):181–186.

Tang L, Lund J, Tache R, Clokie C, Feine J. 1997. A within-subject comparison of mandibular long-bar and hybrid implant-supported prostheses: Psychometric evaluation and patient preference. *J Dent Res* 76(10):1675–1683.

Tawse-Smith A, Payne AG, Kumara R, Thomson WM. 2002. Early loading of unsplinted implants supporting mandibular overdentures using a one-stage operative procedure with two different implant systems: A 2-year report. *Clin Implant Dent Relat Res* 4(1):33–42.

Thomason JM, Heydecke G, Feine JS, Ellis JS. 2007. How do patients perceive the benefit of reconstructive dentistry with regard to oral health-related quality of life and patient satisfaction? A systematic review. *Clin Oral Implants Res* 18(Suppl 3):168–188.

Thomason JM, Lund JP, Chehade A, Feine JS. 2003. Patient satisfaction with mandibular implant overdentures and conventional dentures 6 months after delivery. *Int J Prosthodont* 16(5):467–473.

Timmerman R, Stoker GT, Wismeijer D, Oosterveld P, Vermeeren JI, Van Waas MA. 2004. An eight-year follow-up to a randomized clinical trial of participant satisfaction with three types of mandibular implant-retained overdentures. *J Dent Res* 83(8):630–633.

Visser A, Raghoebar GM, Meijer HJ, Batenburg RH, Vissink A. 2005. Mandibular overdentures supported by two or four endosseous implants. A 5-year prospective study. *Clin Oral Implants Res* 16(1):19–25.

Walton JN. 2003. A randomized clinical trial comparing two mandibular implant overdenture designs: 3-year prosthetic outcomes using a six-field protocol. *Int J Prosthodont* 16(3):255–260.

Walton J, MacEntee M, Glick N. 2002. One-year prosthetic outcomes with implant overdentures: A randomized clinical trial. *Int J Oral Maxillofac Implants* 17(3): 391–398.

Wismeijer D, Van Waas M, Vermeeren J, Mulder J, Kalk W. 1997. Patient satisfaction with implant-supported mandibular overdentures—a comparison of three treatment strategies with ITI-dental implants. *Int J Oral Maxillofac Implants* 12:263–267.

Wismeijer D, Vermeeren JI, Van Waas MA. 1992. Patient satisfaction with overdentures supported by one-stage TPS implants. *Int J Oral Maxillofac Implants* 7(1): 51–55.

Zitzmann N, Marinello C. 2000. Treatment outcomes of fixed or removable implant-supported prostheses in the edentulous maxilla. Part I: Patients' assessments. *J Prosthet Dent* 83(4):424–433.

Zitzmann N, Marinello C, Sendi P. 2006. A cost-effectiveness analysis of implant overdentures. *J Dent Res* 85(8):717–721.

Zitzmann N, Sendi P, Marinello C. 2005. An economic evaluation of implant treatment in edentulous patients—preliminary results. *Int J Prosthodont* 18(1):20–27.

Dental Implants in the Habilitation of Young Patients

George K.B. Sándor

Both the predictability and success of dental implants in adult patients depend on the quality and quantity of alveolar bone, treatment planning, sound surgical technique, optimal prosthodontic restoration, and long-term oral hygiene (Brahim 2005). The same factors also apply to the success of implants placed in children, adolescents, or young adults—referred to in this chapter as "young patients." The unique and critical difference between treatment of pediatric and adult patients is that the wildcard of craniofacial growth and dento-alveolar development may affect outcome unpredictably (Brahim 2005; NIH 1988).

Growth is modulated by a complex interaction of many factors including, to name a few, familial and genetic factors, trauma, endocrine influences, acute and chronic illnesses, and exposure to radiation therapy. Determining the cessation of growth is difficult (Bjork 1963; Brahim 2005; Carmichael and Sándor 2008). In the author's center a combination of serial clinical examinations, wrist carpal radiographs, and serial lateral cephalograms taken 6 months apart are used to assess the degree of skeletal maturity of the jaws. The issue of growth and

estimation of its progress remains a complex issue to this day (Carmichael and Sándor 2008).

Placing implants in young patients is more complicated than in adults. For one thing, young patients may require general anesthesia in order to manage their behavior. Moreover, compliance with home-care instructions and a child's dexterity can constitute serious impediments to the maintenance of a satisfactory level of oral hygiene, which is critical in most situations to ensure the long-term health of the reconstructed dentition.

Recognition that dental implants can inhibit growth (Kuröl and Ödman 1996; Ödman et al. 1991; Thilander et al. 1995) and adaptation of the jaws (Bernard et al. 2004) have led to dialogue in the literature surrounding the earliest possible time at which implants can be placed into a patient (Bishara et al. 1996; Carmichael and Sándor 2008; Forsberg et al. 1991; Oesterle and Cronin 2000; Tarlow 2004). The author's center has adopted a number of general treatment planning principles governing management of young patients requiring dental implants (Sándor and Carmichael 2008). They include the following:

1. Young patients who require dental implants to replace single or a few teeth receive dental implants only after they attain skeletal maturity in order to avoid perturbing growth of the jaws.
2. Patients with oligodontia are treated with dental implants following the completion of orthodontic therapy and the cessation of skeletal growth.
3. Patients with global growth perturbations such as those having been treated with ablative surgery or having suffered severe traumatic loss of multiple teeth, surrounding tissues, and extensive scarring may have dental implants placed prior to skeletal maturation. Under circumstances such as these, growth is abnormal and likely to result in maladaptive compensatory growth of undamaged parts of the maxillofacial complex.
4. Implant treatment in young patients proceeds only if parent and child demonstrate significant motivation to undergo complex long-term treatment and a willingness to maintain proper oral hygiene.

Clinicians should not underestimate the weight of the psychological burden borne by a child with a severe dental malformation (Forsberg et al. 1991). Management must include a humane understanding of the psychological and socioeconomic impact of such conditions on a patient and his or her family, particularly when more than one child is afflicted.

A common denominator of many dental and craniofacial anomalies is congenital absence of teeth or oligodontia. To the extent that many acquired dental anomalies also involve missing teeth, it is instructive therefore to anyone with an interest in the treatment of congenital and acquired anomalies to have an understanding of the subjective and objective consequences of oligodontia or acquired partial edentulism in young patients (Fig. 23.1).

These consequences complicate therapy and must be understood by the treating practitioner (Table 23.1). Severe oligodontia may

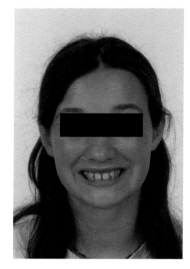

Figure 23.1. Clinical photograph of a 14-year-old girl with oligodontia with undermined aesthetics, poor self-image, and a resultant lack of socialization. There is also loss of lower vertical face height. The patient looks older than her age.

Table 23.1. Consequences of oligodontia.

Undermined cosmesis
Poor mastication
Malocclusion
Hypoplasia of crowns
Poor orthodontic anchorage
Ankylosis of primary teeth
Disruption of alveolar growth
Agenesis of alveolus
Resorption of alveolus
Depleted periodontium
Periodontal trauma
Attrition with dentine and pulp exposure
Extrusion
Insufficient vertical dimension of occlusion
Insufficient intermaxillary space

reduce masticatory efficiency, resulting in decreased alimentation and impaired nutrition (Fig. 23.2).

A variety of malocclusions may present together with oligodontia including retrognathism, deficiency of vertical lower face height, or prognathism. Such malocclusions are

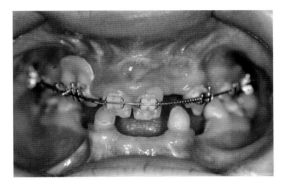

Figure 23.2. Severe loss of vertical height due to attrition in this oligodontia patient complicated by over-eruption of the unopposed permanent teeth. Such over-eruption makes implant hardware difficult to position, not allowing the prosthodontist the opportunity to camouflage metal and hardware.

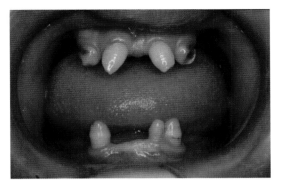

Figure 23.4. Oligodontia may be accompanied by teeth that have hypoplastic crown forms, presenting a variety of restorative and treatment planning challenges.

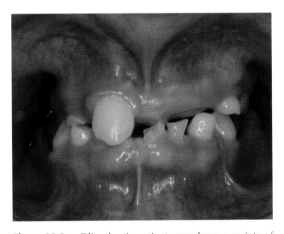

Figure 23.3. Oligodontia patients may have a variety of malocclusions with severe attrition of both the remaining deciduous teeth and what permanent teeth may exist in the mouth.

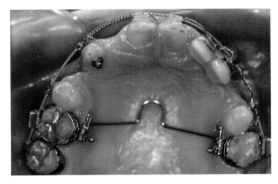

Figure 23.5. Patterns of oligodontia may result in severely reduced orthodontic anchorage, which may greatly prolong treatment time and could result in compromised results.

subject to excessive wear of both the mixed dentition and the depleted permanent dentition (Fig. 23.3).

Tooth crown form in patients with severe oligodontia may be hypoplastic (Fig. 23.4).

Oligodontia may result in severely deficient orthodontic anchorage, which may greatly prolong treatment time and compromise outcome (Fig. 23.5).

Traumatic loss of maxillary teeth is common in young patients. Restoration of edentulous spaces left by traumatic tooth loss should be delayed until skeletal maturity is attained (Ledermann et al. 1993). In a study of 42 implants in 34 growing patients with a mean age of 15.1 years, there was a 90% rate of successful osseointegration, while the major complication noted was the failure of the ankylosed dental implant to match the vertical growth of the alveolus of the adjacent teeth, resulting in submergence and infraocclusion of the restored dental implants (Ledermann et al. 1993). The patient in Figure 23.6 demonstrates submergence of an implant placed at the site of the maxillary left central

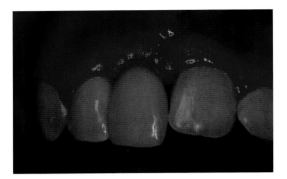

Figure 23.6. A 17-year-old male demonstrating sub-mergence of an implant-supported crown at the site of the maxillary left central incisor placed at 15 years of age.

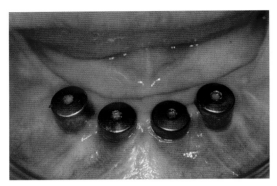

Figure 23.7. Dental implants placed into the anterior mandible of an 8-year-old patient with hypohydrotic ectodermal dysplasia.

Table 23.2. Clinical protocol.

Multidisciplinary assessment
Orthodontic treatment
  Orthodontics alone
  Orthognathic surgery
Grafting of cleft alveolus in alveolar cleft
  patients
Determination of skeletal maturity
Peri-implant alveolar bone grafting
Implant placement
Prosthodontic habilitation
Follow-up

Table 23.3. Some syndromes managed with dental implants.

Binders Syndrome
Cleidocranial Dysplasia
Crouzon's Syndrome
Ectodermal Dysplasias
Epidermylosis Bullosa
Fibrous Dysplasia
Familial Odontodysplasia
Gorlin Syndrome
Hemifacial Microsomia
Lateral Facial Dysplasia
Long Face Syndrome
Pierre Robin Sequence
Singleton-Merton Syndrome
Trisomy 21
Turette's Syndrome
Incontinentia Pigmenti
Treacher Collins

incisor before the cessation of skeletal growth. The resulting discrepancy of gingival margins, between the natural tooth, which has continued to erupt, and the implant, which tends to relatively submerge as would an ankylosed tooth, is very difficult to treat (Sàndor and Carmichael 2008).

The author endeavors to adhere to a standard protocol in the management of complex anomalies involving missing teeth and requiring dental implants as part of his overall treatment (Table 23.2). These cases have responded well to such interdisciplinary management and include many conditions complicated by the agenesis or loss of teeth (Table 23.3).

Growth must always be considered when implant-supported prostheses are inserted into growing children. Patients with severe oligodontia such as in ectodermal dysplasia may be treated at a young age with dental implant-supported fixed prostheses (Brahim 2005; Guckes et al. 1991, 2002). One past attempt to minimize potential growth disturbance was to section the prosthesis placed across the anterior mandible in the region of the symphysis of the lower jaw (Figs. 23.7–23.11), especially in patients with resections for tumor ablation.

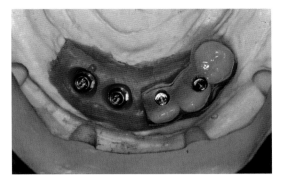

Figure 23.8. The planned restoration is one of a sectional nature with a gap at the midline of the mandible. This photograph shows the left part of the restoration on the model. This represents an attempt to avoid interference of mandibular growth by not crossing the midline of the lower jaw. The author's centers have stopped using prosthesis that were sectioned solely for the reasons of growth.

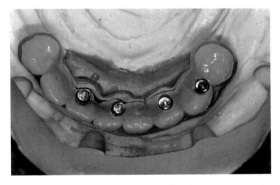

Figure 23.9. The implant-borne fixed restoration in its entirety on the dental cast.

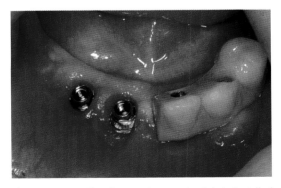

Figure 23.10. The first section on the left is installed into the mouth.

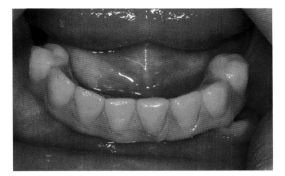

Figure 23.11. Labial view of the installed mandibular anterior prosthesis 2 years after delivery.

These children can be severely debilitated by their tumor resections and so are subsequently treated with implant-supported restorations during the mixed dentition phase, which is a period of intense growth (Bjork 1963; Brahim 2005; Sándor et al. 2008). It was assumed that the prosthesis could be split in the midline to accommodate mandibular growth in the transverse dimension. Subsequent experience has shown this to be unnecessary (Fenton et al. 2007; Sándor et al. 2008). Not a single patient treated with an implant-supported suprastructure that was split in the midline of the mandible has developed a diastema in the midline, even if he or she was actively growing. The author's center has therefore stopped splitting suprastructures in the midline of the mandible solely for the reasons of growth.

The alveolus where the dental implants are placed is not expected to grow vertically (Ödman et al. 1991). As the deciduous molars exfoliate and the permanent molars erupt, the alveolus will grow vertically in the areas of permanent tooth eruption. This may result in a vertical discrepancy between the heights of the posterior and anterior mandible where the resection has been performed and the implants were placed. This growth discrepancy may necessitate serial remakes of the implant-borne prosthesis to accommodate the differential vertical growth in the alveoli and the dynamically erupting dentition in the maxilla and posterior mandible. In the meantime these prostheses help the child adapt functionally and aesthetically, which is especially important to the development of self-esteem in the pediatric patient, both at school and socially (Fenton et al. 2007; Hunt et al. 2005).

Growth following implant placement may occur at the dental alveolus or in other areas of the mandible, for example, in cases of mandibular asymmetry and prognathism. Mandibular growth in such patients is aberrant and may occur once growth is assumed to be complete. Figures 23.12–23.21 illustrate the

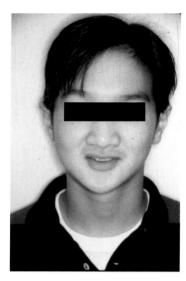

Figure 23.14. Frontal photograph of patient from Figure 23.12 now 18 years of age and restored with implant-supported prostheses.

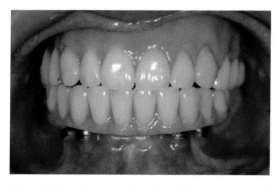

Figure 23.15. Anterior view of occlusion at the time of prostheses insertion and delivery.

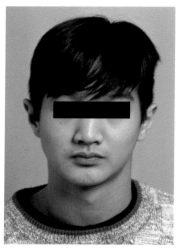

Figure 23.12. Frontal facial photograph of 16-year-old male with anhydrotic ectodermal dysplasia at the time of presentation.

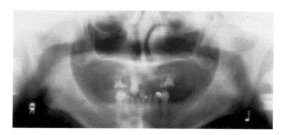

Figure 23.13. Panoramic radiograph of patient in Figure 23.12 showing severe attrition of teeth in patient with severe oligodontia.

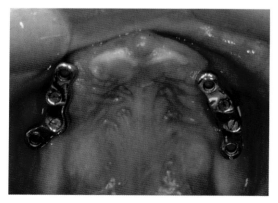

Figure 23.16. Occlusal view of maxillary implant-supported suprastructure.

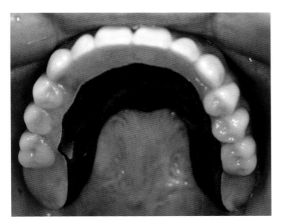

Figure 23.17.   Occlusal view of maxillary overdenture prosthesis.

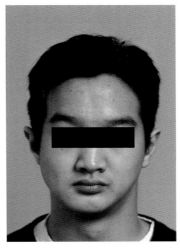

Figure 23.19.   Frontal photograph of patient at 21 years of age with newly developed mandibular asymmetric prognathism. Note the deviation of the chin to the right.

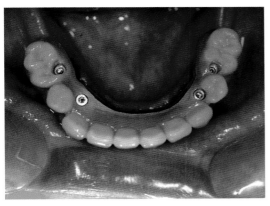

Figure 23.18.   Occlusal view of mandibular fixed prosthesis.

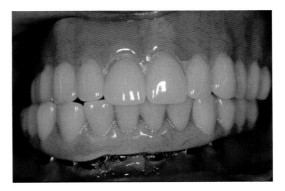

Figure 23.20.   Anterior view of asymmetric malocclusion of the prostheses with skeletal and dental midlines of the mandible shifted to the right with a right buccal segment crossbite, due to late mandibular growth.

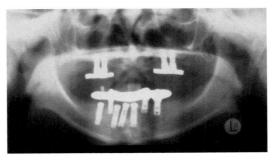

case of a 19-year-old male who developed an asymmetric mandibular prognathism with laterognathia due to late mandibular growth.

Some of the dental implants in the right mandible became overloaded due to the asymmetric malocclusion and were lost. Late mandibular growth can result in implant overload and consequent implant fixture failure.

Figure 23.21.   Panoramic radiograph showing four newly placed implants to replace those fixtures failing from occlusal overload from the newly developed malocclusion.

References

Bernard JP, Schatz JP, Christou P, Belser U. 2004. Long-term vertical changes of the anterior maxillary teeth adjacent to single implants in young and mature adults. A retrospective study. *J Clin Periodontol* 31(11):1024–1028.

Brahim JS. 2005. Dental implants in children. *Oral Maxillofac Surg Clinics of North America* 17(4):375–381.

Bishara SE, Treder JE, Damon P, Olsen M. 1996. Changes in the dental arches and dentition between 25 and 45 years of age. *Angle Orthodontics* 66(6):417–422.

Bjork A. 1963. Variations in the growth pattern of the human mandible: Longitudinal radiographic study by the implant method. *J Dent Res* 42:400–411.

Carmichael RP, Sàndor GK. 2008. Dental implants, growth of the jaws and determination of skeletal maturity. In: *Dental Implants in Children, Adolescents and Young Adults*. GK Sàndor and RP Carmichael (eds.). Atlas of the Oral and Maxillofacial Clinics of North America. Philadelphia: Elsevier 16(1):1–10.

Fenton C, Nish IA, Carmichael RP, Sàndor GK. 2007. Metastatic mandibular retinoblastoma in a child reconstructed with soft tissue matrix expansion grafting. *J Oral Maxillofac Surg* 65(11):2329–2335.

Forsberg CM, Eliasson S, Westergren H. 1991. Face height and tooth eruption in adults—a 20-year follow-up investigation. *Eur J Orthodontics* 12(4):249–254.

Guckes AD, Brahim JS, McCarthy GR. 1991. Using endosseous implants for patients with ectodermal dysplasia. *J Am Dent Assoc* 122(1):59–62.

Guckes AD, Scurria MS, King TS. 2002. Prospective clinical trial of dental implants in persons with ectodermal dysplasia. *J Prosthet Dent* 88(1):21–27.

Hunt O, Burden D, Hepper P, Johnston C. 2005. The psychosocial effect of cleft lip and palate: A systematic review. *Eur J Orthodontics* 27:274–285.

Kuröl J, Ödman J. 1996. Treatment alternatives in young patients with missing teeth. Aspects on growth and development. In: *Consensus Conference on Oral Implants in Young Patients: State of the Art*. G Koch, T Bergendal, S Kvint, and UB Johansson (eds.). Jönköping, Sweden: Institute for Postgraduate Dental Research. 77–107.

Ledermann PD, Hassell TM, Hefti AF. 1993. Osseointegrated dental implants as an alternative to bridge construction or orthodontics in young patients: Seven years of clinical experience. *Pediatr Dent* 15:327–330.

National Institutes of Health (NIH). 1988. Consensus development conference statement on dental implants. *J Dent Educ* 52:824–825.

Ödman J, Gröndahl K, Lekholm U, Thilander B. 1991. The effect of osseointegrated implants on the dento-alveolar development. A clinical and radiographic study in growing pigs. *Eur J Orthodontics* 13(4):279–286.

Oesterle LJ, Cronin RJ, Jr. 2000. Adult growth, aging, and the single-tooth implant. *Int J Oral Maxillofac Implants* 15(2):252–260.

Sàndor GK, Carmichael RP. 2008. Rehabilitation of trauma using dental implants. In: *Dental Implants in Children, Adolescents and Young Adults*. GK Sàndor and RP Carmichael (eds.). Atlas of the Oral and Maxillofacial Clinics of North America. Philadelphia: Elsevier 16(1):60–82.

Sàndor GK, Carmichael RP, Binahmed A. 2008. Reconstruction of ablative defects using dental implants. In: *Dental Implants in Children, Adolescents and Young Adults*. GK Sàndor and RP Carmichael (eds.). Atlas of the Oral and Maxillofacial Clinics of North America. Philadelphia: Elsevier 16(1):110–126.

Tarlow JL. 2004. The effect of adult growth on an anterior single-tooth implant: A clinical report. *J Prosthet Dent* 92(3):213–215.

Thilander B, Ödman J, Gröndahl K, Friberg B. 1995. Osseointegrated implants in adolescents. A three year study. *Nederlandse Tijdschrift Tandheelkunde* 102(4):383–385.

Minimum Competency for Providing Implant Prosthodontics— What Should Be the Educational Requirements?

24

GUARANTEEING TREATMENT FOR EVERYONE: CHANGING EDUCATIONAL CRITERIA FOR "GARDEN VARIETY" CASES TO MAJOR BONE GRAFTS

Kenneth W.M. Judy

Lest we forget, the reality is that dental implants were initially developed in many countries by intrepid clinicians in the 1950s and 1960s without substantive input from the specialties of oral surgery, periodontics, or prosthodontics as then constituted. In fact, implants were routinely condemned by these communities in spite of substantial positive clinical research. In 1968 the American Dental Association's (ADA) position was that implants were highly experimental and that practitioners had to provide extensive informed consent to protect potential patients. In 1978 the National Institutes of Health (NIH) organized its first dental implant consensus conference.

What had happened to motivate the NIH to hold this conference? Simply put, implant therapists were achieving a more than acceptable level of success and the public was being

made aware of the procedures and benefits. Shortly thereafter, in 1982, the first Toronto Osseointegration Conference was held and the profession witnessed the beginning of a bona fide transition to evidence based dentistry vis-à-vis implantology. In 1988 a second NIH consensus conference reinforced the level of success of implant therapy (Judy 1989).

The reality is that in the last 2 decades dental implants have become "big business," not only for implant manufacturers and those manufacturers of related materials and devices but also for engaged generalist and specialist clinicians.

Concurrent with expanded implant usage, at least four applications for specialty status were submitted to the ADA: two by the International Congress of Oral Implantologists (ICOI) U.S. division, the American College of Oral Implantologists (ACOI), and two by the American Academy of Implant Dentistry (AAID). All applications were denied by the Council on Dental Education (CDE), the rationale being that dental implantology could be readily subsumed into existing specialties. Needless to say, an intense lobbying effort by at least one specialty group against an oral implantology specialty contributed to its denial. Ironically, only very recently the ADA has required training to the level of competence in oral implantology for the specialties of oral and maxillofacial surgery, periodontics, and prosthodontics. In the author's opinion the ADA denial of specialty status was flawed, resulting in the creation of very few substantial university-based graduate programs, particularly on the departmental level, an unfortunate situation that persists today. Clearly the field was set to grow dramatically with expanded clinical use and applications, research, and multi-level educational needs. The ADA either had blinders on or their processes were too rigid.

During the past 2 decades the field of aesthetic dentistry has blossomed, so that today patients want spectacular smiles—and implants are just a hidden method of securing them. Consequently the reality is that implant education, especially when coupled with aesthetic concepts, has also become big business. Because of this coupling there appears to be an endless supply of patients globally, not only in developed economic areas but also in emerging markets. It is apparent that for postgraduate degree program teaching purposes there is a need for practice, long continuing education, and methodology for triaging patients into simple and complex cases and cases needing major bone grafts and other procedures (Judy 2008; Perel 2007).

Before addressing the educational requirements relating to minimum competency for implant restoration, it might be useful to look at individual countries to obtain a more realistic perspective relating to need. Keep in mind the fact that the World Health Organization (WHO) seems to be encouraging a position that patients with traditional full denture prostheses are to be viewed as "handicapped" in many instances and that the implant-supported overdenture should become a new "standard of care." There are multi-level disparities that cannot be ignored. The reality is that China, for example, currently has less than 120,000 practicing university-trained dentists, approximately the

same number as the United States. There is a large difference in population and average income. The situation in Nigeria is much worse medically as well as dentally, with a population of one-fifteenth that of the United States. With a current population of 80 million and a 2070 projected population of 150 million, today's 20,000 Egyptian practitioners have trouble delivering suitable basic services, particularly if average income per person (a negative) is factored in with unemployment rates (a negative) and the small percentage of Egyptians that avail themselves of dental care (a tragic positive).

While the profession should not forget Dr. Douglas Atwood's early call for specialty status for implantology as well as that of others (Judy 1986; Judy and Misch 1985), dental education policy makers should also be mindful of trying to bring valid clinical benefits to the neediest and to the largest segments of the world's population. Any educational criteria for placing, restoring, and maintaining dental implants should have this altered mindset as a significant basis for establishing educational criteria and goals.

In pre-doctoral curricula there is a wide range of recommended educational hours and little agreement on practical case loads. Two years ago at a consensus conference sponsored by the ICOI, the Deutsche Gesellschaft für Orale Implantologie (DGOI), and New York University College of Dentistry, the range for recommended pre-doctoral hours varied from 8 to 300. One helpful piece of educational advice that emerged was that whatever hours were established, they had to be made requirements or they would possibly be ignored by students.

During the developmental period of the last 50 years, there was an uncompromising search for scientific truth in all aspects of implantology. The reality is that even today there is very little credible reportage that legitimately compares one company's implant system to another over a meaningful period of time—let alone to several companies' systems. It might be a reasonable conclusion that restorative competency should be initially restricted to perhaps only two or three systems. The intensity and duration of system-specific learning then becomes a legitimate concern.

Further, the reality is that those clinicians placing implants should have extensive diagnostic and treatment planning skills; that is, have considerable prosthodontic knowledge. Likewise, the restoration of implants will usually be done by clinicians who have directed their placement; that is, also having considerable diagnostic and treatment planning skills. Recent advances in CT-based planning, for example, are not just for surgical placement but also for pre-surgical prosthodontic planning. Again we have a clear need for triaging patients prior to placing as well as prior to restoring implants.

The implant societies gathered here in Toronto do not singularly or collectively in any country constitute a specialty board in the same manner or with the same responsibilities as those in the United States. The granting of a dental license there is a state issue and no dentist is restricted from placing, restoring, and/or maintaining dental implants and related prostheses. In the author's opinion, individual dentists should commit early to a surgical method of training for diagnoses, treatment plans and placement, restoration, and maintenance of dental implants (Judy 1990). Specifically, each practitioner should study, observe, assist, and then practice whatever aspect of implantation that he or she is comfortable with.

Didactic study alone cannot possibly be completed on the pre-doctoral level, so substantial commitments to continuing education, manufacturer-specific courses, and/or "institute" training are necessary. A very high percentage of needed implants would then be legitimately placed as well as restored by generalists. Complex cases, needing graduates of specialty training programs, would then become the responsibility of appropriate specialists.

The reality is that the challenge the profession faces is not generalist education vis-à-vis implants but increased specialty education directed toward solving global health care needs. No matter what balance of generalist versus specialist placement and restoration of implants one proposes, the current and future answer is effective education on all levels.

Hopefully, in 2008 the Toronto Osseointegration Conference Revisited will mark the coup de grace to anecdotal or unproven claims and associated devices. Hopefully, the profession will be able to utilize reliable devices and proven prosthodontic concepts so that each clinician can bring his or her skill set to bear and produce consistent, elegant results. Hopefully . . .

References

Judy K. 1986. Implantology as a dental specialty: A moral and educational focus. *Implantologist* 4(1):15–19.

———. 1989. The impact of implants on dental practices: A review of the 1988 NIH Consensus Development Conference. *NY State Dent J* 55(4):24–27.

———. 1990. Treatment planning for the complex implant prosthodontic cases. In: *Implant Prosthodontics: Surgical and Prosthodontic Techniques for Dental Implants*. M. Fagan (ed.). Littleton, MA: Yearbook Medical Publishers. 22–37.

———. 2008. Guaranteeing treatment for everyone: The need for educational triage. *Implant Dentistry* 17(1). In press.

Judy K, Misch C. 1985. An imperative context for recognition of oral implantology as a dental specialty. *NY State Dent J* 55(1): 33–35.

Perel M. 2007. No excuses: Continuing education. *Implant Dent* 16(4):327.

The Toronto Osseointegration Conference Revisited, May 9–10, 2008

Program

Friday 9:00–10:30

Implant Dentistry: A Technology Assessment

Marco Esposito
Senior Lecturer in Oral and Maxillofacial Surgery, School of Dentistry, University of Manchester, Manchester, United Kingdom
What Have We Learned from Clinical Randomized Controlled Trials on Oral Implants?

Michael I. MacEntee
Professor, University of British Columbia, Vancouver, British Columbia, Canada
Putting People into Clinical Outcomes

Bjarni E. Pætursson
Professor, Department of Prosthodontics, University of Iceland, Reykjavik, Iceland
What Have We Learned from Clinical Non-randomized Controlled Trials on Oral Implants?

Comprehensive Treatment Planning Strategies

Luca Cordaro
Professor and Head, Department of Periodontology and Implant Dentistry, Eastman Dental Hospital, Rome, Italy
Complete Arch Rehabilitation in Complex Cases: Technical Innovations May Reduce Patient Discomfort during Treatment?

David Felton
Professor, Department of Prosthodontics, University of North Carolina, Chapel Hill, North Carolina, United States
We Will Not Outlive the Need for Implant-Retained Overdentures!

Carl E. Misch
Clinical Professor, Oral Implantology, Temple University School of Dentistry, Philadelphia, Pennsylvania, United States
Treatment Planning: A Biomechanical Rationale

Pre-implant Surgical Interventions

Nikolaos Donos
Professor and Head, Periodontology, UCL Eastman Dental Institute, London, United Kingdom
Guided Bone Regeneration/Augmentation with or without Bone Grafts. From Experimental Studies to Clinical Application

Burton Langer
Certified Periodontist, specialty private practice, New York, New York, United States
The Horizontal and Vertical Bone Regeneration in Both the Maxilla and Mandible

E. Todd Scheyer
Certified Peridontist, specialty private practice, Houston, Texas, United States
Tissue Engineering for the Oral Cavity: Hard- and Soft-Tissue Applications and Our Influence upon Osseointegration

Friday 11:00–12:30

Comprehensive Treatment Planning Strategies of Complex Patients

James D. Anderson
Professor, Department of Prosthodontics, University of Toronto, Toronto, Ontario, Canada
The Challenging Patient and Implant Therapy—Facial Deformities

Birgitta Bergendal
Head, Senior Consultant; National Oral Disability Centre, the Institute for Postgraduate Dental Education, Jönköping, Sweden
The Challenging Patient and Implant Dentistry—Rare Disorders

Frauke Mueller
Professor, Department of Geriatrics and Prosthodontics, University of Geneva, Geneva, Switzerland
Risks and Benefits of Implant Therapy in Compromised Elderly Adults

Surgery Phase Planning

Jay R. Beagle
Certified Periodontist, specialty private practice, Indianapolis, Indiana, United States
Immediate Implants in Infected Sites: Contraindications Reconsidered

Scott D. Ganz
Maxillofacial Prosthodontist, specialty private practice, Fort Lee, New Jersey, United States
Advances in Diagnosis and Treatment Planning Utilizing CT Scan Technology for Improved Surgical and Restorative Implant Reconstruction: Tools of Empowerment

Homah Zadeh
Associate Professor, University of Southern California, Los Angeles, California, United States
Computer-Aided Implant Surgery: Current Status

Pre-implant Surgical Augmentation Interventions

Karl-Erik Kahnberg
Professor and Chairman, Department of Oral and Maxillofacial Surgery, Institute of Odontology, the Sahlgrenska Academy at University of Göteborg, Göteborg, Sweden
Onlay and Inlay Grafting in the Reconstruction of the Resorbed Maxilla

Craig M. Misch
Certified Oral and Maxillofacial Surgeon and Prosthodontist, Misch Implant Dentistry, Sarasota, Florida, United States
Is Autogenous Bone Still the "Gold Standard" for Grafting? Current Opinion on the Use of Autograft in Implant Dentistry

Friedrich W. Neukam
Chairman and Head, Department of Oral and Cranio-Maxillofacial Surgery, Erlangen-Nuremberg University Dental School, Erlangen, Germany

Hard Tissue Augmentation to Osseointegrate Implants

Friday 2:00–3:30

Oral and Systemic Inflammation and Comprehensive Treatment Planning Strategies

Øystein Fardal
Certified Periodontist, specialty private practice, Egersund, Norway
Profiles and Treatment Options for Refractory Patients in a Periodontal Practice

Myron Nevins
Certified Periodontist, specialty private practice, Boston, Massachusetts, United States
Osseointegration for the Periodontally Compromised Patient

Howard Tenenbaum
Professor and Associate Dean for Biological and Diagnostic Sciences, University of Toronto, Toronto, Ontario, Canada
Oral and Systemic Inflammation; What Is the Impact of Endosseous Implants?

Pre-implant Surgical Interventions with Focus on the Maxilla

Stuart J. Froum
Clinical Professor, Department of Periodontology and Implant Dentistry, New York University Dental Center, New York, New York, United States
The Sinus Augmentation Procedure 1982/2008/and Beyond

Lars Rasmusson
Professor and Maxillofacial Surgeon, Sahlgrenska Academy and Hospital, University of Göteborg, Göteborg, Sweden
Bone Augmentation in the Severely Resorbed Maxilla

Stephen S. Wallace
Associate Professor, Department of Implant Dentistry, New York University, New York, New York, United States

Will Today's State-of-the-Art Sinus Grafting Technique Become Tomorrow's Evidence-Based Therapy?

The Implant Design and Biological Response

Jan Gottlow
PhD, Department of Biomaterials, University of Göteborg, Göteborg, Sweden
Influences of Implant Design and Surface Properties on Osseointegration and Implant Stability

Jaime L. Lozada
Professor and Director, Graduate Program in Implant Dentistry, Loma Linda University, Los Angeles, California, United States
Clinical Outcomes from the Evolution of the Dental Implant Geometry and Surface Topography

Robert M. Pilliar
Professor Emeritus, Faculty of Dentistry and Institute of Biomaterials and Biomedical Engineering, University of Toronto, Toronto, Ontario, Canada
Implant Surface Design and Local Stress Fields—Effects on Peri-implant Bone

Friday 4:00–5:30

Implant Surgical Interventions

Michael S. Block
Professor, Department of Oral and Maxillofacial Surgery, LSU School of Dentistry, New Orleans, Louisiana, United States
The Art of Healing—Using Implant-Related Technology to Reconstruct the Complex Patient

Axel J.A. Wirthmann
Adjunct Professor, Department of Implant Dentistry, New York University, New York, New York, United States, and Klinik Berner Stieg, Hamburg, Germany
Cell Physiology and Molecular Biology of Bone Regeneration, Then and Now

Michael A. Pikos

Certified Oral and Maxillofacial Surgeon, Pikos Implant Institute, Palm Harbor, Florida, United States
Digitally Guided Bone Augmentation: A Three-Dimensional Synergy of Interactive CT Planning/Soft- and Hard-Tissue Grafting for Optimal Esthetic Zone Rehabilitation

The Implant Surface and Biological Response

Lyndon Cooper

Professor, Department of Prosthodontics, University of North Carolina, Chapel Hill, North Carolina, United States
Molecular and Cellular Biology: New Instruments for Improving Osseointegration

John E. Davies

Professor, Faculty of Dentistry and Institute of Biomaterials and Biomedical Engineering, University of Toronto, Toronto, Ontario, Canada
Implant Surface Design: Evolution and Future Challenges

Peter Schüpbach

Professor, Research Institute for Microscopy and Histology, Zurich, Switzerland
Osseointegration and Soft-Tissue Integration: Impact of the Surface

Biomaterials and Substances for Site Optimizing

Michael Reddy

Associate Professor and Chairman, Department of Periodontology, University of Alabama School of Dentistry, Birmingham, Alabama, United States
Dental Implant Regenerative Medicine: Past, Present, and Future

Massimo Simion

Professor, Department of Periodontology and Implant Restoration, University of Milan, Milan, Italy

Ridge Augmentation Using rh-PDGF: Preclinical and Clinical Results

Ulf Wikesjö

Professor and Director, Medical College of Georgia School of Dentistry, Augusta, Georgia, United States
Bone Morphogenic Proteins and Osseointegration

Saturday 9:00–10:30

Restorative Phase Treatment Planning

Peter Scheer

Certified Oral Maxillofacial Surgeon, specialty private practice, Rancho Mirage, California, United States
Intricacies of Anterior Preprosthetic Surgery and Immediate Provisionalization

Clark M. Stanford

Professor, Dows Institute for Dental Research, University of Iowa, Iowa City, Iowa, United States
Integration of Biological Principles to Achieve Stable Esthetics

Paul Weigl

Assistant Professor, Department of Prosthetic Dentistry, J.W. Goethe-University, Frankfurt am Main, Germany
Changing Rationales Connecting Teeth with Implants by a Suprastructure

The Implant and Biological Response

John B. Brunski

Professor, Department of Biomedical Engineering, Rensselaer Polytechnic Institute, Troy, New York, United States
The Healing Bone-Implant Interface: The Role of Micromotion and Related Strain Levels in Tissue

David L. Cochran

Professor and Chair, Department of Periodontics, the University of Texas Health

Science Center at San Antonio, San Antonio, Texas, United States
Does the Body React to All Implant Interfaces the Same Way?

Niklaus P. Lang
Professor, Periodontology and Fixed Prosthodontics, University of Bern, Bern, Switzerland
Early Healing Sequences in Tissue Integration of Oral Implants

Beyond the Mouth—Habilitation and Rehabilitation

Steve Parel
Professor, Center for Maxillofacial Prosthodontics, A&M University System Health Science Center, Houston, Texas, United States
Implant Options for the Restoration of the Compromised Maxillofacial Patient

George Sàndor
Professor and Director, Graduate Program in Oral and Maxillofacial Surgery, University of Toronto and Mount Sinai Hospital, Toronto, Ontario, Canada
Use of Dental Implants in Habilitation of Children, Adolescents, and Young Adults

R. Gilbert Triplett
Regents Professor, Department of Oral and Maxillofacial Surgery, Baylor College of Dentistry, Baylor University Medical Center, Dallas, Texas, United States
Reconstruction of the Severely Debilitated Maxillofacial Patient Using Principles of Osseointegration

Saturday 11:00–12:30

Restorative Phase Treatment Planning Using Early Loading Protocols

Roland Glauser
Certified Prosthodontist, specialty private practice, Zurich, Switzerland

Shortened Clinical Protocols—The Revolution Is Still Ongoing

Maurice A. Salama
Certified Periodontist and Orthodontist, specialty private practice, Atlanta, Georgia, United States
Success by Design: Integrating Biology, New Implant Design, and Esthetics in Simplified and Complex Therapy

Thomas D. Taylor
Professor, Professor and Head, Department of Oral Rehabilitation, Skeletal Development and Biomaterials, University of Connecticut, Farmington, Connecticut, United States
The Stability of Implant/Abutment Connections

The Implant Design and Clinical Outcomes

Shadi Daher
Assistant Clinical Professor, Boston University Goldman School of Dental Medicine, Boston, Massachusetts, United States
A Scientific Basis for the Success, Longevity, and Predictability of Plateau-Designed Short Implants

Antonio Ruiz Sanz
Professor, Periodontal and Implant Department, University of Los Andes, Santiago, Chile
Internal Connection: A Contribution to Esthetic Results

John K. Schulte
Associate Professor, Department of Restorative Sciences, University of Minnesota School of Dentistry, Minneapolis, Minnesota, United States
Is Clinical Performance of an Implant Influenced by Its Design?

Patient Focus on Neurophysiology

Iven Klineberg
Professor and Head, Jaw Function and Orofacial Pain Research Unit, University of Sydney, Sydney, Australia
Clinical Implications of Neuroplasticity

Barry J. Sessle
Professor and Canada Research Chair, Faculties of Dentistry and Medicine, University of Toronto, Toronto, Ontario, Canada
Neural Mechanisms Underlying "Osseoperception" and Sensorimotor Adaptation to Dental Implants and Related Intraoral Procedures

Peter Svensson
Professor and Chair, Department of Clinical Oral Physiology, University of Aarhus, Aarhus, Denmark
Nerve Lesions—A Problem for Oral Implants?

Saturday 2:00–3:30

Loading Protocols and Biological Response

Peter K. Moy
Associate Clinical Professor, Department of Oral and Maxillofacial Surgery, University of California, Los Angeles, California, United States
Understanding Loading Principles for Implant Dentistry to Optimize Clinical Outcome. A Prosthetic and Surgical Decision-Making Algorithm for Delayed, Early, and Immediate Loading

Mario Roccuzzo
Lecturer in Periodontology, University of Torino, Torino, Italy
A View from the Future: Predictable and Safe Early Loading in Posterior Maxilla

Georgios E. Romanos
Professor of Clinical Dentistry, Divisions of Periodontology and General Dentistry, Eastman Department of Dentistry, Rochester, New York, United States

Prerequisites and Clinical Opportunities Using Immediate Occlusal Loading in the Maxilla and Mandible

Patient Focus on Expected and Unexpected Outcomes

Klaus Gotfredsen
Professor, Department of Oral Rehabilitation, University of Copenhagen, Copenhagen, Denmark
Subjective and Objective Evaluation of Implant-Supported Reconstructions

Kent L. Knoernschild
Co-Director, Comprehensive Dental Implant Center, University of Illinois, Chicago, Illinois, United States
Dental Implant Innovations: Best Decisions for Patient Benefit

Alan M. Meltzer
Certified Periodontist, specialty private practice, Voorhees, New Jersey, United States
Tissue Changes on the Mid-facial of Implant Crowns within the Esthetic Zone

The Transmucosal Component and the Supra-construction Revolution

Steven E. Eckert
Professor, Department of Prosthodontics, Mayo College of Medicine, Rochester, Minnesota, United States
CAD/CAM Abutments: From Rescue to Routine

Robert L. Schneider
Professor, Hospital Dentistry Institute, University of Iowa Hospitals and Clinics, Iowa City, Iowa, United States
Relative Illumination of an All-Ceramic and Implant Abutment System

Jörg-R. Strub
Professor and Chair, Department of Prosthodontics, Albert-Ludwig University, Freiburg, Germany
CAD-CAM in Implant Dentistry

Saturday 4:00–5:30

Loading Protocols and Clinical Outcomes

Asbjorn Jokstad
Professor and Head, Department of Prosthodontics, University of Toronto, Toronto, Ontario, Canada
What Have We Learned from Clinical Trials about Early Loading of Implants?

Ignace Naert
Professor, Department of Prosthodontics, University of Leuven, Leuven, Belgium
What Have We Learned about the Influence of Loading on the Quality and Maintenance of Osseointegration?

Hans-Peter Weber
Professor and Chair, Restorative Dentistry and Biomaterials Sciences, Harvard School of Dental Medicine, Boston, Massachusetts, United States
The Concept of Early Loading

Patient Focus on Function and Quality of Life

Jocelyne S. Feine
Professor and Director of Graduate Studies, McGill University, Montreal, Quebec, Canada
1982's Edentulous Patients Are Now Oral Health Care Consumers—What Is Important to Them?

Mark Thomason
Chair of Prosthodontics and Oral Rehabilitation, Newcastle University, Newcastle, United Kingdom
From Professional to Patient Satisfaction—25 Years of Change?

Daniel Wismeijer
Professor, Oral Implantology and Implant Prosthodontics, ACTA, Amsterdam, the Netherlands
Keeping It Simple but Efficient

Minimum Competency for Providing Implant Prosthodontics—What Should Be the Educational Requirements?

Kenneth W.M. Judy
Director, International Congress of Oral Implantologists and Private Practice, New York, New York, United States
Guaranteeing Treatment for Everyone: Changing Educational Criteria for "Garden Variety" Cases to Major Bone Grafts

Steven E. Eckert
Professor, Department of Prosthodontics, Mayo College of Medicine, Rochester, Minnesota, United States
On the Provision of Implant Dentistry

Biographies of Speakers

James D. Anderson
Dr. James D. Anderson is a professor at the Faculty of Dentistry, University of Toronto, where his responsibilities include teaching in the graduate program in prosthodontics. He is also a consultant for maxillofacial prosthetics at several Toronto area teaching hospitals. He is director of the Craniofacial Prosthetic Unit at Sunnybrook Health Sciences Centre, a multidisciplinary unit devoted to the treatment of patients with congenital and acquired facial deformities. He speaks and publishes internationally on prosthetics and clinical epidemiology.

Jay R. Beagle
Dr. Jay R. Beagle, DDS, MSD, maintains a private practice where he specializes in periodontal plastic, reconstructive, and dental implant surgery. Having authored and co-authored numerous articles in the dental literature, Dr. Beagle has primarily focused on advanced surgical concepts in periodontics and implant dentistry. These concepts include but are not limited to immediate implant placement, sinus grafting, complex regenerative procedures, and

periodontal plastic and reconstructive surgery utilizing the surgical microscope. He has lectured extensively both nationally and internationally, and is actively committed to education, training, and clinical research.

Birgitta Bergendal
Dr. Birgitta Bergendal graduated from Karolinska Institute, Stockholm, in 1971, and became a specialist in prosthetic dentistry in 1978. Beginning in 1982 she was a tutor in the specialist program at the Institute for Postgraduate Dental Education, Jönköping, Sweden. Ten years ago she established the National Oral Disability Centre for rare disorders in dentistry. One focus area of research is diagnosis and rehabilitation in disorders where teeth and jaws are affected and the use and outcome of dental implants in rare disorders.

Michael S. Block
Dr. Michael S. Block graduated from the University of Rochester in 1975, attaining both a BA in biology and a BS in biomedical engineering. He completed his dental training at the Harvard School of Dental Medicine in 1979. He completed his residency program in oral and maxillofacial surgery at the LSU School of Dentistry in 1983. He remained at the LSU School of Dentistry and is currently professor in the Department of Oral and Maxillofacial Surgery and maintains a private practice in the Center for Dental Reconstruction in Metairie, Louisiana. Dr. Block is the editor in chief of four textbooks and he is a past president of the Academy of Osseointegration.

John B. Brunski
Dr. John B. Brunski's research has focused on bioengineering aspects of dental implant design. He has authored numerous papers and textbook chapters on oral implants and has given over 150 presentations on these subjects at national and international meetings. Dr. Brunski serves as section editor for biomechanics and biomaterials for the *International Journal of Oral and Maxillofacial Implants*; assistant editor of the *Journal of Biomedical Materials Research/Journal of Applied Biomaterials*; and is a member of the editorial board of *Clinical Oral Implants Research*. In his teaching and research, Dr. Brunski has received a number of awards for innovation and excellence in engineering.

David L. Cochran
Dr. David L. Cochran received his DDS and PhD in biochemistry from the Medical College of Virginia. Dr. Cochran is a member of many professional dental organizations, currently serving as vice president of the American Academy of Periodontology. Dr. Cochran has published numerous scientific articles and abstracts on various periodontal biochemistry and implant topics. He has received awards for his research work at both the national and international levels. Dr. Cochran is an active basic science and clinical researcher who has received funding from both the NIH-NIDR and private industry.

Lyndon Cooper
Dr. Lyndon F. Cooper, DDS, PhD, graduated from the New York University College of Dentistry in 1983 and obtained a PhD in biochemistry at the University of Rochester in 1990. He trained as a prosthodontist at the Eastman Dental Center, Rochester, New York. He has held numerous appointments in national and international committees, including in IADR, AO, and ACP, and holds consultant positions for both industry and academia. Dr. Cooper has published more than 70 peer-reviewed publications in research journals and has had more than 200 national and international presentations.

Luca Cordaro
Dr. Luca Cordaro, MD, DDS, PhD, was appointed assistant in the Department of Periodontology at the Eastman Dental

Hospital in Rome in 1993. He has lectured in Italy, Europe, and the United States. In 2007 he won the Harry Goldman Prize of the Italian Society of Periodontology. His professional interests are periodontology, implant dentistry, and oral surgery with a special interest regarding the reconstructive treatment of alveolar atrophies. Dr. Cordaro serves as a member of the Education Core Group of the ITI. Dr. Cordaro is on the editorial board of *Clinical Oral Implants Research*.

Shadi Daher

Dr. Shadi Daher received his BS degree in mathematics from the American University of Beirut, his DMD degree from Boston University Goldman School of Dentistry, and his oral and maxillofacial training from Boston University and Tufts University. Additionally, he is a diplomate of the American Board of Oral Surgeons and a fellow of both the AAOMS and IAOMS. Dr. Daher is an assistant clinical professor at Boston University Goldman School of Dental Medicine and surgical director of the Bicon Institute.

John E. Davies

Dr. John E. Davies, BDS, PhD, DSc, FBSE, is a professor of dentistry and biomaterials at the University of Toronto. Trained as an oro-maxillofacial surgeon in Wales, he was awarded a degree of doctor of science from the University of London in 1998 for his sustained contributions over 20 years to the field of biomaterials. He was elected as a fellow of biomaterials science and engineering in 2000 and was the recipient of the Society for Biomaterials Clemson Award for Basic Research in 2002.

Nikolaos Donos

Dr. Nikos Donos is the head and chair of periodontology and the director of the Division of Clinical Research at the UCL Eastman Dental Institute, London. His research track record is mainly on GTR and GBR and clinical trials in implantol-

ogy. He has published extensively and is a member of the editorial board of the leading peer-reviewed journals. He is the director of the ITI Scholarship Centre at the UCL Eastman Dental Institute and the education delegate of the ITI UK and Ireland section.

Steven E. Eckert

Dr. Steven E. Eckert is a diplomate of the American Board of Prosthodontics and a fellow of multiple prosthetic associations. He serves on the board of directors for the American Academy of Maxillofacial Prosthetics, the Academy of Osseointegration, and the Academy of Prosthodontics. He is an examiner for the American Board of Prosthodontics. He has served in editorial capacities for a variety of prosthodontic journals and is now editor in chief of the *International Journal of Oral and Maxillofacial Implants*. He has published extensively in the scientific literature and presents at numerous scientific meetings.

Marco Esposito

Dr. Marco Esposito is senior lecturer in oral and maxillofacial surgery, director of the MSc courses in dental implantology, editor of the Cochrane Oral Health Group (University of Manchester), associate professor in biomaterials (University of Göteborg), and editor in chief of the *European Journal of Oral Implantology*. Marco graduated with honors in dentistry at the University of Pavia, Italy, in 1990, was awarded a PhD in biomaterials from the University of Göteborg in 1999, and is a specialist in periodontics.

Øystein Fardal

Dr. Øystein Fardal, BDS, MDS, PhD, is a certified peridontist and has worked in a specialty practice limited to periodontics and implants since 1986. He completed his BDS in 1981, and completed the graduate program in periodontology at the University of Toronto in 1985, MDS in 1987, and PhD in 2002. He has been a president of the Norwegian Society of Periodontology and of the Scandinavian Society of Periodontology. Dr. Fardal's research and publications have focused mainly on patients' preconceptions and perceptions of therapy as well as treatment outcomes of periodontal and implant therapy.

Jocelyne S. Feine

Dr. Jocelyne S. Feine, DDS, MS, HDR, is professor and director of graduate studies at McGill University, Faculty of Dentistry, and associate member, Departments of Epidemiology and Biostatistics and Oncology, McGill University, Faculty of Medicine. Professor Feine's research involves technology assessment studies and randomized clinical efficacy trials of oral rehabilitation. She has published book chapters and books and over 150 articles in peer-reviewed dental and medical journals. Her work is supported by the Canadian Institutes of Health Research and the Fonds de Recherche en Santé du Québec. Dr. Feine is the associate editor for clinical sciences of *The Journal of Dental Research*.

David Felton

Dr. David Felton completed his DDS (1977) and MS (1984—prosthodontics) degrees at the University of North Carolina School of Dentistry in Chapel Hill, North Carolina. He served as director of graduate prosthodontics from 1989 to 1992, and as chair of prosthodontics from 1992 to 2002. He is a past president of the American College of Prosthodontists. He has over 40 published journal articles and 120 abstracts and has presented at the national and international levels. His research interests include dental implants, all ceramic crowns and fixed partial dentures, and biological responses to restorative dental procedures.

Stuart J. Froum

Dr. Stuart J. Froum is a diplomate of the American Board of Periodontology. He is the director of clinical research at the Department of Periodontology and Implant Dentistry, NYU Dental Center, and in private practice limited to periodontics and implant dentistry in New York City. He has served as past president of the Northeast Society of Periodontics and the Research Committee Academy of Osseointegration. He is a trustee of the American Academy of Periodontology and has won numerous educational and research awards.

Scott D. Ganz

Dr. Scott D. Ganz graduated from the New Jersey Dental School, University of Medicine and Dentistry. Dr. Ganz has published over 50 articles in various scientific and professional journals. He has delivered presentations both nationally and internationally on the prosthetic and surgical phases of implant dentistry and is considered one of the world's leading experts in the field of computer utilization for diagnostic, graphical, and treatment planning applications in dentistry. He currently serves as assistant editor for the peer-reviewed journal *Implant Dentistry* and on the editorial staff of *Practical Procedures and Esthetic Dentistry*.

Roland Glauser

Dr. Roland Glauser received his DDS from the University of Zurich. From 1997 to 2006 Dr. Glauser was assistant professor and senior lecturer at the Department for Fixed Prosthodontics and Dental Materials, University of Zurich. In 2006, he became director of the Zurich Dental Center. He has published more than 50 articles and textbook chapters on the subject of restorative dentistry and osseointegrated implants. His research activities mainly focus on tissue integration of oral implants and shortened clinical protocols.

Klaus Gotfredsen

Dr. Klaus Gotfredsen is professor and head of the Department of Oral Rehabilitation, Faculty of Health Sciences, University of Copenhagen. He received a Danish PhD degree in 1990 and a Swedish PhD degree in 2001. He has mainly researched in clinical and experimental implant dentistry and has published more than 65 scientific papers in the fields of implant dentistry and prosthetic dentistry. He is reviewer for a number of clinical and scientific journals and has lectured extensively in the field of implant dentistry.

Jan Gottlow

Dr. Jan Gottlow is DDS, PhD (Dr. Odont.), and licensed specialist in periodontics. Currently he is associate professor at the Department of Biomaterials, Institute for Surgical Sciences, University of Göteborg, Sweden, and at the Brånemark Clinic, Public Dental Health Service, and Faculty of Odontology, Göteborg, Sweden. He is a member of the editorial board of *Clinical Implant Dentistry and Related Research*. He has published extensively and is a well-known international lecturer.

Asbjorn Jokstad

Dr. Asbjorn Jokstad is a DDS graduate from 1979, PhD in 1992, and specialist in prosthodontics in 1994. He became professor at the University of Toronto Faculty of Dentistry in Canada in September 2005 and has the Nobel Biocare Chair in Prosthodontics. He is a former professor in cariology/conservative dentistry and later in prosthodontics at the University of Oslo in Norway. Dr. Jokstad has produced approximately 150 research and teaching publications, book chapters, and abstracts with emphasis on evidence-based dentistry, clinical trials in restorative dentistry and prosthodontics, toxicology, and TMD.

Kenneth W.M. Judy

Dr. Kenneth Judy is the co-chair of the International Congress of Oral Implantologists. He is a clinical professor, Department of Implant Dentistry, New York University College of Dentistry, and a clinical professor, Department of Periodontology and Implantology, Temple University, Kronberg

School of Dentistry, Philadelphia. He has authored or co-authored over 100 articles, textbook chapters, or editorials related to dental implant therapy. Dr. Judy maintains a private practice in New York City.

Karl-Erik Kahnberg

Dr. Karl-Erik Kahnberg is a DDS since 1966 and Odont. Dr. since 1976. He became a specialist in oral and maxillofacial surgery in 1977 and has been professor and chairman of the Department of Oral and Maxillofacial Surgery at the University of Göteborg since 1988. Dr. Kahnberg has published about 100 scientific papers in oral and maxillofacial surgery with emphasis on orthognathic, temporomandibular joint, and implant surgery. He currently supervises the postgraduate OMS specialty training in Göteborg and conducts craniofacial surgery and implant surgery that often involves bone transplant combined with orthognathic surgery repositioning and implant installation.

Iven Klineberg

Dr. Iven Klineberg received his BDS from the University of Sydney (1963), MDS (clinical training and research) (1966), and BSc (major in physiology) (1968). He was a 1967–1968 Dental Health Education and Research Foundation Scholar, and earned his PhD from the University of London in 1971. In a specialist practice in prosthodontics from 1971, he is a board-registered prosthodontist, with emphasis on temporomandibular disorders, orofacial pain, and implant rehabilitation. His research has been focused on occlusion and orofacial pain: occlusion and temporomandibular joint neurology—reflex contributions to jaw muscle function, and studies of jaw muscle electromyography and jaw kinematics.

Kent L. Knoernschild

Dr. Kent L. Knoernschild is a diplomate of the American Board of Prosthodontics and has a private practice limited to prosthodontics. Dr. Knoernschild has lectured internationally and published numerous papers addressing biocompatibility of prosthodontic restorations. Lectures have also focused on an evidence-based decision-making strategy for clinicians that help them make the best decisions in practice. He actively serves in several prosthodontics organizations. He is vice president of the American Academy of Fixed Prosthodontics and a past president for the International Association for Dental Research Prosthodontics Group.

Niklaus P. Lang

Dr. Niklaus P. Lang is professor and chairman of the School of Dental Medicine at the University of Bern, Switzerland. His special research interests include oral microbiology, prevention, epidemiology, pathogenesis, and therapy of periodontal and peri-implant diseases; clinical research; diagnostic procedures and risk assessment; and biology of wound healing around dental implants. He has published nearly 400 articles in peer-reviewed scientific journals and has delivered more than 1,500 lectures on five continents. Dr. Lang serves as editor in chief of *Clinical Oral Implants Research* and editor of *Oral Health and Preventive Dentistry.*

Burton Langer

Dr. Burton Langer is a diplomate of the American Board of Periodontology. He was one of the first periodontists trained in osseointegration by Professor Per-Ingvar Brånemark in 1983. Dr. Langer has lectured extensively throughout the world and has written more than 30 articles. He is the 1997 recipient of the American Academy of Periodontology Master Clinician Award.

Jaime L. Lozada

Dr. Jaime L. Lozada has been instrumental in training residents and fellows in the latest techniques in oral implant surgery and prosthodontics at the Center for Implant Dentistry at Loma Linda University School of Dentistry. Dr. Lozada has been involved with implant dentistry for 20 years. He is an active member of many prosthodontic and implant organizations. Dr. Lozada has published and lectured nationally and internationally on implant dentistry. He maintains an intramural private practice limited to implant surgery and prosthodontics.

Michael I. MacEntee

Dr. Michael I. MacEntee, PhD, LDS(I), Dip. Prosth., FRCD(C). Professor of prosthodontics and dental geriatrics, Faculty of Dentistry, University of British Columbia; and past president of the Association of Prosthodontists of Canada, the International College of Prosthodontists, and the Royal College of Dentists of Canada. His research addresses oral health and quality of life, with a particular focus on frailty, and on the identification, distribution, impact, and management of oral disorders in old age.

Alan M. Meltzer

Dr. Alan M. Meltzer received his dental degree from the University of Pennsylvania and his master's in periodontics and oral medicine from Boston University, School of Graduate Dentistry. He is a diplomate of the American Board of Periodontology and a fellow of the Academy of Osseointegration, where he serves on its Research and Education Committees. He is a featured speaker for the New Jersey Society of Periodontists, New York University Department of Implantology, and the University of Milan, Milan, Italy. Dr. Meltzer maintains a private practice in Voorhees, New Jersey.

Carl E. Misch

Dr. Carl E. Misch holds appointments at the University of Michigan, University of Alabama, University of Detroit, and Loma Linda University. Dr. Misch has been president of many implant organizations and is currently the co-chairman of the board of directors of the International Congress of Implantologists, the world's largest implant organization. He is also co-inventor of the BioHorizons Dental Implant System. He has published over 200 articles and has repeatedly lectured in every state in the United States as well as 47 countries.

Craig M. Misch

Dr. Craig M. Misch received postgraduate certificates in prosthodontics and oral implantology and an MSc from the University of Pittsburgh. He continued completing specialty training in oral and maxillofacial surgery. Dr. Misch is a diplomate of the American Board of Oral and Maxillofacial Surgery. Dr. Misch is a clinical associate professor at both New York University and the University of Florida. He is on the board of directors of the Academy of Osseointegration and serves on the editorial board for the *International Journal of Oral and Maxillofacial Implants*.

Peter K. Moy

Dr. Peter K. Moy received his dental degree from the University of Pittsburgh, a certificate in general practice residency from Queen's Medical Center in Honolulu, Hawaii, and his certificate in oral and maxillofacial surgery from UCLA Hospital. Dr. Moy has written numerous articles related to implant dentistry and osseointegration, specifically on bone grafting and augmentation procedures. He maintains his private practice in the West Coast Center for Oral and Maxillofacial Surgery, located in Brentwood, California. Dr. Moy is the director of implant dentistry at UCLA and director, UCLA Surgical Implant Clinic.

Frauke Mueller

Dr. Frauke Mueller has been professor and chair for gerodontology and removable prosthodontics at the University of Geneva, Switzerland, since 2003. She has a DDS from the University of Bonn, Germany, and later worked in the Prosthetic Department of the University of Mainz. She further spent several years at the London Hospital Medical College in England in a research program in gerodontology. Professor Mueller served on the board of many professional associations: German Society of Gerostomatology, European College of Gerodontology, and the Geriatric Oral Research Group of the IADR. She is associate editor of *Gerodontology*. Her research activity is mainly related to gerodontology and oral function as well as complete dentures.

Ignace Naert

Dr. Ignace Naert graduated from the Catholic University of Leuven in 1977 and became a doctor in dental sciences in 1991. He became a full professor lecturing in fixed prosthodontics in 1995. Dr. Naert is a member of the editorial boards of numerous scientific journals. He is the current president of the Implantology Research Group of the IADR and received the IADR Distinguished Award in Prosthodontics and Implants Research in 2005. He has more than 150 publications and has co-edited several textbooks. His research interests are clinical follow-up studies related to implant-supported restorations and all-ceramics, dynamic force transmission between implants, and bone remodeling.

Friedrich W. Neukam

Prof. Dr. med. Dr. med. dent. Friedrich W. Neukam completed his dental studies at Mainz University in 1976. He was a trainee in oral and maxillofacial surgery and senior staff at Hannover University Medical School between 1979 and 1984, obtained a PhD in 1990, and became associate professor in 1994. He is the current president of EAO and since 2001 the editor in chief of *Deutsche Zeitschrift für Mund-Kiefer-Gesichtschirurgie*. Dr. Neukam's work focuses on lip and palate clefts, orthodontic surgery, tumor surgery, implantology, and bone grafts in combination with implants.

Myron Nevins

Dr. Myron Nevins, DDS, is the editor of the *International Journal of Periodontics and Restorative Dentistry* and associate clinical professor of periodontology at the Harvard School of Dental Medicine. Dr. Nevins is a past president of the American Academy of Periodontology, where his contributions have been recognized with the Gold Medal and the Master Clinician Awards. He is a professor of periodontics at the University of Pennsylvania School of Dental Medicine, a clinical professor at the Temple University School of Dentistry, and adjunct professor of periodontics at the University of North Carolina. He maintains a private practice limited to periodontics and implantology.

Steve Parel

Dr. Steve Parel received his DDS from the Medical College of Virginia in 1969. Dr. Parel is a diplomate of the American Board of Prosthodontics. His literature contributions include over 45 scientific articles and multiple textbook chapters. He was editor and co-author of *Esthetics and Osseointegration,* a landmark reference source for implant dentistry. He was co-founder of Osseointegration Seminars, Inc., is a board member and treasurer of the Osseointegration Foundation, and is a past president of both the American Academy of Maxillofacial Prosthetics and the Academy of Osseointegration. Dr. Parel serves currently as a board examiner for the American Board of Prosthodontics.

Bjarni E. Pætursson

Dr. Bjarni E. Pætursson obtained a DDS from University of Iceland in 1990 and received a specialist certificate in periodontology (EFP and SSP) and doctorate in dentistry from the University of Bern, Switzerland, in 2004. He has been assistant professor and senior lecturer at the Department of Periodontology and Fixed Prosthodontics, University of Bern, and is presently the chairman of the Department of Prostho-

dontics, Faculty of Odontology, University of Iceland. Dr. Pætursson is an ITI fellow and member of the editorial board of *Clinical Oral Implants Research*.

Michael A. Pikos

Dr. Michael A. Pikos is a diplomate of the American Board of Oral and Maxillofacial Surgery, the American Board of Oral Implantology/Implant Dentistry, the International Congress of Oral Implantologists, and the American Society of Osseointegration. He serves as an adjunct assistant professor of oral and maxillofacial surgery at the University of Miami, Ohio State University, and Nova Southeastern University, and as a courtesy clinical associate professor of periodontology at the University of Florida. Dr. Pikos has written and lectured nationally and internationally on dental implants and maintains a private practice limited to implant surgery in Palm Harbor, Florida.

Robert M. Pilliar

Dr. Robert M. Pilliar graduated from the University of Toronto in Engineering Physics in 1961 (BASc) and then went on to obtain his PhD degree from Leeds University, England, in 1965. Subsequently, he worked as a research scientist in industry before returning to the University of Toronto, where he has held cross-appointments in the Faculty of Dentistry and Faculty of Applied Science and Engineering. Dr. Pilliar's research since the early 1970s has focused on development of implants for orthopedic and dental applications.

Lars Rasmusson

Dr. Lars Rasmusson received his DMD in 1990 at the University of Göteborg, Sweden. From 1995 to 2000, he accomplished the training program in oral and maxillofacial surgery at the Sahlgrenska University Hospital. He defended his thesis "On Implant Integration in Membrane Induced and Grafted Bone" at the Faculty of Medicine in 1998. His clinical work is concentrated in orthognatic surgery and reconstructive implant surgery, and in TMJ surgery at the clinic. His scientific work is focused on healing and integration of bone grafts. Dr. Rasmusson is a frequent lecturer at national and international congresses and courses.

Michael Reddy

Dr. Michael Reddy, DMD, DMSc, is professor and chairman of the Department of Periodontology at the University of Alabama at Birmingham School of Dentistry. He has published numerous scientific manuscripts and has been the recipient of research grants from the NIH/NIDCR and industry. He is actively involved as a scientist in the UAB Center for Aging and the UAB Center for Metabolic Bone Disease, where his efforts are currently being applied to the development of dental implants and surgical techniques aimed at the regeneration of bone.

Mario Roccuzzo

Dr. Mario Roccuzzo is lecturer in periodontology at the postgraduate school of oral and maxillofacial surgery of the University of Torino, Italy. He has done extensive research in the field of mucogingival surgery and guided bone regeneration. He is an active member of the Italian Society of Periodontology and fellow of the International Team for Implantology. Dr. Roccuzzo serves on the editorial board of *Clinical Oral Implants Research* and the *European Journal of Esthetic Dentistry*. He has lectured extensively in Europe, Russia, Japan, and the United States and maintains a private practice limited to periodontology and implantology in Torino.

Georgios E. Romanos

Dr. Georgios Romanos, DDS, Dr. med. dent., PhD, has full training in periodontics, prosthodontics, and oral surgery in Germany. He has a doctoral degree in connective tissue research and a post-PhD in immediate loading of oral implants. Between 2004 and 2007 he was a clinical professor of periodontology and implant dentistry at New York University. He is an editorial board member in different peer-reviewed journals and has more than 170 publications and book chapters. He is the author of three books and has lectured in more than 300 presentations worldwide.

Maurice A. Salama

Dr. Maurice A. Salama completed his undergraduate studies at the State University of New York at Binghamton in 1985, where he received his BS in biology. Dr. Salama received his DMD from the University of Pennsylvania School of Dental Medicine (Penn), where he later also received his dual specialty certification in orthodontics and periodontics, as well as implant training at the Brånemark Center at Penn. He is currently on the faculty of the University of Pennsylvania and the Medical College of Georgia as clinical assistant professor of periodontics, and is visiting professor of periodontics at Nova University in Florida.

George Sàndor

Dr. George Sàndor received his dental and medical degrees from the University of Toronto. He trained as an oral and maxillofacial surgeon at the University of Washington in Seattle and in plastic surgery at the University of Toronto. He trained as a craniofacial surgeon in Paris, France, and Bern, Switzerland. Dr. Sàndor completed his PhD at the University of Oulu in Finland. He received his doctor of habilitation from Semmelweis Medical University in Budapest, Hungary.

Antonio Ruiz Sanz

Dr. Antonio Ruiz Sanz is a specialist in periodontics from Universidad de Chile, Santiago, Chile, and in oral implantology from Universidad Complutense, Madrid, Spain. He is the head of the Periodontal and Implant Department and the graduate programs in periodontics and oral implantology in the Faculty of Dentistry at

Universidad de los Andes, Santiago, Chile. Dr. Sanz is an international speaker and active member of many professional organizations. He is past president of the Chilean Periodontal Society.

Peter Scheer
Dr. Peter M. Scheer, DDS, MS, is the founder of the Mirage Center. He is the primary tenant in the Oral and Maxillofacial Surgery Department. He is a well-established expert in both implant dentistry and orthognathic surgery. He received his oral and maxillofacial surgery training from Loma Linda University, where he is on the faculty. Dr. Scheer has lectured internationally on implant dentistry and bone healing, as well as conducting seminars for medical and dental professionals. He is on staff at Eisenhower Hospital and a member of the trauma team at Desert Hospital. Dr. Scheer is a fellow of the American Academy of Cosmetic Surgery.

E. Todd Scheyer
Dr. E. Todd Scheyer received his certificate in periodontics, conscious sedation and a master's degree from the University of Texas Health Science Center at San Antonio focusing on perio-prosthetic reconstruction. Dr. Scheyer was awarded the John F. Prichard Award for graduate research in February 2001. He is a diplomate of the American Board of Periodontology and a member of many dental organizations. He currently serves as an officer and committee member for many outstanding dental organizations. He continues to be involved with clinical research and publications within the private practice setting, sharing his research and perspectives through national and international lecturing.

Robert L. Schneider
Dr. Robert L. Schneider works at the University of Iowa Hospitals and Clinics, Institute of Hospital Dentistry, Division of Prosthodontics and holds the rank of professor, where he has a full-time private practice.

Dr. Schneider received his DDS from the University of Southern California and practiced general dentistry in Arizona for 5 years before earning his MS and certificate in prosthodontics from the University of Iowa in 1983.

John K. Schulte
Dr. John K. Schulte is co-director of graduate prosthodontics and director of the oral implantology program for graduate students at the University of Minnesota. Dr. Schulte graduated in 1973 from the University of Nebraska College of Dentistry. He received a certificate in prosthodontics and a master's degree in dentistry from the University of Washington in Seattle in 1978. He has contributed to the dental literature in the areas of occlusion and dental implantology.

Peter Schüpbach
Dr. Peter Schüpbach studied natural sciences at the Federal Technical High School of Switzerland and in 1979 obtained his doctoral degree. He spent over 20 years at the Dental Institute of the University of Zurich as a head of a histological group. He has a PhD in biology and was lecturer at the Faculty of Medicine of the University of Zurich for "Oral Biology and Pathophysiology." He is a member of several international organizations and author of over 50 publications in the fields of implantology, bone substitutes, tissue regeneration, cariology, and oral microbiology. He is an international lecturer in implantology. Today he runs a research center for microscopy and histology.

Barry J. Sessle
Dr. Barry J. Sessle, MDS, PhD, was dean of the Faculty of Dentistry at the University of Toronto from 1990 to 2001. He is an elected fellow of the Royal Society of Canada and member of the Canadian Academy of Science. He is currently president of the Canadian Pain Society and a past president of the International Associa-

tion for the Study of Pain and of the IADR. He is editor in chief of the *Journal of Orofacial Pain*, has co-authored/edited 11 books, and has published 300 journal articles and book chapters. His orofacial pain and neuromuscular research has been continuously supported for 33 years by both the Canadian Institutes of Health Research and the U.S. National Institutes of Health.

Massimo Simion

Dr. Massimo Simion has had a degree in medicine and surgery since 1979. He specialized in odontostomatology and dental prosthodontics in 1982. He was a member of the board of EAO in 1998–2005 and president for the years 2001–2003. He is the founder of the Italian Society of Osseointegration and an active member and past vice president of the Italian Society of Periodontology (SidP). He is a referee of several scientific journals and has published many scientific papers. He lectures internationally about periodontology, osseointegration, and bone regeneration.

Clark M. Stanford

Dr. Clark M. Stanford received his BS (1984), DDS (1987), certificate in prosthodontics, and PhD (cell biology; 1992) from the University of Iowa. His research areas deal with the areas of osteoblastic gene expression. He manages the Office for Clinical Research in the College of Dentistry and is the associate director for the NIH General Clinical Research Center at the University of Iowa Hospitals and Clinics. Dr. Stanford is the author of 12 book chapters, 74 published papers, and more than 140 published research abstracts. He currently serves on multiple national and international committees. He is the recipient of 16 academic awards, on the review board for 9, and associate editor for 3 journals.

Jörg-R. Strub

Dr. Jörg-R. Strub, born in 1948 in Olten, Switzerland, received his DDS, Dr. med.

dent., and Dr. med. dent. habil. (PhD equiv.) degrees from the University of Zurich, Switzerland. He was a visiting assistant professor of biomaterials at Tulane University and Louisiana State University, New Orleans, 1982–1983, and was formerly associate professor and co-director of the Graduate Programme in Periodontal Prosthetics at the University of Zurich. Since 1988 Dr. Strub has been professor and chair of the Department of Prosthodontics at the Albert-Ludwig University in Freiburg, Germany. He was a visiting clinical professor of fixed prosthodontics at the Osaka University in Osaka, Japan, in 1996.

Peter Svensson

Dr. Peter Svensson graduated as a DDS in 1987 and earned his doctor of odontology in 2000. His research has focused on orofacial pain, physiology, and TMD with more than 200 contributions to peer-reviewed journals and book chapters. He has given more than 150 presentations around the world on orofacial pain mechanisms and TMD problems. He has received multiple awards in pain research and education and is an editorial board member and reviewer for several international dental and neuroscience journals. He has supervised about 20 completed and ongoing PhD projects and has an extensive network of national and international collaborations.

Thomas D. Taylor

Dr. Thomas Taylor is currently professor and chairman, Department of Reconstructive Sciences at the University of Connecticut. He is involved in both clinical and laboratory research and has published extensively in the prosthodontic literature. Dr. Taylor is past prosthodontic editor and abstract editor for the *International Journal of Oral and Maxillofacial Implants*. He is a diplomate and past president of the American Board of Prosthodontics and currently serves as the board's executive director. He is a fellow and past president of the

American College of Prosthodontists and past president of the International Team for Implantology.

Howard Tenenbaum

Dr. Howard Tenenbaum received his DDS from the University of Toronto in 1978 and then completed his specialty in periodontology as well as a PhD in bone cell biology by 1982. Dr. Tenenbaum is a professor of periodontology, and was head of that discipline for 8 years (1997–2005) at the Faculty of Dentistry, University of Toronto. He is a cross-appointed professor in the Department of Laboratory Medicine and Pathophysiology, Faculty of Medicine, University of Toronto and is the head of periodontics at Mount Sinai Hospital.

Mark Thomason

Dr. Mark Thomason qualified BDS in 1983, was made a fellow of the Royal College of Surgeons of Edinburgh in 1985, and completed a PhD in 1995. He is the director of clinical studies in Newcastle and holds an appointment as adjunct professor at McGill University, Montreal, Canada. His research interests are focused on an assessment of factors influencing patient acceptance of prostheses largely through the use of RCTs, including the impact on food choice, nutritional status, and the wider social impact of treatment choice. Professor Thomason is the current president of the Prosthodontic Research Group of the IADR.

R. Gilbert Triplett

Dr. R. Gilbert Triplett served 21 years in the United States Navy, where he completed an internship at Portsmouth Naval Hospital and residency in oral and maxillofacial surgery at the National Naval Medical Center in Washington, D.C., and Boston Naval Hospital in Chelsea, Massachusetts. He received his PhD at Georgetown University in 1982. He was director of residency education in oral and maxillofacial surgery at San Diego Naval Hospital and the University of Texas Health Science Center in San Antonio, Texas.

Stephen S. Wallace

Dr. Stephen S. Wallace is a 1971 graduate of Boston University School of Graduate Dentistry with a certificate in periodontics. He has been on the faculty of the New York University Department of Implant Dentistry for 14 years. He is a diplomate of the ICOI and a fellow of the Academy of Osseointegration. Dr. Wallace is the author of over 25 journal articles and textbook chapters. In addition to his faculty appointment, Dr. Wallace maintains a practice for periodontics, bone regeneration, and implant dentistry in Waterbury, Connecticut.

Hans-Peter Weber

Dr. Hans-Peter Weber is the Raymond J. and Elva Pomfret Nagle Professor of Restorative Dentistry and Biomaterials Sciences at the Harvard School of Dental Medicine and serves as the chair of that department. His current work consists of clinical and translational research, teaching, and intramural practice of all aspects of implant dentistry. He is a co-editor of *Clinical Oral Implants Research* and serves as a reviewer of several other dental journals. He publishes regularly on implant dentistry–related topics and lectures nationally and internationally.

Paul Weigl

Dr. Paul Weigl specializes in the field of prosthetics on implants and is also a senior specialist at the Department of Oral Surgery and Implant Dentistry, University of Frankfurt. Additionally, he runs an R&D project to develop a fully automatic working CAD/CAM process to manufacture complete crowns and bridges and to develop a new fs-laser based device for diagnosis and minimally invasive therapy of caries.

Ulf Wikesjö

Dr. Ulf Wikesjö has developed and characterized unique discriminating models to evaluate the biologic and clinical potential of bone biomaterials/devices and biologic factors including bone morphogenetic proteins for craniofacial tissue engineering with emphasis on alveolar augmentation, to evaluate oral implant/bone interface biology, and for periodontal wound healing/regeneration. Dr. Wikesjö is the author of more than 165 original articles in refereed scientific journals and texts, and he has made more than 180 invited presentations at international scientific workshops and conferences, academic institutions, and to learned societies.

Axel J.A. Wirthmann

Dr. Axel Wirthmann is a 1972 dental and 1973 medical graduate of the University of Göttingen School of Dentistry and Medicine. His PhD thesis from the University of Göttingen Women's Hospital dealt with hormones and cytokines. He specialized in molecular biology of the cell with respect to bone and cartilage metabolism to be applied in the field of oral implantology. He is past president of the German Society for Implantology (DGZI). Besides his faculty appointment at NYUCD, Dr. Wirthmann is head and chief consultant of a private hospital in Hamburg, Germany, specializing in oral implantology.

Daniel Wismeijer

Dr. Daniel Wismeijer received his DDS in 1984. He worked as a prosthodontist in the Department of Oral Function, section of maxillo-facial prosthodontics of the KUN till 1994. He worked as a part-time prosthodontist in the Amphia Teaching Hospital in Breda, the Netherlands, from 1985 till 2006. Since 1989 he has a referral practice for oral implantology. He received his PhD on his research, the Breda Implant Overdenture Study, in 1996. He has been professor of oral implantology and prosthetic dentistry at ACTA since 2006.

Homah Zadeh

Dr. Homa Zadeh, DDS, PhD, received his DDS from USC School of Dentistry. He has also completed advanced clinical education in periodontology and a PhD degree in immunology from the University of Connecticut. Dr. Zadeh directs the Laboratory for Immunoregulation and Tissue Engineering. He has an extensive publication track and serves as editorial reviewer for several scientific journals. He also serves on an advisory panel to the Center for Scientific Review of the National Institutes of Health. Dr. Zadeh is the director of USC periodontal and implant symposium.

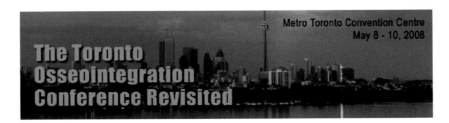

The University of Toronto, Faculty of Dentistry wishes to extend its special thanks to the following sponsors for their partnership in organizing the conference:

Platinum Sponsors

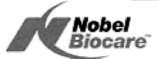 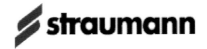

Gold Sponsor

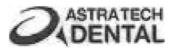

Silver Sponsors

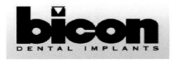 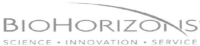 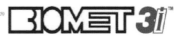

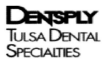 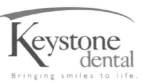

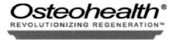 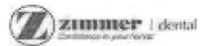

Index

Page references followed by f stand for figures; page references followed by t stand for tables.